KU-541-458

HEALTH EDUCATION
RESEARCH TRENDS

HEALTH EDUCATION RESEARCH TRENDS

PETER R. HONG
EDITOR

Nova Biomedical Books
New York

Copyright © 2007 by Nova Science Publishers, Inc.

All rights reserved. No part of this book may be reproduced, stored in a retrieval system or transmitted in any form or by any means: electronic, electrostatic, magnetic, tape, mechanical photocopying, recording or otherwise without the written permission of the Publisher.

For permission to use material from this book please contact us:
Telephone 631-231-7269; Fax 631-231-8175
Web Site: http://www.novapublishers.com

NOTICE TO THE READER

The Publisher has taken reasonable care in the preparation of this book, but makes no expressed or implied warranty of any kind and assumes no responsibility for any errors or omissions. No liability is assumed for incidental or consequential damages in connection with or arising out of information contained in this book. The Publisher shall not be liable for any special, consequential, or exemplary damages resulting, in whole or in part, from the readers' use of, or reliance upon, this material. Any parts of this book based on government reports are so indicated and copyright is claimed for those parts to the extent applicable to compilations of such works.

Independent verification should be sought for any data, advice or recommendations contained in this book. In addition, no responsibility is assumed by the publisher for any injury and/or damage to persons or property arising from any methods, products, instructions, ideas or otherwise contained in this publication.

This publication is designed to provide accurate and authoritative information with regard to the subject matter covered herein. It is sold with the clear understanding that the Publisher is not engaged in rendering legal or any other professional services. If legal or any other expert assistance is required, the services of a competent person should be sought. FROM A DECLARATION OF PARTICIPANTS JOINTLY ADOPTED BY A COMMITTEE OF THE AMERICAN BAR ASSOCIATION AND A COMMITTEE OF PUBLISHERS.

LIBRARY OF CONGRESS CATALOGING-IN-PUBLICATION DATA

Health education research trends / Peter R. Hong (editor).
    p. ; cm.
 Includes bibliographical references and index.
 ISBN-13: 978-1-60021-871-2 (hardcover)
 ISBN-10: 1-60021-871-7 (hardcover)
 1. Health education. 2. Health promotion. I. Hong, Peter R.
 [DNLM: 1. Health Education--trends. 2. Health Personnel--education. 3. Health Promotion--trends. 4. Research--trends. WA 590 H4352 2008]
RA440.5.H385 2008
613--dc22
                        2007030069

Published by Nova Science Publishers, Inc. ✦ *New York*

CONTENTS

PREFACE

The field of health education is of prime importance in a rapidly changing world where computers and the internet make the possibilities almost limitless. The areas of dynamic impact include education and training of health professionals, patients, medical and other institutions of other higher learning, families of ill people, and the public at large. This book presents new and important issues in this field.

Expert Commentary A - Health education is defined as the process by which individuals and groups of people learn to behave in a manner conducive to the promotion, maintenance or restoration of health. Its aim is to develop in them a sense of responsibility for health conditions, as individuals and as members of families and communities. A health education program consists of planned learning experiences, which will assist clients and/or their families to achieve desirable understandings, attitudes and practices related to critical health issues according to clients' expressed needs (Tones & Tilford, 2001). Targeted health issues may include, but not limited to, appreciation and care of the human body and its vital organs; physical fitness, nutrition and weight control, and effects of exercise on the body as well as general well being; health issues of alcohol, tobacco and drug abuse; psychological health and a positive self-image; sexual relationships, social and economic issues in community health; communicable and sexually transmitted diseases; disaster management and safety maintenance; and choices of professional medical and health services. Recently, an increasing attention and research in different countries on application of health informatics signifies a global movement of the use of computer-assisted or internet-based health care interventions and education for clients with diverse health and illness conditions.

Expert Commentary B - "Continuing medical education (CME) in the United States and Canada is a substantial and seemingly disorganized enterprise with over half a million physician consumers." [1]. In general, programs are limited in scope, implemented on a very limited scale and there is no evaluation or evaluation is limited to individual knowledge. Thompson, Oxman, and Haynes (1995) reviewed 99 educational intervention trials, containing 160 interventions [2]. They concluded that widely used CME delivery methods such as conferences had little direct impact on improving professional practice [3]. In this commentary the authors describe the creation of a national education program developed to improve the management of hypertension with a goal of reducing morbidity and mortality associated with elevated blood pressure. It is their hope that the program may be used as a model for the development of other educational programs in areas of significant public health importance. Further, the authors propose that major health professional education programs be developed based on a national public health agenda created by assessing major health risks and care gaps.

Expert Commentary C - With the shift towards consumerism in health care, the advent of shared treatment decision-making and copious amounts of health material available on the Internet, information that can improve quality of life no longer resides solely within the medical profession. One understudied concept in patient education is the importance of collaborative learning. Knowledge is power and knowledge learned collaboratively with others in similar situations is even more powerful. Information exchange or apprenticeships in which experts mentor those newly diagnosed have existed for many years with in-person support groups. Online collaboration also allows those with an illness who have become experts in their condition to share their anecdotal or experiential information with others. Thus far, however, first generation Internet applications such as newsgroups or message boards have not always been successful at facilitating this endeavor. Recently developed Web 2.0 technology supports bottom-up content development and information exchange such as the consumer product reviews found at Amazon.com. In one successful application of this concept, top-down content delivery associated with Britannica Online is now being replaced by collaboratively-generated bottom-up content like Wikipedia. Internet applications supported by Web 2.0 technology now have even more potential to educate patients and foster collaborative learning.

Expert Commentary D - Eight minority low-income young males who participated in a school-based youth development program to prevent pregnancy, were successful in transitioning to post-secondary education. Following their first year of college they were asked to identify program components that facilitated this transition. They identified personal, social, and academic competencies that they developed with the support of caring adults in the program. Feedback from these young males suggests that a multifaceted youth development approach with caring staff can be effective in building positive behavior.

Expert Commentary E - Advances in the science of HIV prevention have been substantial in the past two decades. Nevertheless, the number of new HIV infections in any given year has remained relatively unchanged during the past decade, indicating that both HIV seropositive and seronegative men and women are still engaging in high risk practices [1-4]. Of concern in the United States (US), half of all new infections occur in people 25 years of age or younger [5-6]. Thus, abstinence-only, sex education targeting youths has proven ineffective in circumventing the HIV/STD epidemics, as the proportion of males 15-19 in the US who ever had heterosexual sex between 1995 and 2002 has virtually remained the same [5-6].

In addition, prevention activities in the US have not necessarily followed rigorous scientific evidence. Sexual transmission of HIV and other pathogens may involve different routes of infection (e.g., anal or vaginal sex) and specific levels of hazard [7-20]. For example, the probability of HIV acquisition by the receptive partner in unprotected vaginal sex is 10 per 10,000 acts, but it greatly increases if it occurs during menses [11-12, 20]. During anal sex, the probability is 50 per 10,000 acts [11, 12, 20]. Furthermore, since condoms are more likely to break during anal sex than during vaginal sex, anal sex can be risky even with a condom [11-12, 20]. Accordingly, anal sex and sex during menses are considered high-risk sexual practices, while oral sex is low-risk [11-20]. It is therefore important to have a clear sense of what has been researched, published, and currently being done (interventions) regarding these high-risk sexual practices. The following sources of data were identified in order to provide a comprehensive analytical review: interviews with leading institutions working in the area of HIV/AIDS and education, such as CDC, NIH, and STD clinics; summaries of research on HIV/AIDS and education by major research organizations; a review of journal-published research on this subject; a synthesis of on-line journal research publications; studies of research proposals representing research in progress, which has not yet been completed for publication; and a review of AIDS conference abstracts. Finally, the authors will highlight the future relevance of the findings and make recommendations for future prevention interventions.

Short Commentary A - Social influence studies of physical activity (PA) and nutrition with regard to children have been mostly focused on parental influence. The purpose of the current study is to explore the correlation between PA and nutrition behaviors of after-school program group leaders, and the children they supervise. Two samples (sample 1, group leader: n=77, 85.7% female; sample 2, children: n=257, 45.1% male) from the same after school program completed Godin's Leisure-Time Exercise Questionnaire and specific questions about inactivity and nutrition. Bivariate correlations revealed large relationships between vegetable consumption (r=.57) of group leaders and children. Small negative correlations were found between mild activity (r=-.25) and fruit consumption (r=-.16) of group leaders and children. No correlation could be found between group leaders and children for strenuous (r=.06) and moderate (r=-.03) PA behavior or inactivity (r=.02). The authors findings indicate that after-school group leaders' health behaviors may be related to some children's health behaviors, which provides another potential avenue of promoting children's health behavior.

Short Commentary B - This communication briefly explores the use of the terms empowerment, self efficacy and health literacy, and suggests that they can be used to define health empowerment in an operationally useful way. It suggests that some of the difficulties in evaluation of empowerment have been the different ways in which the concept has been conceptualised. One particular problem is that discussion of the concept of empowerment often relies solely on issues of power, ignoring the dimension of health decision-making. It is suggested that health empowerment can usefully be considered as a combination of two key concepts Self Efficacy and Health Literacy. The widespread availability of scales for measurement of both self efficacy and health literacy is discussed and it is suggested that a measurement of health empowerment can be made by the combination of existing scales.

Chapter I - Schizophrenia is a disruptive and distressing illness for both patients and their family members who find their caregiving responsibility a heavy burden. Studies demonstrate that family-centered intervention for schizophrenia sufferers is essential and effective. However, little is known about the effects of such interventions for family members, particularly in non-Western populations.

An exploratory qualitative study was conducted to explore from the participants' perspective the benefits and limitations of a mutual support group for Chinese family caregivers of people with schizophrenia. Thirty-four family caregivers, who had participated in a 12-session mutual support group over six months, were interviewed and twelve group sessions were audio-taped for content analysis. The analysis of the interview and group session data indicated that most of the participants indicated positive personal changes during group participation and had progressively undergone the five phases of group development. The results also elicited three therapeutic mechanisms of the mutual support group. They included: reconstructing a new positive self-image in relation to caregiving; the psychological empowerment of caregivers through the acquisition of knowledge and skills for care-giving; and extending the social support networks both within and outside the group.

The study shows that a mutual support group can provide benefits for Chinese families of people with schizophrenia that go beyond those provided by routine family support. The three therapeutic mechanisms of the support group provide insights that might be drawn upon by health professionals when designing family group interventions. Further research is recommended to explore whether these five-phase development and therapeutic components of the group intervention identified in this study apply also to mutual support groups in families with different socio-economic backgrounds and across cultures.

Chapter II - Individuals with intellectual/developmental disabilities (I/DD) are known to have both health and healthcare disparities. The health disparities are related to the general aging process and to health problems typical of individuals with intellectual/ developmental disabilities. Healthcare disparities are experienced by these individuals because historically either these individuals did not survive childhood or they were placed in institutions. Thus, community medical providers, especially adult providers, have had little experience caring for the health of these individuals. As for anyone, healthcare education is important. But, for individuals with I/DD, unique health educational approaches are needed.

As many of the health problems experienced by individuals with I/DD are related to diet, nutrition education is important. One health educational approach is to use a variation of the Plate Method. The Plate Method is a commonly used visual method to show the proportions of a dinner plate that should be used to contain each of the various food groups. This Plate Model could be adapted for use by individuals with I/DD as a way to teach healthy eating.

In addition to a healthy diet, it is important for individuals with I/DD to incorporate into their daily routine activities to promote health. Social stories have been a means of positive behavior supports for children with autism. These social stories could be adapted for use by individuals with I/DD. Each individual would have their own *All About Me Healthy Lifestyle Story* in a book individually tailored to their needs. Pages of the book would cover their day from getting up in the morning to going to bed at night. Various pages would have a picture depicting the desired healthy lifestyle and simple words. Health behaviors that could be promoted include washing hands, brushing teeth, exercising, and taking medications.

In summary, health education for individuals with I/DD presents a unique challenge. Both the Plate Method and the *All About Me Healthy Lifestyle Story* present unique methods of health education for this population.

Chapter III - Health education research is a predominantly Western construct. Problems frequently arise in regards to idea communication and project ownership when investigations are implemented among vulnerable populations, particularly when researchers are from non-vulnerable backgrounds. Participatory Action Research (PAR) is a relevant methodology in health education research involving vulnerable populations because of its fundamental tenets that power be equally shared between the researchers and the researched, that data and information not be removed from their contexts, and that the data collection process be directly influenced by history, culture and local environment. Contemporary health behaviour models, such as the PRECEDE-PROCEED planning model and the Diffusion of Innovation model, suggest that health education interventions among vulnerable populations have much to gain from embracing more holistic, PAR approaches, which in turn are more likely to result in a sustained reduction in harmful health behaviours among vulnerable populations.

Chapter IV - Much has been written about consumers using the Internet for health care purposes, including those individuals with HIV/AIDS. Many of those with HIV/AIDS have engaged in self care and are often involved in decisions about their treatment. Yet little is understood about the ways Internet technologies are used to support learning about treatment information or how this resource is used in conjunction with other more traditional sources of information. In this qualitative inquiry twenty three participants attended four focus groups and shared what HIV treatment information sources they used and their means of collaboration. Using Wenger's (1998) Communities of Practice framework as a theoretical lens it was indicated that novice and intermediate learners are apprenticed by those with more experience. Participation is taking place but with little reification, especially within computer mediated communication technologies. Others relying on this technology as a primary source of information may suffer as a result.

Chapter V - Interest in exploring what is effective in health education and promotion initiatives has increased over the last decade leading to more evaluative research in the health promotion field. This article outlines some of the contemporary debates about measuring effectiveness in health promotion and examines the unique characteristics and features of community-based health promotion programs and what makes them challenging to evaluators. The paper then discusses the emergence and value of mixed method approaches in health promotion research and outlines some of the potential benefits and barriers in using mixed method approaches including opportunities for innovation, time, cost, expertise and strength of evidence. The paper presents a framework for conducting mixed method research in health promotion and discusses the lessons learned from two evaluation studies utilising a mixed method approach: the evaluation of a youth suicide intervention project and the evaluation of a smoking cessation program for marginalised and disadvantaged groups.

Chapter VI - The study was designed to increase organized school sports participation among middle school Latina girls. Two schools in a rural community were matched on important characteristics and recruited to serve as an intervention or control school. Thirteen Latina girls were identified by school personnel and nine were trained as peer leaders. Following training, the peer leaders implemented intervention strategies involving material development and distribution, and interpersonal communication with school personnel, peers, and parents. The primary outcome was sports participation among Latina girls. Data on participation were obtained from the school athletic directors and verified by observation. Secondary outcomes included peer leader knowledge, confidence and self-esteem measured at pre-training, post-training, and post-intervention activities using self-administered questionnaires and interviews. At the intervention school, the percentage of spring athletes who were Latina rose from 15% in 2004 to 27% in 2005 versus a drop in participation in the comparison school (10% in 2004 to 0% in 2005). Significant changes in peer leader knowledge and confidence were observed after training. This study reveals that peer leaders are able to implement an intervention to change sports participation patterns. Increasing participation in organized school sports may be an underutilized area for increasing adolescent physical activity levels.

Chapter VII - The over all objectives of this study was to map factors of importance for breastfeeding such as maternal perception of breastfeeding support, breastfeeding attitudes of health care professionals, and to investigate whether a training intervention within the team of the antenatal care (ANC) and child health centers (CHC) would improve maternal perception of support.

Material and method: A questionnaire was sent to mothers when their babies were 9-12 months old with questions regarding mothers perception of support and duration of breastfeeding (n=540). Thereafter an attitudinal instrument was developed to measure breastfeeding attitudes in health care professionals (n=168). Thereafter ten municipalities was paired and randomized to intervention or control. Thus, all midwives and postnatal nurses working at the ANC or CHC in a randomized municipality were asked to participate in the study (n=81). Health professionals in the intervention group had a process-oriented training in breastfeeding counseling including planned continuity in family education and development of a common breastfeeding policy within the caring team. Thereafter mothers were recruited from the maternity and were allocated to intervention- or control group according to the randomization of municipalities in an earlier study (n=565). Questionnaires were sent out at three days, 3 and 9 months post partum to investigate how the care and counseling skills acquired by the health care professionals would be reflected in maternal perception of breastfeeding support.

Results: Mothers were dissatisfied with the breastfeeding information they got from the ANC and CHC. This induced the idea to develop an attitude instrument and start a training intervention for the care team at ANC and CHC. The attitudinal dimensions identified by the factor analysis were: The regulating factor comprising statements scheduling breastfeeding; the facilitating factor comprising statements showing confidence in the ability of the mother-infant dyad to breastfeed on their own; the disempowering factor comprising statements that objectified the woman and ascribed her no ability to breastfeed without guidance of the health care professional and the breastfeeding hostility factor comprising statements that showed unwillingness and failing knowledge about breastfeeding. After training the health care professionals became less regulating and more facilitating. Family classes provided the intervention mothers with better breastfeeding information, more knowledge about their social rights, the needs of the baby and a stronger social network than the control mothers. The postnatal nurse gave a better over all support, was a better listener, showed more understanding and provided the mother with better information about breastfeeding and the needs of the baby.

Chapter VIII - Written health education materials are frequently used as a method of educating patients, and offer unique benefits. For health education materials to be effective, their readability level and design characteristics must be appropriate and they need to provide information that the patients want. Conventional written health education materials are generally designed to include as much information as possible for as many potential readers as possible. Because of this, the resulting material can be long and complex, and is likely to contain information that is irrelevant to many readers. In recent years, the application of computer technology to health education has led to the expanding use of computer-generated written health education materials that are tailored to the individual.

The majority of studies that have examined the effectiveness of tailored print information have had a health promotion focus and have been attempting to change participants' health-related lifestyle behaviours. A small number of recent studies have evaluated the effectiveness of using computer-generated tailored written information with people with chronic conditions such as arthritis and stroke. Heterogeneity in the patient populations studied, purpose of the interventions, study designs, and the outcome measures used prevents overall conclusions about the effectiveness of tailored health education materials from being drawn. It appears that patients prefer to receive information that is tailored to their individual situation, are more satisfied with tailored information, and are more likely to read and remember tailored information than non-tailored information. In some studies, patients who received tailored information were more likely to alter certain health behaviours than patients who received non-tailored information, however, in other studies, the provision of tailored information had no effect on health behaviours or other patient outcomes.

Overall, evidence regarding the effectiveness of tailored health education materials is inconclusive and it appears that tailored materials are only more effective than non-tailored materials under certain circumstances. What these circumstances are and the reasons why tailored materials are sometimes effective remain unclear. The potential for tailored materials to enhance patient health and well-being is high, however further studies that rigorously evaluate the effectiveness of well-designed tailored materials with various patient populations are urgently needed.

Chapter IX - The purpose of this descriptive study was to analyze longitudinally health risk behaviors of young males who were enrolled in a pregnancy prevention program. The Rites of Passage (ROP) project included 177 adolescent males between the ages of 12-22 and used a culturally grounded approach. Outcomes for the program included sexual and contraceptive behaviors, cigarette smoking, substance use, and antisocial behavior. The study also included open-ended questions that captured participants' expectations from the program and perceived benefits. Data were collected at intake, three months, and six months. Changes over time occurred in several risk behaviors. The results of the open-ended questions also indicated that participants felt that the program benefited them in the areas of self development, heritage awareness and risk reduction. Implications for future culturally grounded interventions are suggested.

In: Health Education Research Trends
Editor: P. R. Hong, pp. 1-5

ISBN: 978-1-60021-871-2
© 2007 Nova Science Publishers, Inc.

Expert Commentary A

COMPUTERIZED AND ONLINE PROGRAMS: A FUTURE TREND OF HEALTH EDUCATION AND PROMOTION?

Wai-Tong Chien[1] and Isabella Y. M. Lee[2]

[1]The Nethersole School of Nursing, Faculty of Medicine, The Chinese University of Hong Kong, Hong Kong;
[2]Department of Medicine & Geriatrics, Tuen Mun Hospital, Tuen Mun, N.T., Hong Kong.

Health education is defined as the process by which individuals and groups of people learn to behave in a manner conducive to the promotion, maintenance or restoration of health. Its aim is to develop in them a sense of responsibility for health conditions, as individuals and as members of families and communities. A health education program consists of planned learning experiences, which will assist clients and/or their families to achieve desirable understandings, attitudes and practices related to critical health issues according to clients' expressed needs (Tones & Tilford, 2001). Targeted health issues may include, but not limited to, appreciation and care of the human body and its vital organs; physical fitness, nutrition and weight control, and effects of exercise on the body as well as general well being; health issues of alcohol, tobacco and drug abuse; psychological health and a positive self-image; sexual relationships, social and economic issues in community health; communicable and sexually transmitted diseases; disaster management and safety maintenance; and choices of professional medical and health services.

Clients (or care recipients) are increasingly involved in participation in their health care decision (Noell & Glasgow, 1999), and health care providers are challenged to educate, motivate and assist their clients to adhere to healthy behaviors and treatment regimens in the community and ambulatory settings. One of the important elements of a successful health education program is an appropriate theoretical framework applied to development of the program, which can guide the changes in health behavior. Studies (Rhodes, Fishbein, & Reis,

1997; Skinner & Kreuter, 1997) indicate that use of health education theories can greatly enhance a patient's motivation to comply with an intervention. For example, the cognitive-behavioral theory focuses more on the individual level of changes (Rhodes et al., 1997) and make use of two key ingredients – cognitions (change of attitude, values and beliefs contributing to behavior change) and behavior (as mediated through cognitions and knowledge). Interpersonal models of health education include the trans-theoretical model (concerned with an individual's readiness; Ogden, 2005), the health belief model (focused on individual perception of the threat of a health problem; Bish, Sutton, & Golombok, 2000), and the theory of reasoned action (regarding individual intention to perform a healthy behavior; Armitage & Conner, 2000).

A client must have a sense of control and self-efficacy about the target behavior; and in addition, personal empowerment should be emphasized in order to increase the client's ability to cope with problem situations (Brug, Campbell, & van Assema, 1999). However, the accessibility, continuity and long duration of most existing education programs often limit the clients' desire and persistence on participation and reduce their commitment in the programs or subsequent behavior change. Enhancement of participation and interest to health education programs are concerned but are found to be achieved by applying information technology and to result from clients' increased computer accessibility and knowledge. This increased computer use by the public has enhanced online interactions between health educators (or the programs) and clients in need of support, and reduced the inconvenience of their face-to-face and time-limited encounters (Dijkstra, De Vries, Roijackers, & van Breukelen, 1998).

Recently, an increasing attention and research in different countries on application of health informatics signifies a global movement of the use of computer-assisted or internet-based health care interventions and education for clients with diverse health and illness conditions. This mode of learning, not limiting to medical and health education, has been developed continuously in parallel with the worldwide trend of computerization and internet use. A literature review by Lewis (2003) on computer use in patient education indicates that the internet users are of different ages and even older clients with little prior computer experience have been successful in obtaining health information in need, using computer software or an online search. At least five characteristics or practical advantages of computer assisted learning are recognized by both clients and health educators (Hebda, Czar, & Mascara, 2005), including:

- Programs can be very interactive, creative and attractive to the users by combining various media such as plain text, graphics, audio and video images;
- There is no limitation on the time each user spends on each topic or access to the program;
- Contents of the programs can be regularly updated and delivered to all users (clients) consistently;
- Programs can be administered in a private and comfortable learning environment; and,
- Users (clients) can choose and focus by themselves on the weak or unfamiliar areas and skip through the familiar contents, thus reducing their learning time.

However, the design of a computerized education program may sometimes reduce its effectiveness in facilitating client learning and these design issues include:

- A poor design with only plain text and nothing more than automatic page turning;
- Lack of control by users who are unable to repeat or review portions of the program or to quit at any point;
- Contents are lack of intellectual stimulation and failed to maintain users' interest by using different audiovisual stimulations or animations; and
- Lack of feedback on any incorrect answers made on tests or games used in the programs.

A recent internet-administered adolescent health promotion program by Mangunkusumo, Brug, Duisterhout, de Koning, & Raat (2007) was successfully implemented in the preventive health-care setting by the municipal health services. It was feasible in terms of attendance, duration, reading of the feedback and administration mode; and the adolescent recipients were satisfied with the mode of learning. Other studies among adolescents conducted in primary preventive-care settings in the United States (Fotheringham et al., 2000; Paperny & Hedberg, 1999; Patrick et al., 2001) also show that computerized adolescent health promotion was feasible and positively evaluated. However, most of the recent studies targeted a single type of health behavior and did not include a clear systematic protocol or guideline for implementation, or a control group to evaluate clients' satisfaction with the intervention.

Moreover, the Internet is an efficient approach to sample data of evaluation because it eliminates manual data entry by researchers thereby reducing transcription errors and workload, and its forced data entry results in complete data collection (Fotheringham et al., 2000; Mangunkusumo et al., 2006). Potentially, once implemented in routine practice, it may be less manpower intensive to deliver the health information or administer evaluation tests. It is recommended that health educators and researchers can further optimize internet application or computer software in relation to health promotion activities, and conduct more evaluation of its use and clients' satisfaction in terms of different health care topics. The feasibility, acceptability and quality as well as the health promotion effects of computer-assisted or online health education programs are highly important and should be further investigated.

Basic quality standards of online health information delivery should be provided for the users in order to judge whether the information in the computerized programs is credible, reasonable, or useful, and to make informed decisions about how to apply this information (Silberg, Lundberg, & Musacchio, 1997). Four aspects of information of an internet-administered program should be made known to the users, including: authorship or expertise of the authors should be known; references and sources for all content should be clearly listed; ownership and potential conflicts of interest should be disclosed; and dates of posting and updating should be indicated. Specific quality control guidelines of online health information can be found in the Code of Conduct developed by the Health on the Net Foundation (1997), a leading non-government organization founded in 1995 and accredited to the Economic and Social Council of the United Nations, which establish eight principles guiding the deployment of useful and reliable online medical and health information, and its appropriate use to the public. These principles are important in considering the quality of a computerized or World-Wide Web health education program.

Another means for enhancing accessibility and practicality of health education programs may be achieved by using mobile devices such as cell phones and digital assistants rather than delivery methods that attach clients to an internet, a computer, telephone, or mailbox. It is because mobile communication devices can offer the benefits of 'anytime and anywhere' communication capability, thus not restricting to any physical environment to send or receive messages; privacy of communication and interaction with others (Klein & Wilson, 2000); and time flexibility for users to access the content when available, interact with the interveners, or postpone interaction if desired (Lewis, 2003). An increasing power and decreasing cost of communication may provide opportunities for educational and counseling purposes that were not feasible before, such as crisis intervention and suicide prevention, and have received considerable attention from health care providers.

Nevertheless, there are potential problems in using these mobile systems, such as the clients' acceptance of these devices, difficulty in operation of the system, intrusiveness of clients' daily life, and economic burden to clients with low income. There are also limited studies evaluating on their relative effectiveness, efficiency and financial implications with routine and/or other modalities of health education interventions (Mangunkusumo et al., 2007). Even though research on these devices currently lags far behind, Friedman, Stollerman, Mahoney, and Rozenblum (1997) suggested that innovative electronic devices that incorporate features of the current telephone, television, video, and computer as well as wireless devices would be carried by clients to seek the health information that they desire.

Friedman (1999) and Mangunkusumo et al. (2007) also proposed that in the future, application of information technology in long distance may strengthen the continuity of care between clients and clinicians by improving access and facilitating the coordination and collaboration of health care services and intervention from a single source. Information technology may reach the point that health behavioral models can be integrated with computer-assisted interventions to provide regular, consistent and interactive community health care. Therefore, it is important to recommend that more research should be focused on evaluation of the effectiveness of these computerized interventions, which has the potential to not only inform the design of appropriate strategies in health education and promotion but also help move the science of health informatics toward the goal of achieving an evidence-based, client-centred health care services.

REFERENCES

Armitage, C. J., & Conner, M. (2000). Social cognition models and health behavior: A structured review. *Psychology & Health, 15*, 173-189.

Bish, A., Sutton, S., & Golombok, S. (2000). Predicting uptake of a routine cervical smear test: A comparison of the health belief model and the theory of planned behavior. *Psychology & Health, 15*, 35-50.

Brug, J., Campbell, M., & van Assema, P. (1999). The application and impact of computer-generated personalized nutrition education: A review of the literature. *Patient Education Counseling, 36,*145-156.

Dijkstra, A., De Vries, H., Roijackers, J., & van Breukelen, G. (1998). Tailored interventions to communicate stage-matched information to smokers in different motivational stages. *Journal of Consulting Clinical Psychology, 66,* 549-557.

Fotheringham, M. J., Owies, D., Leslie, E., et al. (2000). Interactive health communication in preventive medicine: Internet-based strategies in teaching and research. *American Journal of Preventive Medicine, 19,* 113-120.

Friedman, C. P. (1999). Toward a measured approach to medical informatics. *Journal of American Medical Informatics Association,*6, 176-177.

Friedman, R. H., Stollerman, J. E., Mahoney, D. M., & Rozenblum, L. (1997). The virtual visit: Using telecommunications technology to take care of patients. *Journal of American Medical Informatics Association, 4,* 413-425.

Health On the Net Foundation (1997). *HON Code of Conduct (HON code) for medical and health websites- Principles.* Retrieved 4 April 2007, from *http://www.hon.ch /HONcode/conduct.html.*

Hebda, T., Czar, P., Mascara, C. (2005). *Handbook of informatics for nurses and health care professionals* (3rd ed.). Upper Saddle River, NJ: Pearson Prentice Hall.

Klein, J. D., & Wilson, K. M. (2000). Delivering quality care: adolescents' discussion of health risks with their providers. *Journal of Adolescent Health, 30,* 190-195.

Lewis, D. (2003). Computers in patient education. *Computers, Informatics, Nursing, 21*(2), 88-96.

Mangunkusumo, R. T., Brug, J., Duisterhout, J. S., de Koning, H. J., & Raat, H. (2007). Feasibility, acceptability, and quality of Internet-administered adolescent health promotion in a preventive-care setting. *Health Education Research, 22* (1), 1-13.

Mangunkusumo, R. T., Duisterhout, J. S., De Graaff, N., et al. (2006). Internet versus paper mode of health and health behavior questionnaires in elementary schools: Asthma and fruit as examples. *Journal of School Health, 76,* 80-86

Noell, J., & Glasgow, R. E. (1999). Interactive technology applications for behavioral counseling: Issues and opportunities for health care settings. *American Journal of Preventive Medicine, 17,* 269-274.

Ogden, J. (2005). *Health psychology: A textbook* (3rd ed.). Berkshire, UK: Open University Press.

Paperny, D. M., & Hedberg, V. A. (1999). Computer-assisted health counselor visits: A low-cost model for comprehensive adolescent preventive services. *Archives in Pediatric & Adolescent Medicine, 153,* 63-67.

Patrick, K., Sallis, J. F., Prochaska, J. J., et al. (2001). A multi-component program for nutrition and physical activity change in primary care: PACE+ for adolescents. *Archives in Pediatric & Adolescent Medicine, 155,* 940-946.

Rhodes, F., Fishbein, M., & Reis, J. (1997). Using behavioral theory in computer-based health promotion and appraisal. *Health Education Behavior, 24,* 20-34.

Silberg, W. M., Lundberg, G. D., & Musacchio, R. A. (1997). Assessing, controlling, and assuring the quality of medical information on the internet: caveant lector et viewer- let the reader and viewer beware. *JAMA, 277*(15), 1244-1245.

Skinner, C. S., & Kreuter, M. W. (1997).Using theories in planning interactive computer programs. In R. L. Street, W. R. Gold, & T. Manning (eds.), *Health promotion and interactive technology* (pp. 39-66). Mahwah, NJ: Lawrence Erlbaum.

Tones, K., & Tilford, S. (2001). *Health promotion: Effectiveness, efficiency and equity* (3rd ed.). Cheltenham: Nelson Thornes.

In: Health Education Research Trends
Editor: P. R. Hong, pp. 7-11

ISBN: 978-1-60021-871-2
© 2007 Nova Science Publishers, Inc.

Expert Commentary B

HEALTH CARE PROFESSIONAL EDUCATION: A 'CASE STUDY' OF A SUCCESSFUL EDUCATION PROGRAM THAT IMPROVED PATIENT OUTCOMES

Norm Campbell[1], Janusz Kaczorowski[2], Rick Ward[3] and Denis Drouin[4]

[1]Departments of Medicine, Community Health Sciences, and Pharmacology and Therapeutics, Libin Cardiovascular Institute of Alberta, University of Calgary, Canada;
[2]Primary Care & Community Research, Child & Family Research Institute and Department of Family Practice, University of British Columbia, Vancouver, Canada;
[3]Department of Family Medicine and of Continuing Medical Education, University of Calgary, Canada;
[4]Continuing Professional Development Centre, Laval University, Quebec, Canada.

"Continuing medical education (CME) in the United States and Canada is a substantial and seemingly disorganized enterprise with over half a million physician consumers." [1]. In general, programs are limited in scope, implemented on a very limited scale and there is no evaluation or evaluation is limited to individual knowledge. Thompson, Oxman, and Haynes (1995) reviewed 99 educational intervention trials, containing 160 interventions [2]. They concluded that widely used CME delivery methods such as conferences had little direct impact on improving professional practice [3]. In this commentary we describe the creation of a national education program developed to improve the management of hypertension with a goal of reducing morbidity and mortality associated with elevated blood pressure. It is our hope that the program may be used as a model for the development of other educational programs in areas of significant public health importance. Further, we propose that major health professional education programs be developed based on a national public health agenda created by assessing major health risks and care gaps.

Hypertension was selected as the target of this Canadian education program because it is a leading risk for death and the most common reason for an adult Canadian to visit a physician [4]. Furthermore, there was a large gap between the desired treatment and control rate of hypertension based on best clinical evidence, and the actual treatment and control of hypertension as illustrated by national surveys and analysis of administrative databases [5-8].

Specifically, in 1985-1992, only 66% of patients who reported a diagnosis of hypertension were treated with medications, and only 16% were treated to the recommended therapeutic targets [9]. In 1998, management had not appreciably changed; only 68.5% of patients who reported a diagnosis of hypertension were treated with medications (there was no assessment of the rate of hypertension control in 1998) [10]. Treatment of hypertension to lower blood pressure by about 10/5 mmHg is estimated to reduce stroke by 42%, and coronary heart disease by about 14% [11]. Repeated clinical practice studies and audits have documented that patients under routine clinical care did not have therapy adjusted to achieve recommended targets [12-19]. It was believed that an extensive and sustained health care professional education program was needed and had the potential to improve the clinical management of hypertension [20].

In 1999, a program was developed to ensure that primary care professionals were up to date on the latest evidence on the management of hypertension [21]. The program was based on a previously developed episodic evidence based recommendations process [22,23]. The new program was enhanced by an annual updating of the recommendations; new procedures to enhance the quality of recommendations and to reduce bias; an extensive program to implement the recommendations through on-going development of diverse educational tools and materials; and the development of an extensive evaluation framework [24-26]. The program was developed under the auspices of the national hypertension organizations (Blood Pressure Canada and the Canadian Hypertension Society), the Heart and Stroke Foundation of Canada, the national Department of Health and later by national primary care professional organizations (family physicians, pharmacists and nurses). The program was developed and run by volunteers. Initially, the program was supported largely by annual donations of equal value from about ten pharmaceutical companies and more recently it has received support from the government agencies such as the Public Health Agency of Canada.

The program identified and integrated the key national and regional opinion leaders in hypertension in the process of developing, disseminating, and evaluating the annual recommendations. "Train the Trainer" sessions on the recommendations and the process were developed for regional and local opinion leaders to assist in the dissemination process. The annual recommendations are prepared in a variety of summery formats and published in peer-reviewed and non-peer-reviewed journals; pocket cards; booklets; and plastic covered office desk mats. Educational material such as case-based interactive workshops and electronic slides sets are developed and widely disseminated. The materials are updated annually and publicized by public and health care professional media releases. An important aspect of the program is advertising and making the material available on the Canadian Hypertension Society website (www.hypertension.ca). Each year, a new theme important to the management of hypertension is selected around which the dissemination strategy is developed. In addition, updated materials are developed and widely disseminated, highlighting important new recommendations and emphasizing the 5 to 7 key recommendations that the program believes are the most important for improving hypertension management

Local and regional education programs as well as health care professional schools are encouraged to utilize the recommendations in their curricula. Other national programs that impact hypertension management are also encouraged to utilize the recommendations. Once the program was demonstrated to be sustainable (3rd year) a process was outlined to develop indicators of hypertension management in Canada [26]. Specifically, numbers of patients reporting a diagnosis and or treatment for hypertension; numbers of prescriptions for antihypertensive drugs; and hospitalizations or deaths from hypertension related complications were monitored.

From the year prior to the start of the program to three years after its initiation (1998-2002): 1.35 million more adult hypertensives were diagnosed (33% increase); 1.26 million more adults were treated (39% increase); the proportion of those aware of having hypertension who were treated with drugs increased from 68.5 to 85%; and there were reductions in deaths and hospitalizations for acute myocardial infarction, stroke and congestive heart failure [10,27]. The observational nature of the data precludes cause and effect relationships from being established and multiple other factors may affect cardiovascular disease rates and hypertension treatment. Nevertheless, the timing and magnitude of the changes in hypertension management and complications and the lack of viable alternative explanations suggests the improvements are at least partly related to the hypertension education program.

To support the goal of preventing hypertension and improving its management, several other programs have also been developed in parallel to the health care professional education program. To increase the uptake of the recommendations and to increase awareness of hypertension by the Canadian public and patients with hypertension, a new initiative was launched to translate the health care professional management recommendations for the public and to broadly disseminate the translated version [28]. This effort is assisted by the development of "Train the Trainer" sessions to aid health care professionals educating the public and patients about hypertension by using standardized educational material [28]. A network of clinics that provide specialized hypertension care and a network of community programs that are designed to prevent hypertension or improve hypertension management are being developed. It is intended that these networks will share resources and best practices and disseminate this knowledge amongst communities across Canada. Further, a separate initiative has been launched to prevent hypertension by reducing the sodium content of Canadian diets through interactions with governments, health care professional organizations, and companies that process foods.

As such, we propose a new paradigm where health care professional educational agendas are developed based on national public health needs and demonstrated gaps between evidence and clinical practice. Once important areas are identified, comprehensive and sustained education programs need to be developed. The education programs need to include those that influence the uptake of the new knowledge; be regularly updated; have extensive implementation; and be evaluated including parameters of importance to the patient. We have demonstrated that such a program can be developed and successfully operated by volunteers with modest, unrestricted financial support from the pharmaceutical industry and the government. We further propose that health care professional programs on important health issues operate in parallel with enhanced public education programs, community health programs, and changes in health policy. The new paradigm is more likely to improve patient management and outcomes than the usual ad hoc, locally initiated, non-sustained, non-evaluated programs relying solely on continuing medical education.

REFERENCES

[1]   Escovitz GH, Davis D. A Bi-national Perspective on Continuing Medical Education. *Acad Med.* 1990;65:545-50.

[2]   Davis DA, Thomson MA, Oxman AD, Haynes B. Changing Physician Performance. A Systematic Review of the Effect of Continuing Medical Education Strategies. *JAMA.* 1995;274:700-705.

[3]   Davis D, Thomson O'Brien MA, Freemantle N, Wolf FM, Mazmanian P, Taylor-Vaisey A. Impact of Formal Continuing Medical Education. Do Conferences, Workshops, Rounds, and Other Traditional Continuing Education Activities Change Physician Behavior or Health Care Outcomes? *JAMA.* 1999;282:867-74.

[4]   Ezzati M, Lopez AD, Rodgers A, Vander Hoorn S, Murray CJLM, Comparative Risk Assessment Collaborating Group. Selected major risk factors and global and regional burden of disease. *Lancet.* 2002;360:1347-60.

[5]   Hemmelgarn BR, McAlister FA, Grover S, Myers MG, McKay DW, Bolli P et al. The 2006 Canadian Hypertension Education Program recommendations for the management of hypertension: Part 1 - Blood pressure measurement, diagnosis and assessment of risk. *Can J Cardiol.* 2006;22:573-81.

[6]   Khan NA, McAlister FA, Rabkin SW, Padwal R, Feldman RD, Campbell NRC et al. The 2006 Canadian Hypertension Education Program recommendations for the management of hypertension: Part II - Therapy. *Can J Cardiol.* 2006;22:583-93.

[7]   Kearney PM, Whelton M, Reynolds K, Whelton PK, He J. Worldwide prevalence of hypertension: a systematic review. *J Hypertens.* 2004;22:11-19.

[8]   Tu K, Campbell NRC, Durong-Hua M, McAlister FA. Hypertension Management in the Elderly Has Improved: Ontario Prescribing Trends, 1994 to 2002. *Hypertension.* 2005;45:1113-18.

[9]   Joffres MR, Ghadirian P, Fodor JG, Petrasovits A, Chockalingam A, Hamet P. Awareness, Treatment, and Control of Hypertension in Canada. *Am J Hypertens.* 1997;10:1097-102.

[10]   Onysko J, Maxwell C, Eliasziw M, Zhang J, Johansen H, Campbell N. Large Increases in Hypertension Diagnosis and Treatment in Canada Following a Health Care Professional Education Program. *Hypertension.* 2006;48:853-60.

[11]   Smith SCJr, Blair SN, Criqui MH, Fletcher GF, Fuster V, Gersh BJ et al. Preventing heart attack and death in patients with coronary disease. *Circulation.* 1995;92:2-4.

[12]   McAlister FA, Teo KK, Lewanczuk RZ, Wells G, Montague TJ. Contemporary practice patterns in the management of newly diagnosed hypertension. *CMAJ.* 1997;157:23-30.

[13]   Wang PS, Avorn J, Brookhart MA, Mogun H, Schneeweiss S, Fischer MA et al. Effects of Noncardiovascular Comorbidities on Antihypertensive Use in Elderly Hypertensives. *Hypertension*. 2005;46:273-79.

[14]   Hicks LS, Fairchild DG, Horng MS, Orav EJ, Bates DW, Ayanian JZ. Determinants of JNC VI Guideline Adherence, Intensity of Drug Therapy, and Blood Pressure Control by Race and Ethnicity. *Hypertension*. 2004;44:429-34.

[15]   Hyman DJ, Pavlik VN. Self-reported Hypertension Treatment Practices Among Primary Care Physicians. Blood Pressure Thresholds, Drug Choices, and the Role of Guidelines and Evidence-Based Medicine. *Arch Intern Med*. 2000;160:2281-86.

[16]   Kotchen TA. From Clinical Trials to Clinical Practice: Why the Gap? *Hypertension*. 2006;48:196-97.

[17]   Berlowitz DR, Ash AS, Hickey EC, Friedman RH, Glickman M, Kader B et al. Inadequate management of blood pressure in a hypertensive population. *N Engl J Med*. 1998;339:1957-63.

[18]   Margolis KL, Rolnick SJ, Fortman KK, Maciosek MV, Hildebrant CL, Grimm RHJr. Self-Reported Hypertension Treatment Beliefs and Practices of Primary Care Physicians in a Managed Care Organization. *Am J Hypertens*. 2005;18:566-71.

[19]   Oliveria SA, Lapuerta P, McCarthy BD, L'Italien GJ, Berlowitz DR, Asch SM. Physician-Related Barriers to the Effective Management of Uncontrolled Hypertension. *Arch Intern Med*. 2002;162:413-20.

[20]   Lenfant C. Reflections on Hypertension Control Rates. A Message From the Director of the National Heart, Lung, and Blood Institute. *Arch Intern Med*. 2002;162:131-32.

[21]   Zarnke KB, Campbell NRC, McAlister FA, Levine M. A novel process for updating recommendations for managing hypertension: Rationale and methods. *Can J Cardiol*. 2000;16:1094-102.

[22]   Campbell NRC, Burgess E, Choi BCK, Taylor G, Wilson E, Cléroux J et al. Methods and an overview of the Canadian recommendations. *CMAJ*. 1999;160:S1-S6.

[23]   Feldman RD, Campbell N, Larochelle P, Bolli P, Burgess ED, Carruthers SG et al. 1999 Canadian recommendations for the management of hypertension. *CMAJ*. 1999;161:S1-S17.

[24]   McAlister FA. The Canadian Hypertension Education Program - A unique Canadian initiative. *Can J Cardiol*. 2006;22:559-64.

[25]   Drouin D, Campbell NR, Kaczorowski J. Implementation of recommendations on hypertension: The Canadian Hypertension Education Program. *Can J Cardiol*. 2006;22:595-98.

[26]   Campbell NR, Onysko J. The Outcomes Research Task Force and the Canadian Hypertension Education Program. *Can J Cardiol*. 2006;22:556-58.

[27]   Campbell NRC, Onysko J, Johansen H, Gao R-N. Changes in cardiovascular deaths and hospitalization in Canada. *Can J Cardiol*. 2006;22:425-27.

[28]   Campbell NR, Petrella R, Kaczorowski J. Public education on hypertension: A new initiative to improve the prevention, treatment and control of hypertension in Canada. *Can J Cardiol*. 2006;22:599-603.

In: Health Education Research Trends
Editor: P. R. Hong, pp. 13-17

ISBN: 978-1-60021-871-2
© 2007 Nova Science Publishers, Inc.

Expert Commentary C

WEB 2.0: COLLABORATION IN WEB-BASED PATIENT HEALTH EDUCATION

Laura O'Grady

Faculty of Information Studies, University of Toronto, Toronto, Ontario, Canada.

ABSTRACT

With the shift towards consumerism in health care, the advent of shared treatment decision-making and copious amounts of health material available on the Internet, information that can improve quality of life no longer resides solely within the medical profession. One understudied concept in patient education is the importance of collaborative learning. Knowledge is power and knowledge learned collaboratively with others in similar situations is even more powerful. Information exchange or apprenticeships in which experts mentor those newly diagnosed have existed for many years with in-person support groups. Online collaboration also allows those with an illness who have become experts in their condition to share their anecdotal or experiential information with others. Thus far, however, first generation Internet applications such as newsgroups or message boards have not always been successful at facilitating this endeavor. Recently developed Web 2.0 technology supports bottom-up content development and information exchange such as the consumer product reviews found at Amazon.com. In one successful application of this concept, top-down content delivery associated with Britannica Online is now being replaced by collaboratively-generated bottom-up content like Wikipedia. Internet applications supported by Web 2.0 technology now have even more potential to educate patients and foster collaborative learning.

INTRODUCTION

Background: Patient Education

Patient education practices were developed over thirty five years ago by health care providers (Redman, 2001). Patient education has most commonly been associated with the field of nursing (Rankin & Stallings, 2000) but physicians also educate their patients when obtaining informed consents (Redman, 1998). Various models and theories have been implemented since its inception, including the health belief model, which focuses on the patients' understanding of their illness and how this impacts their decision-making process, or the self-efficacy theory, which consists of four core ways of improving health: promoting the ability to maintain one's health (personal mastery); learning about self care by observing others, including health care professionals, family and those with the same illness (vicarious experiences); obtaining support from others (verbal persuasions); and receiving acknowledgment that interventions are working (physiological feedback) (Rankin & Stallings, 2000).

Future Directions in Patient Education: Collaborative Learning

Although self-efficacy theory acknowledged that anecdotal information obtained from those with the same illness (vicarious experiences) is an important part of the recovery process, this form of learning is limited in that it is conducted solely through direct observation. An example of learning by vicarious experiences could involve a newly diagnosed diabetic watching another diabetic successfully injecting themselves with insulin. Opportunities for this kind of direct observation may therefore be limited to location (Does the newly diagnosed patient live where he or she can access other patients with the same condition to support vicarious learning? Where would this process take place?), participation (Are there patients willing to provide instruction on potentially sensitive procedures for the benefit of others?), availability (What medical staff are required to facilitate this type of learning?), and cost (How much time of the medical staff is required? Are there costs associated with this process? Do the patient "educators" require payment or reimbursement?) to name just a few of the many potential issues with the vicarious experiences model.

In formal education, a more comprehensive model of learning that promotes collaboration has long been considered desirable. First introduced in the early 1900s, the concept was promoted by John Dewey as a democratic means by which to promote learning. Collaboration is defined as the process by which group members work together on a common goal or assignment. An example of collaborative learning would include a situation in which learners are working collectively on the same assignment or project rather than assigning different tasks to different people (Brandon & Hollingshead, 1999). It is believed that the process of preparing and sharing one's knowledge in a group setting improves learning ("two heads are better than one"). However, little of what are considered the core components of collaborative learning have moved into the formal field of patient education. This may be due to the fact that the classroom-based format in formal education more readily provides an environment more conducive to supporting collaborative learning than do the venues where patient education has traditionally taken place (Woolfolk-Hoy, 2006). Individuals with a shared interest in learning about an illness are not likely to be in contact with each other in a group setting like a classroom.

In-person support groups provide the potential to promote collaborative learning, but participation is limited to those who are geographically close and well enough to travel. One of the most successful applications of in-person support groups is Alcoholics Anonymous or AA. The premise behind this model is a system of enculturation in which newcomers are instructed by old-timers (Lave & Wenger, 1991). Unfortunately, for reasons that will subsequently be made clear, this model did not translate well to the computer mediated communication (CMC) based interventions initially available on the Internet.

Background of Internet use in Health Care

Early applications on the Internet included gopher sites (repositories of information) and gopher search mechanisms such as Veronica. WAIS (Wide Area Information Servers) were used for searching online databases (Gilster, 1996). These technologies were created to support the dissemination of information in a "one to many" model – one person or organization created content for distribution to many people. Later, newsgroups, web-based message boards, and mailing lists proliferated as means of exchanging information (Krol, 1992). This second model of information dissemination, "many to many," allows information to be created and distributed by all those involved. A wide variety of information, including hobby-based, recreational, sports, financial, and health care content, is exchanged using these CMC mechanisms.

Perhaps surprisingly, one of the most successful aspects of the Internet has been its use for health care. Even more surprising is the focus on consumer-driven efforts to create and maintain health-related content on the Internet. Unlike previous patient education efforts formally instigated by health care professionals, many educational web sites found online today have been developed by consumers with an illness. In many cases newsgroups and mailing lists, also often started or facilitated by lay persons, are filled with message postings by health care consumers with only a small number of postings by health care professionals. Over time however, many of these initially extremely effective means of communication have degenerated into repositories for spam (unsolicited advertisements for goods or services), flaming (posting messages that are deliberately offensive or insulting in nature), and baiting (posting messages with the goal of soliciting a response that will be embarrassing the poster but humorous to others). Unfortunately, as a result of this deterioration in content, many CMC efforts, including health-related initiatives, did not reach their full potential as a means of supporting collaborative learning.

Future Directions in Patient Education: Web 2.0 and Collaborative Learning

In 2004 a new concept related to Internet technologies, Web 2.0, was first conceptualized. It was defined as *"...a set of economic, social, and technology trends that collectively form the basis for the next generation of the Internet – a more mature, distinctive medium characterized by user participation, openness, and network effects."* (Musser & O'Reilly, 2006, p. 4). These concepts are manifested in such technologies as blogging, keeping an online diary of personal thoughts and reflections; tagging and social bookmarking, the practice of sharing personalized bookmarks that contain self-made labels called tags to categorize content; and read-write web, which are web sites that can be edited by users (Anderson, 2007). At the core of these technologies is the concept of bottom-up delivery of content, or the "many to many" model. Read-write web, for example www.wikipedia.org, has great potential to support collaborative learning due to its capacity for mutual (and bottom-up) exchanges of information. This is especially relevant to supporting patients' efforts to find answers to questions they are unlikely to obtain from their health care provider (Deshpande & Jadad, 2006). Over time the newly-diagnosed patients will become experts and in turn can provide support in the form of advice to novices, much like the AA support group model.

Patients are now more responsible for making their own health care decisions (Charles, Whelan & Gafni, 1999), therefore more information about one's illness is likely required in order to be confident in one's decision making abilities. Questions remain as to how technologies can be better leveraged to support this need in a collaborative fashion, especially given the apparent failures of past efforts online. Recent web sites such as www.wikipedia.com or http://del.icio.us/. that use collaboration to build content may be indications that the culture of the Internet has changed. Wikipedia shows how read-write web can operate relatively successfully without flaming, baiting, or spamming. While there are cases in which incorrect information has been posted or even deliberate vandalism of the site, other Wikipedia contributors are available to change incorrect contributions or rollback content to the previous version. There is great potential to support health-based collaborative learning using Web 2.0 technologies. Patient education now has the mechanisms to facilitate collaborative learning in an online environment.

CONCLUSION

Patient education was previously the domain of nurses and other health care professionals. In many cases instruction was provided in isolation with little opportunity for patients to learn from others in similar circumstances. Education theories suggest that collaborative efforts have the potential to improve learning. Many individuals with an illness discovered mechanisms to share information about their health care using collaborative Internet technologies, but initial efforts to support collaborative learning online using newsgroups, message boards, and mailing lists were often not successful. More recent movement towards Web 2.0, bottom-up and collaboratively-driven content development have positioned the Internet to better support learning amongst various patient advocacy and health movements. These new technologies may signal a change to the culture of the Internet that could provide opportunities for the development of successful collaboratively-built patient education sites online.

ACKNOWLEDGEMENTS

The research reported herein was supported by a Canadian Institutes of Health Research (CIHR)/Ontario Women's Health Council (OWHC) post doctoral training award. Funding was also provided by the CIHR training program Health Care, Technology, and Place (HCTP).

REFERENCES

Anderson, P. (2007). *What is Web 2.0? Ideas, technologies and implications for education* (No. TSW0701). London, England: Joint Information Systems Committee.

Brandon, D. P., & Hollingshead, A. B. (1999). Collaborative learning and computer-supported groups. *Communication Education, 48*, 109-126.

Deshpande, A., & Jadad, A. (2006). Web 2.0: Could it help move the health care system in the 21st century? *The journal of men's health & gender, 3*(4), 332-336.

Charles, C., Whelan, T., & Gafni, A. (1999). What do we mean by partnership in making decisions about treatment? *British Medical Journal, 319*(7212), 780-782.

Gilster, P. (1996). *Finding it on the Internet: the Internet Navigator's guide to search tools and techniques* (Rev. and expanded, 2nd ed.). New York: Wiley.

Krol, E. (1992). *The whole Internet user's guide & catalog.* Sebastopol, CA: O'Reilly & Associates.

Lave, J. & Wenger, E. (1991). *Situated learning: legitimate peripheral participation.* Cambridge [England]; New York: Cambridge University Press.

Musser, J., & O'Reilly, T. (2006). *O'Reilly Radar Report: Web 2.0 Principles and Best Practices.* O'Reilly Media.

Redman, B. K. (1998). *Measurement tools in patient education.* New York: Springer Pub.

Redman, B. K. (2001). *The practice of patient education* (9th ed.). St. Louis, Mo.: Mosby.

Rankin, S. H., & Stallings, K. D. (2000). *Patient education: principles & practices* (4th ed.). Philadelphia, PA: Lippincott.

Woolfolk-Hoy, A., Winne, P. H., & Perry, N. E. (2006). *Educational psychology* (Custom for the Ontario Institute for Studies in Education of the University of Toronto ed.). Boston, MA: Pearson Custom Publishing.

In: Health Education Research Trends
Editor: P. R. Hong, pp. 19-24

ISBN: 978-1-60021-871-2
© 2007 Nova Science Publishers, Inc.

Expert Commentary D

YOUNG MINORITY MALES WHO PARTICIPATED IN A YOUTH DEVELOPMENT PROGRAM: THEIR PERCEPTIONS OF PROGRAM IMPACT ON THEIR TRANSITION TO POST SECONDARY EDUCATION

Peggy B. Smith[1], Maxine L. Weinman[2], Ruth S. Buzi[1] and Gilbert Chavez[3]

[1]Baylor College of Medicine, Houston, TX 77030, USA;
[2]Graduate School of Social Work, University of Houston, Houston, TX 77204, USA;
[3]Office of Attorney General, State of Texas, USA

ABSTRACT

Eight minority low-income young males who participated in a school-based youth development program to prevent pregnancy, were successful in transitioning to post-secondary education. Following their first year of college they were asked to identify program components that facilitated this transition. They identified personal, social, and academic competencies that they developed with the support of caring adults in the program. Feedback from these young males suggests that a multifaceted youth development approach with caring staff can be effective in building positive behavior.

Keywords: Inner city males, teen pregnancy prevention, risk reduction, theoretical models.

INTRODUCTION

Traditional programs to prevent pregnancy include sex education in schools, provide improved access to family planning services, and access to condoms (Vincent, et al., 2000). Recently, initiatives have targeted the specific needs of young males such as education, training, and employment (Sonenstein, Stewart, Lindberg, Pernas, & Williams, 1997). For example, the Department of Health and Human Services, Office of Population Affairs/ Office of Family Planning (OPA/OFP) supports male initiatives that focus on preventing pregnancies and other related risk behaviors. Moreover, researchers are now suggesting that prevention programs for at-risk youth should use an approach that focuses on enhancing a variety of protective factors such as positive values, social abilities, and positive identity in addition to reducing risk behavior (Resnick, et. al, 1997; Roth, Brooks-Gunn, Murray, & Foster, 1998; Epstein, Botvin, Griffin, & Diaz, 2001).

The present paper provides information on the experiences of eight young males who participated in a school-based youth development program to prevent pregnancy. These young males were successful in making the transition to post-secondary academic education. Following a year in college they were asked to participate in a group discussion and identify components of the program that supported this approach.

METHODS

Program Description

The resiliency theoretical framework suggested by Rutter (1985, 1987, 1999) was used to guide this program. The objectives of this program were to develop personal, educational, and social competency in addition to reinforcing messages of prevention of pregnancy. Core components in the program included case management, peer support groups, mentoring, community service activities, and life skills training.

The program was conducted at a high school in an inner city area in the Southwest United States. This school was selected for the program because youth in this area were defined as high-risk based on indicators such as high rates of teenage pregnancy and school dropout. A total of 245 minority young males 14 to 19 years of age were enrolled during the five years of the program. Although assistance with entry to post secondary education was available to all program participants, only eight young males showed an interest and received assistance with their college application.

Subjects

The sample for this study was comprised of all the eight males who enrolled in post secondary education. This included 5 African American (62.5%) and 3 (37.5%) Hispanic males. Their mean age at entry to the program was 15.86 (*S.D.* =1.0, range=14-17). These young males who began the program as freshmen or sophomores were accepted into post high school educational institutions.

Instrument and Procedures

At the completion of the first year in post-secondary academic education, all eight students who graduated from the program were invited to participate in a group discussion to reflect on various aspects of program effectiveness. Following a group discussion, they were asked to respond in writing to five questions examining their experience with the program. These questions are used by the research team as an evaluative instrument in male involvement programs to obtain participants' input on program implementation.

Data Analysis

Two members of the research team, who were not involved in conducting the group discussion, independently summarized the themes that emerged in the written responses. They then compared the themes and reached a consensus. The research team member who was involved in the group discussion reviewed and verified the themes based on notes taken during the group discussion.

RESULTS

The results are organized around the five questions presented to study participants. A summary of the main themes from responses to these written questions and selected quotes to illustrate the ideas are presented as follows:

Question 1: In what ways do you Consider Yourself Successful?

Eight young men responded to the question. All of their statements reflected the importance of education as the way they defined their success. In addition, two identified the ability to avoid early fatherhood as success. An example of a response is as follows:

> "The program pushes its' participants to reach for their goals. The program encouraged me to go to college and become what I always wanted to be, a doctor. On the plus side, without the program's help on contraception and awareness, I'd probably had kids now."

Question 2: What were some of the Barriers you Faced?

Eight young men responded to this question. Two stated they did not face any barriers, two stated peer pressure as barriers, and the other four identified various barriers. While no major theme emerged, most barriers were related to social issues such as family trouble, racism and being stereotyped, and low self-esteem.

Question 3: What was Helpful in the Program to You?

Eight young men responded to the question. All of them identified social support they received from the program staff as helpful. Aspects of social support were feedback, helpful insight, mentoring, and skill acquisition. An example of a response is as follows:

"Everything from the people, the feedback, and the helpful insight that they provided to help us along the way from boys into manhood."

Question 4: How did the Changes Change Your Family Relationships?

Seven young men responded to this question. Four of the seven participants did not identify any changes in family relationships. They felt things were about the same and were positive. The three who identified changes stated that it helped with either family communication or community connectedness. An example of a response is as follows:

"My family is more in touch with the community now than ever before. Every month the Program would send out a post card of what was happening in the community and with that postcard also came a question. The questions would normally be about family bonding. Questions like, parents should ask their kids on what their into these days, stuff like that."

Question 5: What Advice would You Give to other Programs that Wanted to Work with Young Men?

Eight young men responded to this question. An essential element that emerged in this question was the importance of program staff building relationships with participants. Aspects of building relationships included listening, patience, respect, and empowerment. An example of a response is:

"I would tell them that to really get in touch with young men, they have to act and feel like them. They have to really bond with every young man that enters the program. It's all about helping young men. So the only real way to know what they really need help on is to ask and to make relationships with. The more bonding that does on the better the outcome."

DISCUSSION

Eight minority students, who participated in a school-based program to prevent pregnancy prevention program, were successful in transitioning to post secondary education. This accomplishment is remarkable as the school they attended has been categorized as "Academically Unacceptable" by the Texas Education Agency for its average scores on the Texas Assessment of Knowledge and Skills (TAKS) scores. Additionally, this school has a graduation rate of only 68% as compared to 83% for the state (Schools Profiles (2004) Great Schools.net. Retrieved on October 25, 2004 from: http://www.greatschools.net/modperl/ browse_school/tx/551).

The reports of these participants suggested that a youth development framework can enhance the potential of minority low-income males and facilitate the development of personal, social, and academic skills that are required for the transition to higher education. This multifaceted approach with its case management, peer support group, mentoring with continuous follow-up provided these young males an opportunity to develop inner resources such as positive self-image, confidence, self-direction, and skills to avoid risk behaviors. This is congruent with Kirby's (2002) conclusion that an intensive youth development program with multiple components can be effective in reducing high risk behaviors among youth. Although a small sample, our data suggest that high risk youth benefit best from a comprehensive youth development program, when appropriate support is given. Consistent follow up, support services and opportunities to address issues pertaining to protective factors are the key elements in successful interventions with this group.

ACKNOWLEDGEMENTS

This project was funded in part by the Department of State Health Services (DSHS), and the Office of Population Affairs/Office of Family Planning (OPA/OFP) Department of Health and Human Services.

REFERENCES

Epstein, J. A., Botvin, G. J, Griffin, K. W., & Diaz, T. (2001). Protective factors buffer effects of risk factors on alcohol use among inner city youth. *Journal of Child and Adolescent Substance Abuse, 11*(1), 77-90.

Kirby, D. (2002). Effective approaches to reducing adolescent unprotected sex, pregnancy and childbearing. *The Journal of Sex Research, 39*(1), 51-57.

Office of Population Affairs/Office of Family Planning. (2000). *Male Involvement Projects-Prevention Services.* Washington, DC: U.S. Department of Health and Human Services.

Resnick, M. D., Bearman, P. S., Blum, R. W., Bauman, K. E., Harris, K., Jones, M. J., Tabor, J., Beuhring, T., Sieving, R. E., Shew, M., Ireland, M., Bearinger, L. H., & Udry, J. R.

(1997). Protecting adolescents from harm. *The Journal of the American Medical Association, 278*(10), 823-832.

Roth, J., Brooks-Gunn, J., Murray, L., & Foster, W. (1998). Promoting healthy adolescence: synthesis of Youth Development Program Evaluations. *Journal of Research on Adolescence, 8*, 432-459.

Rutter, M. (1985). Resilience in the face of adversity: protective factors and resistance to psychiatric disorder. *British Journal of Psychiatry, 147*, 598-611.

Rutter, M. (1987). Psychosocial resilience and protective mechanisms. *American Journal of Orthopsychiatry, 57*(3), 316-331.

Rutter, M. (1999). Resilience concepts and findings: implications for family therapy. *Journal of Family Therapy, 21*(2), 119-145.

Sonenstein, F.L., Stewart, K., Lindberg, L.D., Pernas, M., and Williams, S. (1997). *Involving males in preventing teen pregnancy-a guide for program planners.* Washington, DC: The Urban Institute.

Vincent, M. L.,Paine-Andrews, A., , Fisher, J., Devereaux, R. S., Dolan, H. G., Harris, K. J., & Reiniger, B. (2000). Replication of a community-based multicomponent teen pregnancy prevention model: realities and challenges. *Family and Community Health, 23*(3), 28-45.

In: Health Education Research Trends
Editor: P. R. Hong, pp. 25-32
ISBN: 978-1-60021-871-2
© 2007 Nova Science Publishers, Inc.

Expert Commentary E

CAN CONTEMPORARY HEALTH EDUCATION PREVENTION PROGRAMS HOLD THE CURRENT HIV/STD EPIDEMIC: A MISSING PIECE IN THE PROGRAM?

Maria Jose Miguez-Burbano and John E. Lewis

University of Miami Miller School of Medicine, Department of Psychiatry and
Behavioral Sciences, USA

ABSTRACT

Advances in the science of HIV prevention have been substantial in the past two decades. Nevertheless, the number of new HIV infections in any given year has remained relatively unchanged during the past decade, indicating that both HIV seropositive and seronegative men and women are still engaging in high risk practices [1-4]. Of concern in the United States (US), half of all new infections occur in people 25 years of age or younger [5-6]. Thus, abstinence-only, sex education targeting youths has proven ineffective in circumventing the HIV/STD epidemics, as the proportion of males 15-19 in the US who ever had heterosexual sex between 1995 and 2002 has virtually remained the same [5-6].

In addition, prevention activities in the US have not necessarily followed rigorous scientific evidence. Sexual transmission of HIV and other pathogens may involve different routes of infection (e.g., anal or vaginal sex) and specific levels of hazard [7-20]. For example, the probability of HIV acquisition by the receptive partner in unprotected vaginal sex is 10 per 10,000 acts, but it greatly increases if it occurs during menses [11-12, 20]. During anal sex, the probability is 50 per 10,000 acts [11, 12, 20]. Furthermore, since condoms are more likely to break during anal sex than during vaginal sex, anal sex can be risky even with a condom [11-12, 20]. Accordingly, anal sex and sex during menses are considered high-risk sexual practices, while oral sex is low-risk [11-20]. It is therefore important to have a clear sense of what has been researched, published, and currently being done (interventions) regarding these high-risk sexual practices. The following sources of data were identified in order to provide a comprehensive analytical review: interviews with leading institutions working in the area of HIV/AIDS and education, such as CDC, NIH, and STD clinics; summaries of research on HIV/AIDS and education by major research organizations; a review of journal-published research on this subject; a synthesis of on-line journal research publications; studies of research proposals representing research in progress, which has not yet been completed for publication; and a review of AIDS conference abstracts. Finally, we will highlight the future relevance of the findings and make recommendations for future prevention interventions.

HETEROSEXUAL RECEPTIVE ANAL SEX

Considering that heterosexuals account for 80% of the 40 million people infected with HIV and that almost half of the new infections are among women, HIV prevention strategies targeting heterosexual men and women are critical.[21] Published reports have established receptive anal intercourse without a condom as one of the most efficient routes of HIV transmission [7-14]. However, anal sex is presumed to not occur among heterosexuals, and many educational programs have neglected to cover what they call an "embarrassing topic" [7-14,22-23]. Although anal intercourse has been primarily associated with same gender transmission of HIV, the numbers of new HIV/AIDS cases due to heterosexual anal intercourse is increasing globally [7 8,18,25-27]. In 1992, 23% of respondents acknowledged having heterosexual anal intercourse within the previous year [25]. In Gross's survey [26] of 1,268 sexually active women, 32% reported having anal sex in the previous 6 months and most did not use condoms. Thus, it has been estimated that in term of absolute numbers women in the US are more likely to engage in unprotected anal intercourse than homosexual men [6, 7, 25-27]. To further add to the risks, anal sex was reported by higher proportions of women who had other risk behaviors associated with HIV/STDs, such as not always using condoms, use of drugs, a male sex partner with a history of injecting use, and having a STD in the previous year [18]. Halperin [8] reported that the risk of transmission for women was 10 times higher for anal sex than vaginal intercourse. Furthermore, Skurnick [27] demonstrated that concordant heterosexual couples were more likely to engage in unprotected anal sex than heterosexual discordant couples (p=0.001). It has become increasingly evident that heterosexual anal sex is an issue that needs to be addressed. In addition, anal intercourse and infection with multiple serotypes of human papillomavirus, the causative agent of precancerous dysplasia, are known risk factors for anal and cervical cancer [24]. The risk for progression of dysplastic lesions increases as the CD4+ cell counts decline, further highlighting concerns associated with high-risk sexual behavior. In sub-Saharan Africa, where an estimated 30 million people have HIV, experts believe that anal sex, both heterosexual and homosexual, is the second biggest cause of HIV transmission. Not surprisingly, heterosexual anal sex is practiced more than vaginal sex because of the mutilating type of cliteredectomies performed on young girls [24, 25]. In the Americas, our results along with others also demonstrated their important role in the transmission of HIV/STDs among the heterosexual population [22].

SEX DURING MENSTRUATION

In the early 1990s, Malamba and colleagues [16] investigated the risk involved in having unprotected sex during the menses. His study *reported that men exposed to menstrual blood were 7 times more likely to become infected with HIV* [16]. Sex during menses carries several compounding risks: 1) Reichelderfer [15] recently demonstrated that the highest HIV RNA levels occur during menses, independent of genital infections or inflammation. In the follicular period, one week after menses HIV levels in the genital tract are at their lowest. HIV levels gradually increase by the luteal phase and rise further by the pre-menstrual period, achieving the peak at menstruation. 2) The presence of blood changes the *pH* of the vagina from acidic to neutral, creating a more favorable environment for the survival of HIV. 3) During menstruation, women are more likely to have bacterial vaginosis, which has also been associated with HIV transmission [28]. 4) Al-Harthi et al. [29] provide evidence of elevated vaginal pro-inflammatory cytokine levels (IL-1beta, IL-4, IL-6, IL-8, IL-10, and MIP 1beta) during menses, which appear to regulate vaginal and not plasma HIV shedding. Elevations of those interleukins are of particular concern, as they have been associated with increased viral replication [30]. In addition, condoms for birth control are often not used.

Our studies in Colombia demonstrated that almost all commercial sex workers (99%) and 50% of the surveyed women from the general population reported having sex during menstruation [22]. Despite the recognized identification of blood as a primary source of HIV transmission (98%), only half of the women recognized the risk associated with menstrual blood. Our published studies in HIV-1 infected chronic drug users indicate that a large proportion (33%) of the Miami cohort engages in unprotected sex during menstruation [23]. These data suggest that additional research needs to be conducted to understand the cultural influences, knowledge, and beliefs involved in these high-risk sexual behaviors.

In a European Study group comprising 563 couples, risk factors for heterosexual transmission of HIV and efficiency of male-to-female and female-to-male transmission were investigated [31]. Results from this study indicated that AIDS in the index patient (odds ratio 17.6) and sexual contacts during menses (3.4) increased the risk of female-to-male transmission and stage of infection (2.7), anal sex (5.1), and age of the female partner (3.9; for age >45 years) increased the risk of male-to-female transmission (1992). To confirm the worldwide practice of unprotected sex during the menses, studies from Africa have shown that sex during menses is prevalent and may be a facilitating factor for HIV transmission in South Africa with an increased odds ratio of six [16-17]. Similar findings have been described among women from the Dominican Republic and Haiti [32].

Interestingly, we have observed that the level of education is not related to the frequency of sexual practices [22-23]. On one hand, unprotected intercourse during menstruation has been described as a frequent practice among commercial sex workers. On the other hand, a behavioral study conducted in Washington suggests that sex during menses is relatively more common among the better educated, young, white women and their sex partners [33]. Despite the fact that sex during menses is most common among women in relatively low-risk groups, the researchers were able to observe a significant association between sexual intercourse during menstruation and self-reported STD history [33], as it is associated with low indices of pregnancy, which is often considered a "safe" sexual practice.

Despite the increased risk for HIV transmission during the menses, few studies have investigated and targeted this high-risk behavior. These findings indicate that important health education issues remain to be fully addressed, and urgency exists to develop and implement prevention programs that include specific education principles targeting high-risk sexual behaviors.

Why Have Recommendations Been Ignored?

Twenty-five years after AIDS was first identified, the taboos that surround an open discussion of sexual behavior are still haunting us in our efforts to contain this pandemic. Studies have shown an increase in reported risk behavior among HIV-positive individuals receiving care, suggesting that primary care providers are not deeply involved in prevention efforts [34]. Studies have shown that primary care physicians do not routinely assess or intervene with their patients regarding their risks for HIV infection [35-36]. In addition, our data suggest that many physicians feel uncomfortable talking about sex [37]. Moreover, the roles of unprotected sex during menstruation and heterosexual anal sex as high-risk sexual practices have been downplayed by arguments that these sex acts are infrequent. However, our findings along with others demonstrate that these behaviors are widespread among members of our community, and more prevalent among some racial/ethnic groups.

Government-supported prevention programs in the US have addressed the drug-using risks of heterosexual men. Few have addressed their sexual behavior and none has targeted the risks posed by heterosexual anal sex and/or sex during menses. Although the CDC summarized the risks of oral sex and mention anal sex regarding same gender sex encounters in their fact sheet [5-7], these data have not been translated into any specific behavioral intervention, including information, education, communication programs, condom promotion, and behavior change initiatives that encourage people, particularly heterosexuals, to specifically reduce these high-risk behaviors [38]. Accordingly, most men and women are oblivious to the health-risk consequences of engaging in these practices without condoms [9,17]. On the contrary in Africa, heterosexual anal sex and sex during menses have recently been cited by researchers as the cause of the spread of the HIV epidemic [39-41].

The other important source of information is the mass media, but unfortunately, the last time major journals reported on the issue was two years ago regarding Africa's epidemic. In the US, the news mainly covers the annual CDC reports and only a handful of local papers make reference to these high-risk sexual practices behind too much text [11]. Disregarding the importance of unprotected anal sex and sex during menstruation for the risk of STD transmission is fueling the spread of HIV in the general population. Unwillingness among doctors, prevention programs, some governments, journalists, and the public in general to acknowledge the issue will continue to undermine prevention and education efforts.

Need for Interventions

Although condoms can prevent viral transmission, large numbers of uninfected men and women who have receptive anal sex do not use condoms consistently; either by choice or due to reasons out of their control. With anal intercourse, more strain is placed on the condom, thus stronger and thicker condoms are recommended. Use of a generous amount of water-based or silicon-based lubricant with a condom when having anal sex is also recommended to reduce friction and condom breakage [42]. Condoms with a lubricant containing Nonoxynol-9 should not be used for anal sex, as Nonoxynol-9 damages the lining of the rectum, which increases the risk of transmitting HIV and other STDs. Due to these limitations, some people use the female condom for anal sex [42]. Although it can work effectively, it is difficult to use and can be painful. The risk of rectal bleeding also increases the risk of contracting HIV.

Rectal microbicides could be a good protection alternative. Efforts have primarily focused on the development and evaluation of mechanism-specific microbicides to be applied intravaginally before sex to prevent transmission of HIV and other sexually transmitted diseases [43]. The first generation of surfactant microbicides had a non-specific mechanism of action and target-specific microbicides are in clinical development [43]. When vaginal microbicides demonstrate effectiveness, they are likely to be used rectally, whether or not data support the safety and efficacy of this application [44]. Understanding the extent to which anal intercourse spreads HIV infection will also become increasingly important as researchers race to devise microbicides, which may be effective only when used vaginally. The development of a rectal microbicide is even more complicated than a vaginal microbicide because the area to be protected from infection is so much larger and the tissues more delicate. It is essential that we substantially increase our knowledge and that microbicide knowledge and design be based on scientific and specific foundations, rather than based upon 'what is available to test or use'.

CONCLUSION

These findings recommend a new generation of behavioral interventions, which provide both factual knowledge and life skills, to promote behavioral risk reduction. As this information is currently unavailable, it is important to develop pertinent educational material for appropriate prevention strategies.

REFERENCES

[1]   Kelly J. A., Kalichman S.C. (1998). Reinforcement value of unsafe sex as a predictor of condom use and continued HIV/AIDS risk behavior among gay and bisexual men. *Health Psychol, 17*(4):328-35.

[2]   Miller M., Meyer L., Boufassa F., et al. (2000) Sexual behavior changes and protease inhibitor therapy. SEROCO Study Group. *AIDS, 14*(4):pF33-9.

[3]   Roffman R. A., Stephen R. S., Curtin L., Gordon J. R., Craver J. N., Stern M., Beadnell B., Downey L. (19980. Relapse prevention as an interventive model for HIV risk reduction in gay and bisexual men. *AIDS Educ Prev, 10*(1):1-18.

[4]   Sherman D. W., Kirton C. A. (1999). The experience of relapse to unsafe sexual behavior among HIV-positive, heterosexual, minority men. *Appl Nurs Res, 12*(2):91-100.

[5]   Vital Statistics. 2007 April 1. Available from: http://www.until.org/statistics.shtml

[6]   Centers for Disease Control and Prevention (CDC). Last time visit: 2007 April 1. Available from: *http://www.cdc.gov/hiv/topics/surveillance/basic.htm#hivaidsage*

[7]   Centers for Disease Control and Prevention (CDC). Last time visit: 2007 April 1. Available from: Can I get HIV from anal sex. *http://www.cdc.gov/hiv/resources/qa/qa22.htm*

[8]   Halperin D. T. (1999). Heterosexual anal intercourse: prevalence, cultural factors, and HIV infection and other health risks, Part I. *AIDS Patient Care STDS, 13*(12):717-30.

[9]   Halperin D. T., Shiboski, et al. USAID. Wash DC. Abst# ThPeC7438. AIDS, Barcelona, 2002.

[10]   Voeller B. (1991). AIDS and heterosexual anal intercourse. *Arch Sex Behav.,* 1991;20(3):233-76.

[11]   William Saletan. (2005).The media's Silence about Rampant Anal Sex Available from: *http://www.slate.com/id/2126643/*

[12]   Centers for Disease Control and Prevention (CDC). Fact Sheet 2003. Last time visit: 2007 April 1. Available at: *http://www.cdc.gov/hiv/pubs/Facts/afam.pdf*

[13]   Kingsley L.A., Detels R., Kaslow R., Polk B.F., Rinaldo C.R., Chmiel J., Detre K., Kelsey S.F., Odaka N., Ostrow D. (1987). Risk factors for seroconversion to human immunodeficiency virus among male homosexuals. Results from the Multicenter AIDS Cohort Study. *Lancet, 1*(8529):345-9.

[14]   Polk B. F., Fox R., Brookmeyer R., Kanchanaraksa S., Kaslow R., Visscher B., Rinaldo C., Phair J. (1987). Predictors of the acquired immunodeficiency syndrome developing in a cohort of seropositive homosexual men. *New Engl J Med,316*(2):61-6.

[15]   Reichelderfer P. S., Coombs R. W., Wright D. J. (2000). WHS 001 Study Team. Effect of menstrual cycle on HIV-1 levels in the peripheral blood and genital tract. *AIDS, 14* (14):2101-7.

[16]   Malamba S. S., Wagner H. U., Maude G., et al. (1994). Risk factors for HIV-1 I infection in adults in a rural Ugandan community: a case-control study. *AIDS, 8*(2):253-7.

[17]   Kalichman S. C. Simbayi L. C. (2004). Sexual exposure to blood and increased risks for heterosexual HIV transmission in Cape Town, South Africa. *African Journal of Reproductive Health, 8*(2):55-8.

[18]   Erickson P. I., Bastani R., Maxwell A. E., Marcus A. C., Capell F. J., Yan K. X. (1995). Prevalence of anal sex among heterosexuals in California and its relationship to other AIDS risk behaviors. *AIDS Education & Prevention. 7*(6):477-93.

[19]   Mayer K. H. Anderson D. J. (1995).Heterosexual HIV transmission. *Infectious Agents & Disease, 4*(4):273-84.

[20]   HIV: How high is your risk?. Last time visit 2007 April 1. Available from: *http://www.health24.com/medical/Condition_centres/777-792-814-1764,35251.asp*

[21]   UNAIDS. AIDS Epidemic Update, (2002).

[22]   Miguez-Burbano M. J., Angarita I., Shultz J. M., Shor-Posner G., Klaskala W., Duque J. L., Lai H., Londoňo B., Baum M. K. (2000). HIV-related high-risk sexual behaviors and practices among women in Bogotá, Colombia. *Women & Health, 30*(4):109-19.

[23]   Miguez-Burbano M. J., Pineda-Medina L., Lecusay R., Page J. B., Castillo G., Burbano X., Rodriguez A., Rodriguez N., Shor-Posner G. (2002). Continued high risk behaviors in HIV infected drug abusers. *J Add Dis., 21*(4):67-80.

[24]   Palefsky J. M. (1996). Anogenital Neoplasia in HIV-positive women and men. *HIV Adv Res Ther, 6*(3):10-17.

[25]   Fullilove M. T., Willie J., Fullilove R. E et al. (1992). Risk for AIDS in multiethnic neighborhoods of San Francisco California. The population based AMEN. *West J Med,157*:32-40.

[26]   Gross M., Holte S. E., Marmor M., Mwatha A., Koblin B. A., Mayer K. H. (2000). Anal sex among HIV-seronegative women at high risk of HIV exposure. The HIVNET vaccine preparedness study 2 protocol team. *JAIDS, 24*(4):393-98.

[27]   Skurnick J. H., Kennedy C. A., Perez G., Abrams J., Vermund S. H., Denny T., Wright T., Quinones M. A., Louria D. B. (1998). Behavioral and demographic risk factors for transmission of human immunodeficiency virus type 1 in heterosexual couples: report from the Heterosexual HIV Transmission Study. *Clin Infect Dis, 26*(4):855-64.

[28]   Quayle A. (1994). Mucose membrane susceptibility to HIV infection. *The AIDS Reader,* 125-27.

[29]   Al-Harthi L., Kovacs A., Coombs R. W., Reichelderfer P. S., Wright D. J., Cohen M. H., Cohn J., Cu-Uvin S., Watts H., Lewis S., Beckner S., Landay A., WHS 001 Study Team. (2001). A menstrual cycle pattern for cytokine levels exists in HIV-positive women: implication for HIV vaginal and plasma shedding. *AIDS, 15*(12):1535-43.

[30]   Lewis H. S., Beckner S., Landay A., WHS 001 Study Team. (2001). A menstrual cycle pattern for cytokine levels exists in HIV-positive women: implication for HIV vaginal and plasma shedding. *AIDS, 15*(12):1535-43.

[31]   Anonymous. (1992). Comparison of female to male and male to female transmission of HIV in 563 stable couples. European Study Group on Heterosexual Transmission of HIV. *BMJ, 304*(6830):809-13.

[32]   Brewer T. H., Hasbun J., Ryan C. A., Hawes S. E., Martinez S., Sanchez J., Butler de Lister M., Constanzo J., Lopez J., Holmes K. K.(1998). Migration, ethnicity and environment: HIV risk factors for women on the sugar cane plantations of the Dominican Republic. *AIDS, 12(14):1879-87.*

[33]   Tanfer K., Aral S. O. (1996). Sexual intercourse during menstruation and self-reported sexually transmitted disease history among women. *Sex Transm Dis., 23*(5): 395-401.

[34]   Erbelding E. J., Stanton D., Quinn T. C., Rompalo A. (2000). Behavioral and biologic evidence of persistent high-risk behavior in an HIV primary care population. *AIDS, 14:* 297–301.

[35]   Gerbert B., Bleecker T., Bernzweig J. (1993). Is anybody talking to physicians about acquired immunodeficiency syndrome and sex? *Arch Fam Med,* 2:45–51.

[36] Gerbert B., Brown B., Volberding P., et al. (1999). Physicians' transmission
      prevention assessment and counseling practices with their HIV positive patients. *AIDS
      Educ Prev, 11*: 307–320.

[37] Miguez-Burbano, M. J., Navas, G., Forero, M.G., Burbano, X., Rodriguez, N., Shor-
      Posner, G. (2002). Evaluation of HIV prevention and counseling practices of
      obstetrician/gynecologists in Bogota, Colombia: Impact on women's knowledge and
      risk practices. *AIDS Education and Prevention, 14* (Suppl. A):68-76.

[38] Compendium of HIV Prevention Interventions with Evidence of Effectiveness.

[39] Last time visit 2007 April 1. Available from: *http://www.cdc.gov/hiv/pubs
      /hivcompendium HIVcompendium.pdf*

[40] AIDS Risk in Africa vastly different from Western countries or the U.S. Available
      from: *http://www.libchrist.com/std/africa.html*

[41] Brady M. (1993). Female genital mutilation: complications and risk of HIV
      transmission. *AIDS Patient Care and STDs, 13*: 709-716.

[42] Africa needs anal sex awareness. Last time visit 2007 April 1. Available from:
      http://www.mask.org.za/article.php?cat=news&id=665 - 36k - Apr 28, 2007 -2010.

[43] AIDSmap. Condoms and lubricants. Last time visit 2007 April 1. Available from:
      http://www.aidsmap.com/en/docs/A85BA23D-6F72-4CD2-90A4-D914A60BEF79.asp

[44] Balzarini J. Van Damme L. (2007). Microbicide drug candidates to prevent HIV
      infection. *Lancet. 369*(9563):787-97.

[45] Elias CJ. Female-controlled methods to prevent sexual transmission of HIV (Abstract
      Tu08). In: Programs and abstracts of the XI International Conference on AIDS,
      Vancouver, Canada, 1996.

In: Health Education Research Trends
Editor: P. R. Hong, pp. 33-41

ISBN: 978-1-60021-871-2
© 2007 Nova Science Publishers, Inc.

Short Communication A

RELATIONSHIP BETWEEN AFTER-SCHOOL GROUP LEADERS' AND CHILDREN'S PHYSICAL ACTIVITY AND FRUIT AND VEGETABLE CONSUMPTION

Stefanie Haas[1] and Claudio R. Nigg[2,]*

[1]University of Karlsruhe, Institute for Sport and Sport Sciences, Karlsruhe, Germany;
[2]University of Hawaii at Manoa, Department of Public Health Sciences,
Honolulu, HI 96822.

ABSTRACT

Social influence studies of physical activity (PA) and nutrition with regard to children have been mostly focused on parental influence. The purpose of the current study is to explore the correlation between PA and nutrition behaviors of after-school program group leaders, and the children they supervise. Two samples (sample 1, group leader: n=77, 85.7% female; sample 2, children: n=257, 45.1% male) from the same after school program completed Godin's Leisure-Time Exercise Questionnaire and specific questions about inactivity and nutrition. Bivariate correlations revealed large relationships between vegetable consumption (r=.57) of group leaders and children. Small negative correlations were found between mild activity (r=-.25) and fruit consumption (r=-.16) of group leaders and children. No correlation could be found between group leaders and children for strenuous (r=.06) and moderate (r=-.03) PA behavior or inactivity (r=.02). Our findings indicate that after-school group leaders' health behaviors may be related to some children's health behaviors, which provides another potential avenue of promoting children's health behavior.

* Correspondence concerning this article should be addressed to: Dr. Claudio R. Nigg, Department of Public Health Sciences, John A. Burns School of Medicine, University of Hawaii at Manoa, 1960 East-West Road, Honolulu, HI 96822. Tel: (808) 956-2862, Fax: (808) 956-5818, Email: cnigg@hawaii.edu.

Keywords: Physical activity, nutrition, adults, children, social support, after school.

Improving physical activity levels of youth is a central public health challenge. On the basis of the decline in physical activity during preadolescence, it is necessary to develop effective interventions to support children and young people in increasing their physical activity levels [1]. Benefits of regular physical activity include a reduced risk of coronary heart disease, diabetes, colon cancer, hypertension and osteoporosis [2]. Additionally, physical activity can enhance physical functioning and aid in weight control [2]. Unhealthy nutrition and lack of physical activity contribute to overweight and obesity. Among children (6-11 years of age) and adolescents (12-19 years of age), the percent overweight has increased from 1976 to 1980. From 1999 to 2002 about 16 percent of children and adolescents were overweight [2].

In addition, trends indicate a continual decrease in physical activity. For example, only 28 percent of high school students, nationwide, engaged in daily physical activity in 2003 [2]. The alarming decline in physical activity during preadolescence and adolescence presents a particular challenge to researchers and professionals in health and physical activity [3]. There are various factors that may influence a young person's level of physical activity. One such factor is the interaction between adults and children.

BACKGROUND / SOCIAL SUPPORT / INFLUENCE

Social support has been defined in numerous ways, commonly referring to any behavior of another that helps a person in achieving desired goals or outcomes [4,5]. Social support is classically divided into subtypes that include emotional, instrumental, appraisal and informational support [6]. Emotional support is often offered by an intimate other, although less intimate ties can provide such support under circumscribed conditions [6]. Instrumental support refers to help, aid, or assistance with concrete needs, for example getting to an appointment [6]. Appraisal support relates to assistance in decision making or giving suitable feedback [6]. Informational support is connected to the provision of advice or information in the service of exacting needs [6].

Social support has been identified to influence social behavior. Different studies examined the influence of parents, teachers, family members, and friends,. The behavior of parents and friends are considered to be among the more important influences on adolescent behavior [7,8,9]. Bandura's *social learning theory* explains that young people tend to imitate the behaviors of parents and peers [9].

Parental influence has been studied across health behaviors. Their use of cigarettes influences the child's smoking behaviors [10,11,12] Children of alcoholic parents are more likely to use substances [13] and have negative effects of their intellectual ability [14]. Some studies examined children's eating attitudes and behaviors, finding significant correlations between parent and child snack food intake [15,16].

Social support has been cited as an essential correlate of physical activity [17,18]. A few studies have examined the impact of family and friend support on youth physical activity and have found initial support for this influence [19,20,21]. However, social factors other than parent modeling have not been broadly studied [22]. There are some studies analyzing teachers' influences among children's social behavior, such as aggression [23,24]. participation [25] and students' motivation [26], but there seems to be limited evidence for physical activity or nutrition. Further, after-school programs provide an opportunity to influence children's health behaviors [27]. However, this environment or after-school group leaders' potential influence on the children they oversee has not been investigated regarding health behaviors.

The purpose of the current study is to examine the relationship between after school program group leaders and the children they supervise, regarding physical activity and nutrition behaviors. It is hypothesized that the group leaders' behavior is related the children's behavior in terms of physical activity level and fruit and vegetable consumption.

METHODS

Design and Procedure

The two data sets used in this investigation involved different study populations associated with the Fun 5 project – a physical activity and nutrition program delivered in an after-school program setting [27,28]. All data collection and consent forms used in this study have been IRB approved. Sample 1 [group leader baseline data of year 1 for Fun 5 dissemination sites in Oahu, Big Island (Hawaii), and Maui] data collection was conducted by study staff on-site during after-school program time. For sample 2 [child baseline data of year 1 for Fun 5 dissemination with same sites in Oahu, Big Island (Hawaii) and Maui],master documents of parent consent and student questionnaires were provided to all of the participating after-school site coordinators. The site coordinators were asked to copy and then collect consent and subsequently administer the survey and returned the complete materials.

Table 1. Frequencies and Percentage of the different samples

| | Groupleader | | | Children | |
	%	n		%	n
Age	**n=77**		**Grade**	**n=258**	
15-20	46.90	23	4	37.20	96
21-30	20.40	10	5	36.80	95
31-40	14.30	7	6	26.00	67
41-50	10.20	5			
51-60	8.20	4			
Gender	**n=77**		**Gender**	**n=257**	
male	14.3	11	male	45.10	116
female	85.7	66	female	54.90	141

Participants

Sample 1: These data were collected in Fall 2004. 77 group leaders of 15 sites (85.7% female, M_{age}=28.20 (SD =12.48)) completed the survey.

Sample 2: These data were collected in Fall 2004. 15 of 72 after school programs returned data with a total of 258 participants (45% male, grade 4-6, M_{grade}=4.89 (SD =.79)).

For this study the two samples were merged into one data set. Data was analyzed at the after school site level and compared the relationship between the group leaders and their students from the same site. Fifteen different sites (n=15) were examined. Table 1 shows the distribution across grade/age and gender for sample 1 (group leader) and sample 2 (children).

Measures

Survey

Physical activity behavior: The Leisure-Time Exercise Questionnaire created by Godin and Shephard was adapted [29]. Participants report how many times during an average week they do strenuous, moderate, and mild physical activity for more than 30 minutes continuously during their leisure time. 30 minutes was used instead of the original 15 minutes, to be congruent with the physical activity guidelines [30]. Strenuous activity was defined as heart beats rapidly, sweating, e.g. jogging, running, vigorous swimming, vigorous long distance bicycling, vigorous aerobic dance classes. Moderate physical activity was defined as not exhausting, light sweating, e.g. fast walking, baseball, easy bicycling, volleyball, hula. Mild physical activity was defined as minimal effort, no sweating, e.g. easy walking, yoga, horseshoes. Jacobs, Ainsworth, Hartman and Leon [31] have reported excellent reliability and validity for this instrument. In addition, one further question was included; addressing sedentary behavior – how many hours the participant watched TV or played video games on an average day [32].

Fruit and Vegetable Consumption was assessed by one item each: "How many servings of fruits do you eat each day?" and the same question for vegetables. A serving was described as ½ cup of cooked vegetables = size of 2 golf balls; 1 cup of salad = size of 1 baseball; 1 piece of fruit = size of 1 baseball; or ¾ cup of 100% fruit juice = 6 ounces.

Analyses

Due to power issues, interpretations for correlations were based on Cohen's guidelines [33] (r=.2 small; r=.5 medium; r=.8 large). Data analysis was conducted via SPSS 14.0. (2005, SPSS Worldwide Headquarters, Chicago, IL).

RESULTS

Table 2 shows the means and standard deviations of group leaders and children for all variables.

Table 2. Mean and Standard deviation of group leader and children

	Groupleader		Children	
Variables	mean	std.	mean	std.
strenuous PA	2.78	1.55	3.99	.62
moderate PA	3.27	1.33	3.28	.65
mild PA	4.19	.96	3.09	.74
inactivity	2.51	1.20	3.53	1.10
fruit consumption	2.36	1.00	3.28	.66
vegetable consumption	2.40	1.10	2.87	.70

Table 3. Correlation between PA and nutrition variables of group leader and children

	1	2	3	4	5	6	7	8	9	10	11	12
group leaders												
strenuous PA (1)	1.0	.91**	.64**	-.40	.28	.34	.06	-.12	.04	.06	-.70**	.19
moderate PA (2)		1.0	.71**	-.51	.17	.16	-.03	-.03	-.04	.11	-.67**	.05
mild PA (3)			1.0	-.13	-.01	.24	.01	-.15	-.25	.21	-.50	.14
Inactivity (4)				1.0	-.32	-.12	-.39	-.08	.14	.02	.28	-.11
fruits (5)					1.0	.73**	-.16	.05	.18	.47	-.16	.16
vegetables (6)						1.0	-.22	-.25	.04	.13	-.17	.57*
Children												
strenuous PA (7)							1.0	.16	-.16	-.07	.00	-.08
moderate PA (8)								1.0	.71**	.31	-.10	-.56*
mild PA (9)									1.0	.18	-.09	-.23
inactivity (10)										1.0	-.36	-.43
fruits (11)											1.0	.27
vegetables (12)												1.0

**Correlation is significant at the 0.01 level (2-tailed).

*Correlation is significant at the 0.05 level (2-tailed).

Table 3 presents the correlations between the physical activity and nutrition variables for children and group leaders. There was a medium correlation between group leaders and children for vegetables consumption ($r=.57$). A small negative correlation between group leaders and children for mild activity ($r=-.25$) and fruit consumption ($r=-.16$). No correlation could be found between group leaders and children for strenuous ($r=.06$) and moderate ($r=-.03$) physical activity behavior, or for inactivity ($r=.02$).

DISCUSSION

The purpose of this study was to investigate if physical activity and nutrition behaviors of after-school program group leaders are related to the same behaviors of the children in their care.

The outcomes of this study show that there is an influence in terms of nutrition. This is primarily driven by vegetable consumption. The results show a medium correlation between vegetable consumption of group leaders and the consumption of vegetables of their students. Both groups eat between 2 and 3 servings a day. Bandura has theorized a plausible mechanism – that behavior of other people can influence an individual's own behavior and observing others can be a source of self-efficacy beliefs [34]. No positive influence emerged in terms of fruit consumption. It seems that group leaders (mean=2.36) eat less fruits than children (mean=3.28). An explanation could be that children are more influenced by parents in terms of fruit consumption.

Between group leaders and children, no significant correlations of physical activity behavior could be found. One reason for this could be a low commitment by the group leaders to their own physical activity, or a lack of interest in children's physical activity. Children are not usually in this after-school program for physical activity or nutrition. The group leaders' primary task is to watch over the children and not to do physical activity or nutrition. Another reason could be that the group leaders do not know how to properly impart their knowledge about physical activity or nutrition to the children. They are not trained teachers.

The results of this study show that the group leaders are related to children more in terms of nutrition than physical activity behavior. The reason for the stronger influence of nutrition could be a lack of physical activity during the after school program, as only 13% of the time in the after school program was committed to physical activity [27]. The group leaders may spend more time having snacks than being active and doing physical activity.

Another reason why the outcomes of this study are not as pronounced as expected could be the limited social support provided by the group leaders. As mentioned earlier, social support is divided into four subtypes [6]. Because of the limited interaction and the fact that the group leaders in the after school programs are not trained teachers, emotional and instrumental support for health behaviors is most likely not provided to the children. Group leaders' social support is restricted to a few hours and only a fraction thereof is health related. In addition, their appraisal and informational support is distributed over their entire group, limiting individual attention.

There are some limitations that need to be considered when interpreting the outcomes of this study. First of all, the sample (15 sites) used in this research is small. With decreasing numbers the chance of random distortion of the results increases (Law of Large Numbers) [35]. Consequently, the significance results have to be considered cautiously. Also, the data were collected by self-report only. Therefore, the results could possibly be influenced by social desirability. In addition, the questionnaire targets the physical activity and nutrition during leisure time. However, exercising in leisure time does not affect children's behavior since the group leaders are not modeling it in front of the children. Social modeling is an important factor for behavior change, when it can be observed [34].

In conclusion, after-school group leaders' health behaviors may be related to some children's health behaviors. This preliminary evidence provides another potential avenue of promoting children's health behavior. More research is necessary to examine the influence of physical activity and nutrition behavior of after school group leaders among children, using larger samples. Further, it would be interesting to examine whether boys or girls are particularly influenced by male or female group leaders. A further focus should also examine the extent, intensity and duration of social support that is necessary to promote children to engage in appropriate physical activity and nutrition behavior.

ACKNOWLEDGEMENT

Funded by the Hawaii Medical Service Association, an Independent Licensee of the Blue Cross and Blue Shield Association. We would like to thank the valuable contributions of: Marisa Yamashita, Jo Ann Chang, Richard Chung, Jackie Battista, Megan Inada, Crystalyn Hottenstein, Nicole Kerr, and Kelley McGee; the private providers (Kama'aina Kids, YMCA and the Hawaii State Department of Education) and the participating sites.

REFERENCES

[1]   Sallis JF, Prochaska JJ, Taylor, WC, Hill JO, Geraci JC. Correlates of physical activity in a national sample of girls and boys in grades 4 through 12. *Health Psychol.* 1999;18(4):410-415.

[2]   Centers for Disease Control and Prevention. Health, United States, *2005 With chartbook on trends in the health of Americans*. Hyattsville, Maryland, U.S.; 2005.

[3]   Pender NJ, Sallis JF, Long BJ, Calfas KJ. Health-care provider counseling to promote physical activity. In R.K. Dishman (Ed.), *Advances in Exercise Adherence* (pp. 213-235). Champaign, IL: Human Kinetics; 1994.

[4]   Caplan RD, Robinson EAR, French JAP, Caldwell JR, Shinn M. *Adhering to medical regimes: Pilot experiment in patient education and social support*. Ann Arbor: University of Michigan, Institute for Social Research; 1976.

[5]   Taylor WC, Baranowski T, Sallis, JF. Family determinants of childhood physical activity: A social-cognitive model. In R.K. Dishman (Ed.), *Advances in exercise adherence* (pp. 319-342). Champaign, IL: Human Kinetics; 1994.

[6]   House JS. *Work stress and social support*. Reading, MA: Addison-Wesley; 1981.

[7]   Sutherland EH, Cressey DR. *Principles of criminology*. 7th ed. Philadelphia: Lippincott; 1966.

[8]   Hirschi T. *Causes of delinquency. Berkeley*, CA: University of California Press; 1969.

[9]   Bandura A. *Social learning theory*. Englewood Cliffs, NJ: Prentice-Hall; 1977.

[10]   Sasco AJ, Kleihues P. Why can't we convince the young not to smoke? *Eur J Cancer*. 1999;35,1933-1940.

[11]   Maziak W, Mzayet F. Characterization of the smoking habit among high school students in Syria. *Eur J Cancer*. 2000;16,1169-1176.

[12]   Bauman KE, Carver K, Cleiter K. Trends in parent and friend influence during adolescence: the case of adolescent cigarette smoking. *Addict. Behav*. 2001; 26(3):349-61.

[13]   Chassin L, Rogosch F, Barrera, M. Substance use and symptomatology among adolescent children of alcoholics. *J Abnorm Psychol*. 1991;100(4):449-463.

[14]   Poon E, Ellis DA, Fitzgerald HE, Zucker RA. Intellectual, cognitive, and academic performance among sons of alcoholics, during the early school years: differences related to subtypes of familial alcoholism. *Alcoholi Clin Exp Res*. 2000;24(7):1020-7.

[15]   Fisher JO, Birch LL. Restricting access to a palatable food affects children's behavioral response, food selection and intake. *Am J Clin Nutr*. 1999;69,1264-1272.

[16]   Brown R, Ogden J. Children's eating attitudes and behavior: a study of the modeling and control theories of parental influence. *Health Ed Res*. 2004;19(3):261-271.

[17]   King AC. Clinical and community interventions to promote and support physical activity participation. In RK Dishman (Ed.), *Advances in Exercise Adherence* (pp. 183-212). Champaign, IL: Human Kinetics; 1994.

[18]   Pender NJ, Sallis JF, Long BJ, Calfas KJ. Health-care provider counseling to promote physical activity. In RK Dishman (Ed.), *Advances in Exercise Adherence* (pp. 213-235). Champaign, IL: Human Kinetics; 1994.

[19]   Sallis JF, Simons-Morton BG, Stone EJ, Corbin CB, Epstein LH, Faucette N. Determinants of physical activity and interventions in youth. *Med Sci Sport Exer*. 1992;24,S248-S257.

[20]   Zakarian JM, Hovell MF, Hofstetter, CR, Sallies JF, Keating KJ. Correlates of vigorous exercise in a predominantly low SES and minority high school population. *Prev Med*. 1994;23(3):314-321.

[21]   Cleland V, Venn A, Fryer J, Dwyer T, Blizzard, L. Parental exercise is associated with Australian children's extracurricular sports participation and cardiorespiratory fitness: A cross-sectional study. *Int J Behav Nutr Phys Act*. 2005;6;2(1):3.

[22]   Sallis JF, Taylor WC, Dowda M, Freedson PS, Pate RR. Correlates of vigorous physical activity for children in grade 1 through 12: Comparing parents-reported and objectively measured physical activity. *Ped Exer Sci*. 2002;14,30-44.

[23]   Hughes JN, Cavell TA, Jackson T. Influence of the teacher-student relationship on childhood conduct problems: a prospective study. *J Clin Child Psychol*. 1999;28(2),173-184.

[24] Chang L. Variable effects of children's aggression, social withdrawal, and prosocial leadership as functions of teacher beliefs and behaviors. *Child Dev.* 2003;74(2):535-548.

[25] Ladd GW, Birch SH, Buhs ES. Children's social and scholastic lives in kindergarten: related spheres of influences? *Child Dev.* 1999;70(6):1373-400.

[26] Wentzel KR. Are effective teachers like good parents? Teaching styles and student adjustment in early adolescence. *Child Dev.* 2002;73(1):287-301.

[27] Battista J, Nigg CR, Chang JA, Yamashita M, Chung R. Elementary After School Programs: An opportunity to promote physical activity for children. *Calif J Health Promot.* 2005;3(4),108-118.

[28] Nigg CR, Inada M, Yamashita M, Battista J, Chang JA, Chung RS. Fun 5: a physical activity and nutrition program - dissemination in elementary after school programs. *Ann Behav Med.* 2005;29,52.

[29] Godin G, Shepard RJ. A simple method to assess exercise behavior in the community. *Can J Appli Sport Sci.* 1985;10,141-146.

[30] Pate RR, Pratt M, Blair SN et al. Physical activity and public health. A recommendation from the Centers of Disease Control Prevention and the American College of Sports Medicine. *JAMA.* 1995;273,402-407.

[31] Jacobs DR, Ainsworth BE, Hartman TJ, Leon AS. A simultaneous evaluation of 10 commonly used physical activity questionnaires. *Med Sci Sport Exer.* 1993;25,81-91.

[32] Buckworth J, Nigg, CR. Physical activity, exercise, and sedentary behavior in college students. *J Am Coll Health.* 2004;53(1),28-34.

[33] Cohen J. *Statistical power analysis for the behavioral sciences.* Hillsdale: Lawrence Erlbaum; 1988.

[34] Bandura A. Self-efficacy: Toward a unifying theory of behavioral change. *Psychol Rev.* 1997;84,191-215.

[35] Boes K, Haensel F, Schott N. *Empirische Untersuchungen in der Sportwissenschaft.* Hamburg: Czwalina; 2000.

In: Health Education Research Trends
Editor: P. R. Hong, pp. 43-48

ISBN: 978-1-60021-871-2
© 2007 Nova Science Publishers, Inc.

Short Commentary B

HEALTH EMPOWERMENT = SELF EFFICACY + HEALTH LITERACY – A *USEFUL* EQUATION

John Hubley[1] and Peter Sternberg[2]

[1]School of Health and Community Care, Leeds Metropolitan University, UK;
Department of Health, Exercise and Rehabilitative Sciences, Winona State University,
Winona, MN 55987, USA.

ABSTRACT

This communication briefly explores the use of the terms empowerment, self efficacy and health literacy, and suggests that they can be used to define health empowerment in an operationally useful way. It suggests that some of the difficulties in evaluation of empowerment have been the different ways in which the concept has been conceptualised. One particular problem is that discussion of the concept of empowerment often relies solely on issues of power, ignoring the dimension of health decision-making. It is suggested that health empowerment can usefully be considered as a combination of two key concepts Self Efficacy and Health Literacy. The widespread availability of scales for measurement of both self efficacy and health literacy is discussed and it is suggested that a measurement of health empowerment can be made by the combination of existing scales.

This communication briefly explores the use of the terms empowerment, self efficacy and health literacy, and suggests that they can be used to define health empowerment in an operationally useful way.

The concept of empowerment has mixed origins. Conceptually, within psychology, it is related to 'Perceived Locus of Control' and also to 'Self Efficacy' from 'Social Learning Theory.' The term also has roots in adult education theory drawing heavily on Brazilian,

Paulo Freire, whose radical adult literacy method was based on the idea of 'conscientisation' - a dynamic process of critical understanding, reflection, action and learning from action (praxis) (Freire 1972). Since the Ottawa conference in 1986, health promotion has been concerned with the operationalizing of empowerment. Much has been written about the concept, which has become almost a holy grail for health promoters. Yet even defining empowerment remains a problematic exercise fraught with semantic and theoretical dangers (Rissel 1994).

Empowerment seems to mean different things not only to different disciplines which use it but also to the individual theorists and practitioners within those disciplines. It is seen by some as a cognitive concept related to self determination and self efficacy (Tones 1991;Wallerstein and Bernstein 1994). It is seen by others as the process of gaining control over material resources (Laverack and Wallerstein 2001). Empowerment is viewed by a number of commentators as a dialectic and dynamic process of change in power relationships (Rappaport 1981; Katz 1983; Gibson 1991; Ryles 1999) and citizen participation (Rich *et al.* 1995). To others empowerment is regarded as the cornerstone of responsible behavior (Ryles 1999). Some regard it as a process, others as an outcome (Wallerstein and Bernstein 1988).

Though the literature around empowerment distinguishes between community empowerment and personal or psychological empowerment, there is a recognition that individual empowerment is a necessary precursor of community empowerment and that making distinctions between the process of empowering individuals and empowering their communities may be a rather academic exercise (Speer and Hughey 1995; McMillan *et al.* 1995). Empowered communities consist of empowered individuals, but, as Wilson (Wilson 2004) points out, in order to be an empowered individual, one needs to connect with others, a product of this connection is community empowerment. That said, the process by which communities become empowered continues to be a focus of research by many as there seems to be a recognition that at least in terms of outcome the effect of community empowerment is more than the sum of its parts (empowered individuals) (Sheill A. and Hawe 1996). For this reason, it is perhaps useful to regard empowerment as ultimately a product of community rather than the sum of empowered individuals. Reading these comments and arguments about the meaning of empowerment, it is easy to come to the conclusion as Laverack and Wallerstein point out (Laverack and Wallerstein 2001), that the concept remains remains "thorny and elusive" and for practitioners rather confusing and difficult to operationalize.

Despite all of the rhetoric and discussion of empowerment over the last twenty years, little evidence exists that empowerment can in fact lead to positive changes in the health of individuals or communities. Given the ill-defined and problematic nature of empowerment it is not surprising that the evidence-base for it remains weak.

In contrast, the concept self efficacy has a well established basis in the health education and psychological literature. Bandura (9301) suggests that a perception of self efficacy (viewed as the perception that one has control over events that affect one's life), is a necessary precursor and motivator to action. Simply put, empowered action is only possible if one has a perception of self efficacy. Bandura (Bandura 1994) observes that self efficacy is created in four ways. It can be the result of successfully completing a task, especially if this success has not come easily. Self efficacy can result from the observation of others who are competent and proficient social models. Self efficacy may result from social persuasion that a person is good enough or 'has what it takes.' Finally self efficacy may be the result of reducing emotional stress and encouraging a positive outlook.

Perceived self efficacy has been shown to be an important predictor of people's abilities to make major lifestyle changes, such as to their nutritional habits (Bagozzi and Edwards 1998; Brug *et al.* 1997; Fuhrmann and Kuhl 1998; Gollwitzer and Oettingen 2004) or to the amount of physical activity that they take (Dzewaltowski et al. 1990; Feltz and Riessinger 1990; McAuley 1992; McAuley 1993). In order to measure self efficacy and in particular to distinguish it from other cognitive predictors of change suggested by the Health Belief Model, self efficacy scales have been developed. An on-line search of Pubmed and Medline data bases found 30 separate self efficacy scales targeting 27 separate health behaviors and conditions.

Evaluations of health education programmes have repeatedly demonstrated that change in knowledge does not result in action and improved health (Hubley 1986). The lesson is clear - knowledge alone is not enough, people need to feel that they have the power to make health promoting changes in their lives. However, though power is self evidently central to an understanding of empowerment, any definition of the concept that restricts itself solely to a discussion of power has serious weaknesses. Health promotion requires not only that individuals and communities are capable of exercising their power to make change but also that they understand the health issues well enough to make informed health decisions. Consequently, an approach to empowerment that concentrates solely on changing power relations without also facilitating understanding of the health issues is seriously flawed.

It is at this point that the concept of health literacy appears of offer real benefits in understanding the concept of empowerment in a way which is useful for practitioners. Health literacy has been variously defined. Originally, the concept was used as a measure of the capacity of individuals to understand instructions about medicines. Nutbeam in his *Health Promotion Glossary* (Nutbeam 1998) broadens the concept from a strictly cognitive domain. In his definition, "health literacy represents the cognitive and social skills which determine the motivation and abilities of individuals to gain access to, understand and use information in ways to promote and maintain good health". In testimony to the growing interest in this area, a comprehensive bibliography of the health literacy literature from January 1990 to October 1999 by the National Library of Medicine (Selden *et al.* 2000) contains 479 citations and provides a useful working definition of self literacy: "the degree to which individuals have the capacity to obtain, process and understand basic health information and services needed to make appropriate health decisions."

Both definitions expand on earlier narrowly-focussed concepts based on reading ability to include including a cognitive element of basic understanding about health issues, interpretation of health information and the ability to apply this to make informed decisions about health. The inclusion of social skills by Nutbeam is of particular interest. It is not just a question of being able to understand and process information, but importantly also of having the communication, assertiveness and negotiation skills to use the information to bring about health promoting change.

In a recent review Tones (Tones 2002) criticises the concept of 'health literacy' calling it "old wine in new bottles." While the substance of Tone's critique is true - many of the elements of health literacy are familiar existing concepts - this does not negate the usefulness of an overarching concept that brings health understandings and decision making skills together in a way that they can be usefully applied to health promotion.

We suggest that Health Literacy and Self Efficacy can be usefully considered as the two key components of Health Empowerment such that Health Empowerment results from the combination of Self Efficacy and Health Literacy as shown below:

Health Empowerment = Self Efficacy + Health Literacy

This understanding of Health Empowerment has some immediate advantages in health promotion. The most important benefit is that it makes the cognitive and affective domains of health empowerment explicit. Conceiving of health empowerment as the combination of Self Efficacy and Health Literacy incorporates what is already known about two well-researched existing concepts each with already validated indicators. The result of using these well researched concepts to define health empowerment is that empowerment becomes measurable and therefore capable of being evaluated through changes in objective indicators. The practical upshot of this is that it is much easier for practitioners to design, implement and evaluate interventions that aim to empower individuals and their communities to make changes that affect their health.

Self efficacy can be achieved in a variety of ways that promote self esteem and develop individual or community power over their lives and surroundings.. In situations where self efficacy has already been developed in members of a community through action on other issues not involving health, health promoters can build upon this and focus on the promotion of health literacy. While scales for self efficacy exist at the individual level, less clear cut is what such scales might look like when applied at the family or community level. To some extent, the work of Rifkin on measurement of participation (Rifkin *et al.* 1988) and more recently Laverack on community capacity (Laverack and Wallerstein 2001) might be interpreted as useful attempts to define self efficacy at a community level.

Promoting health literacy involves appropriately designed health education, which seeks to develop understanding of health issues and how to apply these to make decisions. Ratzen , one of the members of the National Library of Medicine team that compiled the literature review cited above, provides a thoughtful review of some of the communication methods required to promote health literacy and discusses the role of strategic scientific communication using formative research (Ratzan 2001). The field manual, *Communicating Health,* applies health literacy and self efficacy to the developing world and provides suggestions on the use of various health education methodologies including patient education, community- and school- based interventions folk and mass media (Hubley 2004). The challenge is to provide this cognitive input through health education methods which reinforce and not undermine individual and community confidence and power.

In conclusion we propose that that a concept of health empowerment that brings together self efficacy and health literacy provides some real benefits for planning and evaluation of health promotion. The challenge ahead is to apply these ideas to real life programmes in community settings to demonstrate that interventions can bring about a change in health empowerment and that this will lead to improvements in health.

REFERENCES

Bagozzi, R. P. and Edwards, E. A. (1998) Goal setting and goal pursuit in the regulation of body weight. *Psychology and Health, 13,* 593-621.

Bandura, A. (1994) Self-efficacy. In Ramachaudran, V. S. (ed), *The encycopaedia of human behaviour.* Academic Press, New York, pp. 71-81.

Brug, J., Hospers, H. J. and Kok, K. (1997) Differences in psychosocial factors and fat consumption between stages of change for fat reduction. *Psychology and Health, 12,* 719-727.

Dzewaltowski, D. A., Noble, J. M. and Shaw, J. M. (1990) Physical activity participation: Social cognitive theory versus the theories of reasoned action and planned behaviour. *Journal of Sport & Exercise Psychology, 12,* 388-405.

Feltz, D. L. and Riessinger, C. A. (1990) Effects of in vivo emotive imagery and performance feedback on self-efficacy and muscular endurance. *Journal of Sport & Exercise Psychology, 12,* 132-143.

Freire, P. (1972) *Pedagogy of the Oppressed.* Penguin Books, London.

Fuhrmann, A. and Kuhl, J. (1998) Maintaining a healthy diet: effects of personality and self-reward versus self-punishment on commitment to and enactment of selfchosen and assigned goals. *Psychology and Health, 13,* 651-686.

Gibson, C. H. (1991) A concept analysis of empowerment. *J Adv.Nurs, 16,* 354-361.

Gollwitzer, P. M. and Oettingen, G. (2004) The emergence and implementation of health goals. *Psychology and Health, 13,* 687-715.

Hubley, J. (2004) *Communicating health - an action guide to health education and health promotion. 2nd Edition.* Macmillan, Oxford.

Hubley, J. H. (1986) Barriers to health education in developing countries. *Health Education Research: Theory and Practice, 1,* 233-245.

Katz, R. (1983) Empowerment and synergy: expanding the community's healing resources. *Prev Hum Serv, 3,* 201-230.

Laverack, G. and Wallerstein, N. (2001) Measuring community empowerment: a fresh look at organizational domains. *Health Promot.Int., 16,* 179-185.

McAuley, E. (1992) The role of efficacy cognitions in the prediction of exercise behavior in middle-aged adults. *J.Behav.Med., 15,* 65-88.

McAuley, E. (1993) Self-efficacy and the maintenance of exercise participation in older adults. *J.Behav.Med., 16,* 103-113.

McMillan, B., Florin, P., Stevenson, J., Kerman, B. and Mitchell, R. E. (1995) Empowerment praxis in community coalitions. *Am J Community Psychol, 23,* 699-727.

Nutbeam, D. (1998) Health promotion glossary. *Health Promotion International, 13,* 349-364.

Rappaport, J. (1981) In praise of paradox: a social policy of empowerment over prevention. *Am J Community Psychol., 9,* 1-25.

Ratzan, S. C. (2001) Health literacy: communication for the public good. *Health Promotional International, 16,* 207-214.

Rich, R. C., Edelstein, M., Hallman, W. K. and Wandersman, A. H. (1995) Citizen participation and empowerment: the case of local environmental hazards. *Am J Community Psychol*, *23*, 657-676.

Rifkin, S. B., Muller, F. and Bichmann, W. (1988) Primary health care: on measuring participation. *Social Science and Medicine*, *26*, 931-940.

Rissel, C. (1994) Empowerment: The Holy Grail of Health Promotion? *Health Promotion International*, *9*, 39-47.

Ryles, S. M. (1999) A concept analysis of empowerment: its relationship to mental health nursing. *J.Adv.Nurs.*, *29*, 600-607.

Selden, C. R., Zorn, M., Ratzan, S. and Parker, R. M. (2000) *Health literacy. Current bibliographies in medicine; no.2000-1*. National Library of Medicine, Bethesda (MD).

Sheill A. and Hawe, P. (1996) Health promotion, community development and the tyranny of individualism. *Health Econ*, *5*, 241-247.

Speer, P. W. and Hughey, J. (1995) Community organizing: an ecological route to empowerment and power. *Am.J Community Psychol.*, *23*, 729-748.

Tones, B. K. (1991) Health promotion, empowerment and the psychology of control. *Journal of the Institute of Health Education*, *29*, 17-26.

Tones, K. (2002) Health literacy: new wine in old bottles? *Health Educ.Res.*, *17*, 287-290.

Wallerstein, N. and Bernstein, E. (1988) Empowerment education: Freire's ideas adapted to health education. *Health Educ.Q.*, *15*, 379-394.

Wallerstein, N. and Bernstein, E. (1994) Introduction to community empowerment, participatory education, and health. *Health Educ.Q.*, *21*, 141-148.

Wilson, P. (2004) Empowerment: Community economic development from the inside out. *Urban Studies*, *33*, 617-630.

In: Health Education Research Trends
Editor: P. R. Hong, pp. 49-94

ISBN: 978-1-60021-871-2
© 2007 Nova Science Publishers, Inc.

Chapter I

THERAPEUTIC MECHANISMS OF A MUTUAL SUPPORT GROUP FOR CHINESE FAMILY CAREGIVERS OF PEOPLE WITH SCHIZOPHRENIA

Wai-Tong Chien[1] and Ian Norman[2]

[1]The Nethersole School of Nursing, Faculty of Medicine, The Chinese University of Hong Kong, Hong Kong SAR, China;
[2]Division of Health & Social Care Research, King's College London, UK.

ABSTRACT

Schizophrenia is a disruptive and distressing illness for both patients and their family members who find their caregiving responsibility a heavy burden. Studies demonstrate that family-centered intervention for schizophrenia sufferers is essential and effective. However, little is known about the effects of such interventions for family members, particularly in non-Western populations.

An exploratory qualitative study was conducted to explore from the participants' perspective the benefits and limitations of a mutual support group for Chinese family caregivers of people with schizophrenia. Thirty-four family caregivers, who had participated in a 12-session mutual support group over six months, were interviewed and twelve group sessions were audio-taped for content analysis. The analysis of the interview and group session data indicated that most of the participants indicated positive personal changes during group participation and had progressively undergone the five phases of group development. The results also elicited three therapeutic mechanisms of the mutual support group. They included: reconstructing a new positive self-image in relation to caregiving; the psychological empowerment of caregivers through the acquisition of knowledge and skills for care-giving; and extending the social support networks both within and outside the group.

The study shows that a mutual support group can provide benefits for Chinese families of people with schizophrenia that go beyond those provided by routine family support. The three therapeutic mechanisms of the support group provide insights that might be drawn upon by health professionals when designing family group interventions.

Further research is recommended to explore whether these five-phase development and therapeutic components of the group intervention identified in this study apply also to mutual support groups in families with different socio-economic backgrounds and across cultures.

INTRODUCTION

In spite of rapid development in pharmacological and psychosocial treatments of schizophrenia, the dissemination of psychosocial interventions as routine practice within the mental health services has been slow and patchy (Penn & Mueser, 1996). Many newly invented neuroleptic drugs can give patients partial protection against environmental stress to patients with schizophrenia and other psychotic illnesses, but they need to be supplemented with a therapeutic social environment, especially a healthy and supportive family. However, the shortcomings of community care have produced many negative consequences for the families of the mentally ill, who are often coerced into the service to compensate for the deficiencies of the community care system (Saunders, 1999). Specialized care and new early intervention services may be a means of engaging patients in community mental health services and reducing patients' re-hospitalizations; however, limited evidence exists because of wide variations in implementation with little guidance, or inadequate funding from the health authorities towards early detection, home treatment and services to prevent relapse (Craig et al., 2004).

Families, particularly those family members who live with their relative with schizophrenia, often face daily stressors including the patient's unpredictable and bizarre behavior, external stressors of social stigma and isolation, emotional frustration such as guilt and loneliness, and family conflicts, which arise during the caring process (Ohaeri, 2003). Studies have shown that family caregivers may report psychological distress, social and family disharmony, and practical problems in living with and taking care of the patient at home. Similarly Canive et al. (1996) and Martens and Addington (2001) describe family caregivers as suffering from depression, anxiety, grief and somatic complaints, as well as disruption to their social and recreational activities and domestic routine, and reduction in their household income. Therefore, caregiving for a relative with schizophrenia or other severe mental illness is extremely stressful and burdensome, with negative consequences for social and psychological health of the caregivers, indicating the importance of health professionals providing family-oriented mental health care (Loukissa, 1995).

Family intervention for schizophrenia sufferers has consistently demonstrated positive effects on improving patients' relapse rates, and enhancing their families' knowledge about the illness and their coping ability in caregiving. Psychological models of family intervention involving psychoeducation, behavioral management, or family-centered psychosocial support (Dixon et al., 2001; Hogarty et al., 1991; Sellwood et al., 2001) are the recent widely used approaches. Review studies suggest that an effective family intervention should include education about the illness and its treatment, and discussion about the skills in caregiving such as communication, problem solving, medication compliance, and information about health care resources (Barbato & D'Avanzo, 2000; Pharoah, Mari, & Streiner, 2001).

However, recent studies have suggested that the effect of such intervention on patient and family-related outcomes, other than the positive effects mentioned above, are inconsistent and inconclusive (Sellwood et al., 2001; Telles et al., 1995).

Nevertheless, the notion of family intervention is multifaceted and complex in nature. Pharoah et al. (2001) have suggested that the widely held belief that family intervention programs that consist of a clearly defined set of psychoeducational and/or cognitive-behavioral techniques following a step-by-step skill-building format do not always indicate significant positive effects on patients and/or their families' health conditions. Increasing research evidence indicates that peer support and practical assistance within family groups associates with considerable improvements in psychological adjustments by families of a relative with chronic physical or mental illness (Heller, Roccoforte, Hsieh, Cook, & Pickett, 1997a).

Mutual support groups for families of people with schizophrenia, which are characterized as client-led, community alternatives to the professional-dominated programs in today's mental health services, have demonstrated apparent benefits. In many qualitative and quasi-experimental studies (Heller et al., 1997; Pearson & Ning, 1997), and recently in two controlled trials with a Chinese population (Chien, 2004; Chien, Norman, & Thompson, 2004), it has been reported that mutual support groups maintain the psychological and social well being of family caregivers, as well as their mentally ill relatives.

Cook, Heller, and Pickett-Schenk (1999) suggest that a mutual support group offers a place for family members to ventilate their feelings, not just of resignation but also of helplessness, pain and fear. Thus, group cohesiveness can be established on the basis of these common concerns and experiences. Chou, Liu, and Chu (2002) also indicate that it is important and essential to establish a trusting relationship between participants in a mutual support group to induce a sense of security and personal respect. As a result, the group participants can face their fears and worries and discuss these feelings without needing to defend their positions. Self-disclosure might help resolve difficulties in getting participants involved and developed in a support group.

It is also noteworthy that little is known about the therapeutic components of mutual support groups, psychoeducation, and other approaches to family intervention for schizophrenia or other chronic mental illnesses, which are perceived as beneficial to the participants. Lehman and Steinwachs (1998) and Brooker (2001) suggested that the hesitation of clinicians to use family intervention might be attributed to inadequate knowledge of researchers of the key elements within family intervention that enhance its therapeutic effects for family caregivers and patients. Increased understanding of the active ingredients of family intervention, such as a mutual support group, would facilitate the design of interventions for family caregivers of patients with schizophrenia and thus produce optimal benefits for patients and their families (Chien & Chan, 2004). This Chapter presents the exploratory study that was one of the relatively few and had sought to identify the group participants' perceived therapeutic benefits and difficulties of a mutual support group for family caregivers of these patients in a Chinese population.

The results of analyses of the interview and group session data in this study identified the therapeutic mechanisms of a mutual support group program, which may reveal possible explanations of its effectiveness on promoting the health of the family members caring for a relative with schizophrenia. The group participants gave their accounts of the psychological and behavioral changes in terms of the five phases of group development, as suggested by Wheelan (1994) and Kimberly (1997). The main themes and sub-themes, which were the factors or mechanisms perceived by the participants as influencing the therapeutic values of the mutual support group, are illustrated with verbatim data; and four therapeutic mechanisms of the mutual support group and their potential outcomes by bringing together the findings are presented. Finally, there is a detail discussion about each of the four therapeutic mechanisms; and in the final section, the limitations and implications of the study for clinical practice and research are presented.

BACKGROUND OF THE STUDY

Importance of Family-focused Intervention for People with Schizophrenia

There are several reasons for providing interventions for families of people with schizophrenia. First, studies on expressed emotion, which refers to the critical or emotionally over-involved attitudes and behavior displayed by one or more family members to their relative with schizophrenia (Kavanagh, 1992), has revealed that family dynamics and emotional climate affect the reoccurrence of positive symptoms and therefore the course of the illness (Butzlaff & Hooley, 1998). While the mechanisms of action of high expressed emotion in the course of schizophrenia are unclear, it is clear that a high level of distress is inevitably experienced by a patient who is in regular and frequent contacts with such family members (Mueser & Gingerich, 1994; Repper & Brooker, 1998). However, the education and involvement of these family members in the planning and implementation of treatment can only benefit the monitoring of progress of treatment and changes in patient's condition. Enhanced ability of family members to detect any warning signs of relapse, and notifying health professionals about such signs, can be crucial in preventing these illness relapses. There have been reports of long delays in treatment due to inadequate family support (Barnes et al., 2000; Drake et al., 2000).

Second, having an intimate relationship with a relative with schizophrenia and providing care for such a person can induce a great burden on family members. Families, if used as a 'dumping ground' for these patients, may be overwhelmed by the challenges and difficulties in managing a patient with schizophrenia, even though there are some positive aspects of caregiving such as a sense of inner strengths and satisfaction, personal growth and enhanced family relationship (Greenberg, Greenley, & Benedict, 1994; Winefield & Harvey, 1994). Reducing caregiver burden is an important goal of family support and care that can help family members remain involved with their loved ones while maintaining their own physical and psychosocial well-being (Mueser, 2003).

Lastly, high levels of stress within a family, which may arise from caregiver burden, can have a negative effect on a patient's illness, increasing their vulnerability to relapse (Butzlaff & Hooley, 1998). The intimate relationship and interactions between patients with schizophrenia and their family members warrants application of family-centred interventions for improving the ability of families to work with their patient to cope more effectively with stress relating to caregiving from within and outside the family (Mueser & Glynn, 1999).

Families were once scapegoated as a major causative factor of the pathogenesis of schizophrenia (Lefley, 1996), but more evidence today is that families can play a vital role in helping their relative with schizophrenia in making good progress towards recovery from the illness (Mueser, 2003). Working with families appears to be one effective way of delivering community-based intervention to the patients. Nevertheless, families need adequate support themselves if they are to support their disabled relative. To enhance family support and care for patients with schizophrenia, there have been increased research studies in developing and testing different modes of family intervention over the past 20 years. The development of various types of family intervention for patients with schizophrenia has brought significant positive changes in psychosocial interventions for these patients, and their families.

Development of Family Interventions for People with Schizophrenia

Treatments for patients with schizophrenia reflect dominant ideas on the causes of the illness. The origins of family intervention can be traced to theories of family causation of the illness, which go back to the 1940s and 1950s. In the 1950s, research on dysfunctional communication in families originated from the idea of the 'double bind' (Bateson et al., 1956), which occurs when an instruction is given overtly to a patient by family members, but is contradicted by a second more covert instruction. As suggested by Bateson, this 'double bind' communication leaves the child able to make only ambiguous or meaningless responses, and schizophrenia was thought to develop when this process persists. Studies of communication in families of patients with schizophrenia have indicated rather inconsistent and conflicting findings (Hirsch & Leff, 1975), the disordered family communication and role relationships are considered to be important factors associated with the course of the illness and patient's recovery.

In the late 1950s, the theory of expressed emotions (EE) was developed in an attempt to describe emotional attitudes of family members towards patients with schizophrenia and its relationship with the illness. The concept of EE was developed by Brown et al. (1962) and measured with a semi-structured interview schedule (Camberwell Family Interview) on three dimensions: criticisms, hostility and emotional involvement. This EE concept has proven useful for understanding the interactions within families with a member suffering from schizophrenia. A meta-analysis of 27 studies of the EE-outcome relationship with schizophrenia in the United States and other Western countries (Butzlaff & Hooley, 1998), confirms that EE is a significant and robust predictor of relapse in schizophrenia (i.e. the weighted mean effect size was 0.31), particularly for those primary family caregivers with high face-to-face contact with the patient. More evidence continues to accumulate highlighting the link between health status of patients and family caregivers and family relationships (Cole & Reiss, 1993; Wearden et al., 2000).

Leff et al. (1985) using a combination of support and education for family members managed to successfully lower expressed emotion in families and thus positively reduce patients' relapse rate (i.e. 14% relapse in family support group vs. 78% in control group with regular medications over two-year follow-up). Since then, EE related research has focused not only on the patient's relapse but also on the effect of caring on the whole family. Karanci and Inandilar's (2002) study of coping and distress of caregivers of Turkish patients with schizophrenia indicated that caregivers' perceptions of their ability to cope with patient's symptom behaviors such as aggression and antisocial behavior, and their reported distress due to these behaviors are closely related to their EE level. Similarly in the United Kingdom, Budd, Oles and Hughes (1998) studied the relationship between caregiver burden and coping style in 91 family caregivers of patients with schizophrenia, and reported that greater extents of emotional involvement and criticism are associated with higher levels of family burden. It has also resulted in various therapeutic and educational strategies aimed at reducing family caregivers' EE in order to improve patients' illness and symptom intensity, and thus reduce their relapse rates.

A long-standing theoretical rationale underlying the use of family-centered intervention comes from studies in the West, which have reported consistently that patients with schizophrenia who live in families that have high levels of EE would have relapse rates three to 10 times greater than those who live in low EE families (Bebbington & Kuipers, 1994; Ivanovic, Vuletic, & Bebbington, 1994). Studies on EE also show that the role of family attitudes and interactions influence the course of schizophrenia, but there is not enough evidence that it influences onset of the illness, as might be predicted by the stress-vulnerability model (Barrowclough & Johnston, 1996; Wearden et al., 2000). Barrowclough and Parle (1997) suggest that critical factors common to successful psychosocial interventions for schizophrenia include helping the family, especially those with high levels of EE, in reducing their negative attitudes towards patient's illness and increasing their confidence in coping with patient's symptoms and bizarre behavior.

Family intervention techniques have developed gradually and become accepted as an alternative to biomedical or pharmacological treatment for changing families' attitudes, relationships and communication patterns. However, even up to the late 1970s, family theories and therapies for schizophrenia were supported by little empirical evidence. Most studies showed disappointing, non-significant or modest results, which contrasted with over-ambitious claims for the efficacy of family therapy. Mueser (2003) suggested that in the West, there are difficulties in employing family interventions in everyday clinical practice with groups of patients with schizophrenia in receipt of community care, due to inadequate mental health care services, staff training and resources. Research in the 1980s has already indicated that information and caregiving skills learning were important but were too frequently unavailable as a community resource for patients and families (Noh & Turner, 1987). A field study in the US (Dixon et al., 1999) also found that less than one-third of patients who have contact with their families reported that their families had received information, support, or advice about their illness and less than 10% said that their families had attended an educational or supportive program. Ma and Yip (1997) suggest similar reasons to explain why family intervention has not been frequently used in community-based treatment for patients with schizophrenia in Chinese and Asian populations.

In spite of inadequately trained therapists, research over the 1980s has established a more sound evidence base on the effects of family environment for schizophrenia, especially for those families with highly critical or emotionally over-involved attitudes towards patients.

With much increased interest and understanding of the importance of the role of the family in caring for patients with schizophrenia in the community, there have been very positive advances in the development of different types of family intervention in parallel to psychosocial intervention for patients with schizophrenia, over the last 15 years (Brooker, 2001; Mueser, 2003).

Continuing Development of and Demands for Family Intervention Programs

Demands for family interventions within the community have also increased substantially as a result of changes in the organization of mental health services over the past decade in Western countries (Budd & Hughes, 1997), and also in Asia, mainland China, or Hong Kong. It is beyond doubt that the current emphasis on community care and caring for the caregivers has made family intervention a crucial component of the treatment plans for patients with schizophrenia. Wide dissemination of an effective model of family intervention is a priority for improvement of contemporary community mental health services.

Pharoah et al. (2001) and Pilling et al. (2002) in their meta-analysis of controlled trials of family interventions involving over 2,000 patients with schizophrenia (from 1980 to 1999), in different countries such as the United States, the United Kingdom, Australia, and mainland China, concluded that all types of family intervention (both single and group format) are more effective in reducing patient relapse up to one year, readmission up to two years and rates of treatment compliance, when compared to standard care. As recommended by the American Psychiatric Association (1997) and Schizophrenia Patient Outcomes Research Team (Lehman, Steinwachs & the Survey Co-investigators of the PORT project, 1998), which was funded by the National Institute of Mental Health in the US, patients who have ongoing contact with their families should be offered a family psychosocial intervention that spans at least six months and provides a combination of education about the illness, family support, crisis intervention, and problem-solving skills training. In addition, the team suggests that family intervention should not be restricted to patients whose families are identified as having high levels of expressed emotion. Similarly, the National Institute for Clinical Excellence in the United Kingdom in its clinical guideline of core interventions in the management of patients with schizophrenia suggested that family intervention should be available to the families who are living with or who are in close contact with patients with schizophrenia (National Collaborating Centre for Mental Health, 2002).

Nevertheless, the past decade has witnessed rapid growth of a variety of family intervention strategies, which have been largely influenced by cognitive-behavioral and stress and crisis theories. Single or multiple-family group intervention programs, and those consisting mainly of education, behavioral and supportive components, have been used in the treatment of people with a variety of chronic mental health problems such as depression, anxiety disorders (Anderson et al., 1986), dementia (McCallion & Toseland, 1995), and eating disorders (Dare & Eisler, 2000). However, different terms are used to refer to work with families, such as psychoeducational, psychosocial, family education, family management, family support, or combinations of these terms. In the absence of agreed terminology, the guidelines suggested by Fadden (1998) in the research update on family interventions may be helpful. Fadden suggested that the terms psychosocial, psychoeducation and behavioral management approaches to family interventions, generally refer to those interventions in an individual or group format, where patient and family members meet together, where there is a component of skills acquisition in addition to a didactic teaching element; and the primary aim of the program is to reduce patient relapse and readmission. He also suggested that family education, consultation, support, and counseling and relatives' groups usually refer to interventions directed at family members (excluding the patient); and their primary focus is on the needs of family members.

Four board modes of family intervention are frequently used in the West and mainland China to address specific treatment outcomes including reduction of patient relapse and family burden and improvement of family and patient functioning. These modes include: family psychoeducation, behavioral family management, multiple-family group intervention, and family consultation or supportive counseling. Of these four types of family intervention, most recently developed programs begin with a few teaching sessions, which cover basic information on the etiology, symptoms, medical and psychological treatments, and prognosis of schizophrenia (Pilling et al., 2002; Hazel et al., 2004). Intervention approaches then differ in subsequent sessions over content, format, duration, and the time intervals between sessions. As suggested by the Schizophrenia Patients Outcomes Research Team in the United States (Lehman et al., 1998), family education and support programs are usually organized around the central theme of providing family members of people with schizophrenia with education about the illness and its treatment, guidance and resources for patient care and for family caregivers during crisis, and training in managing common problems in caregiving.

Even though different techniques or approaches are used, family interventions for schizophrenia aims to achieve some common goals, including: (1) working in alliance with families who care for the person with schizophrenia to identify stressors associated with family dysfunction and patient relapse; (2) enhancement of problem anticipation and problem solving; (3) improvement of family atmosphere by reduction of high emotional involvement and critical attitudes towards the patient by their family such as hostility and criticism; (4) setting realistic expectations on patients' social, vocational and performance in the home; (5) helping families improve communication and relationship with patients; and (6) attainment of desirable change in family members' behavior and understanding of the illness and its care (Pharoah et al., 2001). However, little is known about the therapeutic value of different components or strategies (Dyck et al., 2002). With better understanding of these crucial therapeutic elements within family intervention, it may be possible to develop a more consistent, reliable and effective family intervention program for patients with schizophrenia.

In addition, two reviews of family intervention studies (Dixon et al., 2000; Solomon, 2000) suggest that there are several characteristics common to the four modes of family intervention mentioned above: (1) being delivered and led by health professionals such as nurses, social workers and psychiatrists; (2) primary focus on patient outcomes such as relapse and medication compliance with family outcomes as secondary; main components, including information about the illness, its medication and treatment and strategies on patient management; (3) involving all interested family members, including the patient; long-term intervention is more effective (e.g. at least six months); and (4) exclusion of any beliefs and concepts which presume families are the causal agent of the development of schizophrenia.

In the last decade, a number of reviews (Barbato & D'Avanzo, 2000; Mari & Streiner, 1996; Pilling et al., 2002) have highlighted the possible advantages of family intervention for people with schizophrenia conducted in several countries such as the United States, the United Kingdom and other European countries, and mainland China. Among the different models of family intervention in schizophrenia, psychoeducation (e.g., Hogarty et al., 1991) and behavioral family management programs (e.g., Falloon & Pederson, 1985) have been the most extensively studied modalities. More recently needs-based psychosocial interventions (e.g., Sellwood et al., 2001) have been established with specific consideration of individual family needs.

However, there were some exceptions, namely trials mostly undertaken in 1970s and 1980s, using models such as crisis intervention model by Goldstein et al (1978) and psychodynamic model by Kottgen et al. (1984). These models demonstrated negative or non-significant effects when compared with standard care (Leff et al., 1982; Levene et al., 1989) or psychoeducation intervention (McFarlane et al., 1995), and evaluations suffered major methodological limitations such as small sample size, non-equivalent or no control group, and case study design.

A relatively recent systematic review of controlled trials between 1978 and 1996 by the Cochrane Schizophrenia Group (Pharoah et al., 2001) suggests that most psycho-education and supportive approaches of family intervention have consistently demonstrated positive effects on reducing patients' relapse rate and improving patients' medication compliance and families' knowledge about the illness. The specific effects of family intervention on family members' psychosocial needs, such as family functioning, coping with caregiving, psychological distress and burden of care, and management of patient within the home environment, have not been studied adequately and so data are few and equivocal. However, those few studies (Falloon & Pederson, 1985; Tarrier, 1991; Xiong et al., 1994), which have included an economic evaluation, suggest that psychoeducational or behavioral family intervention is more cost-effective than the conventional mental health services.

When comparing the effects of different models of family intervention on patient and family-related outcomes, studies in mainland China (Xiong et al., 1994; Zhang et al., 1994), the United Kingdom (Tarrier et al., 1994) and other Western countries (Dixon et al., 2001; McFarlane, Dixon, Lukens, & Lucksted, 2003), have consistently demonstrated that family psycho-education and/or behavioral approaches of intervention spanning at least 10 sessions over six months is more effective and shows relatively long-lasting effect (more than three years) on the prevention of relapse among people with schizophrenia, than individual psychosocial treatment or medication alone. However, the psychoeducation and behavioral approaches of intervention, as described by researchers in previous studies, consisted of a variety of content, format and techniques. The common elements in several approaches of effective family psychoeducation programs include social support, education about the illness and its treatment, guidance and resources during crisis, and training in problem solving (Dixon et al., 2001; Lehman & Steinwachs, 1998). However, little is known about the major therapeutic components of psychoeducation and other psychosocial models of family intervention for schizophrenia (Barbato & D'Avanzo, 2000).

Methodological Limitations of Studies of Family Intervention for People with Schizophrenia

In spite of inconsistent findings from research on family intervention for people with schizophrenia, the superiority of family intervention programs over routine outpatient care has been demonstrated and some significant effects such as relapse rate and medication compliance have been maintained for as long as two years. Recent reviews of more than 20 clinical trials of family interventions for people with schizophrenia conducted in Western countries and mainland China (Dixon et al., 2000; Solomon, 2000; Pharoah et al., 2001), highlighted questions about the effectiveness of family interventions, which remain unanswered and require further research. First, there is a lack of conclusive evidence about the effects of commonly used models of family intervention on health outcomes of family caregivers of people with schizophrenia. With much responsibility and burden put onto family members caring for their relative with schizophrenia under the trend of community care, more preparation of family caregivers in terms of knowledge and skills of caregiving as well as coping with the illness and problems in caregiving should be provided within the family intervention program. The family caregivers' psychosocial health conditions, which are significantly associated with the care of their ill relatives and the treatment outcomes, should be emphasized and treated as important indicators for the effectiveness of a family-focused intervention. Assessment of family-related outcomes of family intervention including family functioning, perceived social support, and health services utilization should be addressed in further research. In addition, as suggested by Pharoah et al. (2002), clinically significant changes in family outcome measures following the intervention were defined and examined in this thesis to understand the significant and meaningful changes in psychosocial health conditions of family caregivers in the direction of functionality, resulting from participation in the specifically designed family group work.

Second, little is known about the therapeutic value of different family intervention components or strategies. The described curative factors and mechanisms of change in the literature consist mainly of subjective accounts by therapists or facilitators of what they believed to be the important factors experienced within their own practice. Major identified factors include learning by analogy and identification of similar experience (Steinglass, 1998; Bishop et al., 2002), establishing a community of shared experiences (Steinglass, 1998), overcoming social stigma to the illness (Asen, 2002), and creating hope and adaptive patterns of coping and perspectives on illness and family life (Bishop et al., 2002). Although education about the illness and provision of social support are consistent ingredients of most models of family intervention for schizophrenia, they do not show any significant effect in isolation. Therefore, it is important to test the effect of family education and social support components in a specific model of family intervention emphasizing their use, for example the mutual support group used in this study. In fact, mutual support groups have been used increasingly with patients with chronic physical diseases, terminal illnesses and enduring mental illness and there is convincing evidence that they can meet caregivers' psychosocial needs (Cook et al., 1999). Further research is also needed to explore the most beneficial and important components of the family intervention used. The exploration of caregivers' perceived benefits and important therapeutic components of the intervention is also one major purpose of the evaluation study of a family mutual support group in this study. With better understanding of these crucial therapeutic elements within the family intervention, it may be possible to develop a more consistent, reliable and effective family intervention program for patients with schizophrenia.

Third, previous studies examined the effects of the highly structured family psychoeducation model such as Anderson et al.'s (1986) family psychoeducation program and the manual driven behavioral model such as Falloon and Pederson's (1985) family behavioral management program. These studies indicated that these prevalent approaches of family intervention for people with schizophrenia did not show consistent immediate or long-term improvements in family members' psychosocial health conditions, when compared with routine care or other simple supportive interventions such as brief crisis-oriented family psychoeducation (Linszen et al., 1996) and supportive family education programs (Bellack et al., 2000). Sellwood et al. (2001) also highlighted that effective family intervention may not require a specific defined set of advanced techniques, delivered through a highly structured model and manual of intervention, or with an intensively trained professional. The positive results of their trial of a needs-based family intervention indicate that family intervention should be designed from a family caregivers' perspective to be more able to recognize and meet their own psychosocial health needs in relation to caregiving, thus showing more positive family-related outcomes. With much increasing empirical evidence on multiple-family group interventions, bringing families together in supportive group intervention can produce specific and beneficial effects to family caregivers on improving their social support and coping with their caregiving role. The burden of care in schizophrenia is an issue that requires recognition, and attempts to ameliorate it, rather than to provide support, may be misplaced (Pilling et al., 2002).

Fourth, the implementation of family intervention techniques in routine practice has been hindered, however, for several reasons. Most importantly inadequate staff training and supervision, scarce resources, and lack of availability of trained staff, and difficulty in maintaining the effectiveness of an intervention delivered over many years compared to a relatively short term intervention which is subject to evaluation. Fadden (1997) shows great concern about implementation of family interventions in routine clinical practice and suggests that many of the difficulties experienced most frequently by trained staff are related to service issues. For cognitive-behavioral family intervention to be effective, staffs who are acting as therapists must be intensively trained and supervised in practice. It is often reported that trained staff cannot use the skills learned in their practice or intervention program following training, without adequate supervision or management support (Kavanagh et al., 1993; Brooker, 2001). Also, therapists need to be able to work flexible hours in order to accommodate evening or weekend appointments. Those therapists who were able to visit families frequently reported that they only managed to do so by working in their own time or working outside regular hours. Dyck et al. (2002) suggested that running family intervention programs with multiple-family groups may be one way of overcoming these staff and resource limitations for individual family treatment.

Finally, most of the studies of family intervention for people with schizophrenia were conducted in Western countries. The results of the evaluation of cross-cultural applicability of Falloon's behavioral management program in a Spanish-speaking population by Telles et al. (1995) did not support the positive findings from previous studies on patients' relapses and symptoms control when applied to a socio-cultural diverse population. This finding indicates that socio-cultural factors may influence caregivers' responses to different types of family intervention. Hence, modes of family intervention, which were originated in the West, should be tested in a variety of patient populations with different cultural backgrounds such as the Chinese patients in this study, thus providing more evidence on their effectiveness across cultures. The perceptions of family members as program participants should be explored to identify their views on the actual benefits and barriers in attending the family intervention program.

Mutual Support Groups for Families of People with Severe Mental Illness

In the 1980s, multiple-family group intervention was increasingly used among families of people with chronic and severe mental illness. Most of the clinical trials on family intervention for people with chronic and severe mental illness in the United States and the United Kingdom were professional-led, didactic education programs with patient participation, and focused on teaching family members how to take care of their patient at home and to prevent patient's relapse (McFarlane, 2002). The use of mutual support groups as an approach to family intervention for these patients was not commonly accepted and used in Western countries until the late 1980s (Lefley, 1996). With increased attention and concerns about the health needs of family caregivers under the trend of family-based treatment for severe mental illness, many clinicians and researchers suggest that family intervention should not only contribute to patient recovery but also meet the families' psychosocial needs in caregiving (Solomon, 2000). Mutual support groups for family caregivers of a relative with severe mental illness, which provide information about mental illness, its treatment and community resources, opportunities to share feelings and experiences without fear of stigma, and emotional support and empathy, has been increasingly established throughout the United States, such as the National Alliance for the Mentally Ill in the early 1990s (Burland, 1998), purporting to meet the needs for social support and other aspects of mental health of these families.

Recent studies indicate significant positive effects of the use of mutual support groups for family-based treatment of patients with chronic mental health problems such as eating disorders, dementia and alcoholic abuse, on some family-related outcomes (Colahan & Robinson, 2002; Doyle et al., 2003; McCallion & Toseland, 1995). Toseland and Rossiter (1989) reviewed 10 experimental or quasi-experimental studies on caregivers of patients with dementia in the 1980s and showed that mutual support group can produce significant positive effects on families' psychosocial outcomes such as burden and distress, and coping with caregiving and social isolation, when compared with routine care. Colahan and Robinson (2002) in their study of family support groups conducted within an eating disorder service centre of a London National Health Services hospital reported that family members are able to gain insight into their young relative's eating problem, improve family communication and, in presenting their experiences from the position of being in a similar predicament, provide support to participants in order to alleviate their sense of isolation and resistance to treatment. Despite the use of mutual support groups expanding into the domain of chronic and severe mental illness, the positive values of this intervention to patients and their families are not conclusive (Heller et al., 1997).

While there are few clinical trials on mutual support group for families of patients with schizophrenia in Chinese and Western countries, the literature is replete with case studies, cross-sectional surveys and qualitative and quasi-experimental approaches of single treatment group, emphasizing the apparent benefits of the group in maintaining the psychological and social well-being of families (Heller et al., 1997; Katz, 1997). However, there is relatively little empirical evidence, which supports any enthusiastic claims of their benefits in improving families' functioning and satisfying their health needs (Citron, Solomon, & Draine, 1999).

The paucity of empirical studies on mutual support groups for families of adult people with schizophrenia over the past two decades may be explained by the suggestions from the literature that: (1) the families tend to be socially isolated by the demands, burden and stigma of the illness, and their feeling of guilt and self blame for the illness; thus, they seldom seek help from professionals and other people outside family (Chien, Chan, Lam, & Kam, 2005); (2) support groups are informal network of individuals depending on the leadership of peer volunteers, and challenges like maintaining momentum, ensuring regular evaluation and addressing individual and group changes are accentuated even more than in professional-led programs (Katz, 1997); (3) the goals, structure and activities of mutual support groups for these families vary as widely as the communities where groups are present, thus it is difficult to replicate a standardized procedure of intervention and investigate its effectiveness and applicability in different settings and across cultures (Chien & Chan, 2004).

However, families caring for a relative with schizophrenia usually experience negative reactions from society towards patients and themselves, and many isolate themselves from their natural helping network due to feelings of shame and stigma. Mutual support tends to be viewed as a replacement support network for those in psychosocial crisis, one that, by its nature, is more appropriately able to provide empathy and support for participants who are 'in the same boat' (Chien et al., 2005). Therefore, all mutual support groups function as informal social support systems in that they promote an enduring pattern of continuous or intermittent ties that play a significant part in maintaining the psychiatric and physical health over time. Social support theories broadly hold that social support and social networks are useful to promote mental health because they: (a) buffer the impact of stressful life events; and (b) directly influence or reduce the occurrence of various mental disorders (Champion & Goodall, 1994; Lakey & Cohen, 2000). Studies demonstrate the influence of life events on the occurrence of various psychiatric and physical disorders, and which appears to be mediated by adequate perceived social support (Champion, 1990; Chou et al., 1999). This finding also echoed by Cohen and Wills (1985) in their reviews of studies on families of mentally ill people; and they concluded that emotional and instrumental support from intimate social interactions can have a potential buffering effect on the impact of stressful events in caregiving.

However, there is evidence that the mutual support group is effective in some chronic physical and mental illnesses. There is preliminary evidence from descriptive studies among people with schizophrenia in Western and non-Western people (Chou, Liu, & Chu, 2002;

Heller et al., 1997) and thus this approach of family intervention needs to be empirically evaluated to establish its effectiveness with families of persons with schizophrenia. Mutual support group programs require only limited training for nurses or other health professionals to serve as facilitators and provide a flexible, interactive client-directed approach to help families cope with their caregiving role. It is therefore interesting and worthwhile to examine whether mutual support group intervention can be an effective alternative model of family intervention for the schizophrenia sufferers. It is also important to test this intervention among Chinese families, as such in this study, who are living in a specific culture characterized by a strong sense of filial responsibility, close interdependence, and mutual support.

Table 1. Content and Phases of Mutual Support Group Program

1st Phase(Engagement) - Who we are; why we need to share our experience (2 sessions; included the patient in the 2nd session):
- Orientation of the group programme (format, duration, content, flexibility, and so forth)
- Introduction of the overall purposes of the group intervention and expectations of each participant;
- Beginning of sharing common concerns and establishing trust and acceptance; ensuring confidentiality;
- Negotiation of goals/objectives, rules and norms, and roles and responsibilities;
- Recognising and clarifying the role of a facilitator in the group;
- Initial discussion of the patients' mental illness, symptoms, behaviours, and their effects on family.

2nd Phase(Recognition of Psychological Needs) - Our feelings and concerns towards patient illness (2 sessions):
- Resolution around power, control and decision making within group; any need of a peer leader;
- Discussion about Chinese culture of their family (e.g. family structure, relationships and communication patterns) and attitude towards mental illness
- Clarifying information and misconceptions by them (and other family members) about schizophrenia and its related illness behaviour;
- Exploring and verbalising the intense emotions and feelings about the difficulties in patient care provision and family interactions; sharing stories of success and difficulties in living and interacting with patient;
- Discuss about the ways to deal with negative feelings and emotions to patient;
- Encouraging members to face powerlessness and limitations and accepting the 'self-as-is'
- Focusing and paying specific attention to: (a) helping members view themselves as 'average' or 'similar as others' among the group members, not exceptional; and (b) reduction of caregivers' dysfunctional sense of shame, by sharing and recognizing unrealistic expectations to self/patient, and externally imposed evaluations.

3rd Phase(Dealing with Psychological Needs of Self & Family) - Understanding themselves and patient's needs and available resources (3 sessions; included the patient in the 6th session):
- Discussion about each carer's bio-psychosocial health needs (how they relate to family culture);
- Information about medications, management of the illness, and available mental health services for patient and family;
- Learning and practice for effective communication skills with patient; seeking social support from others e.g. family members and friends;
- Exploration of appropriate home management strategies e.g. finance and budgets, social support network, living environment and hygiene.

4th Phase (Adopting New Roles & Challenges) – Recognizing and adapting to new roles and challenges in caregiving (3 sessions):
- Sharing their coping skills for demands of care, family dysfunctions and conflicts, and their positive things/experience with patient;
- Identifying the supporting persons to their burden of care in their social environment;
- Enhancing problem solving skills in caregiving and minimising family conflicts and burden, by working on some individual patient management situations;
- Conducting behavioural rehearsals of interactions with patient and other family members within group;

Table 1. (Continued)

- Practicing coping skills learned during the sessions to real family life (in-between group sessions) and evaluate the results;
- Re-evaluating their family role and responsibility and shared responsibility of caregiving among family members.

5th Phases (Ending) – Conclusions: Where will we go from here? (2 sessions):

- Preparation and discussion on termination issues e.g. separation anxiety, independent living and use of coping skills learned;
- Evaluation of learning experiences and goals achievement;
- Discussion about the continuity of care after this group programme and the utilisation of community supporting resources
- Explanation of post-intervention assessment and follow-up taken in the following months.

The mutual support group used in this study met biweekly at a psychiatric outpatient clinic within the residential district of the family caregivers, for 12 two-hour sessions. A registered psychiatric nurse who was an experienced group worker, acted as the group facilitator and assisted and encouraged the development of the group. One or two peer leaders, elected by the group members themselves, agreed to coordinate and plan the group sessions and outside group activities in collaboration with the facilitator. The peer leaders received three two-hour briefing and discussion sessions on skills and experiences in coordinating and leading group meetings, which followed a mutual support group protocol. This protocol was designed by the research team to guide development of the mutual support group across five phases of development (see Table 1), as modified from the support group handbooks by Galinsky & Schopler (1995) and Wilson (1995).

The protocol was based on evidence from other support group intervention studies for family caregivers (Chien & Chan, 2004; Chou et al., 2002; Gidron & Chesler, 1995), with the phased development reflecting accepted good practice (Wilson, 1995). It was preferred to the identification of definite tasks or topics for each group session; however, this also allowed flexibility in time, task achievement, and the development of trust, autonomy, closeness, interdependence, and termination of the group (Wilson, 1995). This study builds upon preliminary evidence for the effectiveness of mutual support groups for Chinese families (Chien & Chan, 2004; Chou et al., 2002), and takes account, in its design, of the methodological limitations of previous studies on family intervention discussed earlier in this chapter. The effectiveness of the mutual support group was evaluated in a group of Chinese families of people with schizophrenia, using a controlled trial. Using the same group of group participants, an exploratory research approach was employed in this study to analyze the process data of the group intervention, and understand the perceptions of the family caregivers concerning their group participation.

In addition, fidelity of the facilitator and peer group leaders to the group intervention protocol was assured by review of the audio-tape of each group session by the research team and giving feedback after each session. In addition, the facilitator received supervision during the first and second group meetings from one member of the research team, at which problems of group facilitation were discussed and strategies for the next group session clarified.

AIMS OF THE STUDY

The aim of this study was to explore the perceived benefits obtained from and difficulties experienced in participating in a mutual support group for a group of Chinese family caregivers of patients with schizophrenia who attended follow-up consultations at one of two regional psychiatric outpatient clinics in Hong Kong. Such perceived benefits and difficulties identified by the group participants might be important in explaining the development of group integrity, the therapeutic mechanisms of the group, and those observable effects in the families themselves.

METHOD

Design and Sample

This was a qualitative exploratory study undertaken between September 2003 and August 2004. A convenience sample of 34 pairs of family caregivers and their patients with schizophrenia was recruited from the 38 pairs of mutual support group participants in a controlled trial conducted by the research team (Chien, Norman, & Thompson, 2006). They were randomly selected from the patient lists of two psychiatric outpatient clinics located in the largest geographical region in Hong Kong, and met the inclusion criteria:

(a) The family caregivers lived with the relative diagnosed with schizophrenia according to criteria of the Diagnostic and Statistical Manual of Mental Disorders, 4th edition (American Psychiatric Association, 1994);

(b) The patients with schizophrenia suffered no co-morbidity of another mental illness during recruitment, because family caregiving to a patient with a dual diagnosis could be quite different from that given to those with schizophrenia only;

(c) The patients had been diagnosed with schizophrenia for not more than five years, because too long duration of the illness might lower their enthusiasm for family caregiving and participation in a mutual support group;

(d) Both the caregivers and their patients were aged at least 18 years and could understand and read Cantonese or Mandarin; and

(e) The family caregivers were agreed to participate voluntarily in the study.

Those caregivers who suffered from any psychiatric disorder themselves, who took care of more than one family member with mental or chronic physical illness, or who were the primary carer for less than 3 months, were excluded from the study.

The first author, who was independent of the support group facilitation process, interviewed the 34 families (family caregivers and their patients). However, only 11 patients agreed to participate in the interview, and they preferred to be interviewed together with their family caregivers, whose prior consent was also obtained. Reasons for the patients' refusal to be interviewed were mainly having a lack of time to attend interview, feeling too anxious and uncomfortable to be interviewed, and/or dislike to reveal or to talk about their mental condition. With their written consent, the caregivers were asked to recall and discuss their experiences of group participation and to explain the aspects or experiences in the group that they found beneficial to their caregiving. The 12 audio-taped group sessions (with participants' prior consent for recording) were another main data sources to examine the group development, and validate and clarify the experiences and feelings expressed by the interviewees.

Procedures and Data Analysis

Ethical approval to conduct this study was obtained from the research ethics committees of the clinics and the university. Patients and their family caregivers were informed about the purpose and procedure of the study and their right to withdraw from the study at any time. Confidentiality of data and personal identity of the study participants and clinics were assured; personal information and interview and group session data were kept safely in the principal investigator's office and could be accessed only by the research team; and identities of the participants and clinics were not revealed in any research publications and documentations. With their consent obtained, data pertaining to the family caregivers and/or patients' experiences and perceived therapeutic and non-therapeutic aspects of group participation were gathered through in-depth semi-structured interviews and examination of the audio-taped group sessions.

We established a tentative agenda for the interviews by reviewing the recent published literature and relevant issues on mutual support group intervention and family intervention for patients with schizophrenia. Specific reference was made to the design and principles of the mutual support group set up for this study and published recently (Chien et al., 2004). Detailed description of the group program can be requested from the first author (i.e., Table 1 indicates an outline of the protocol). Draft interview questions were reviewed and agreed on by an expert panel comprising two psychiatrists, one clinical psychologist, two nurse educators, and two psychiatric nurse specialist clinicians. Examples of the interview questions are presented in Table 2. One 60-minute interview was conducted in Cantonese by the first researcher in the outpatient clinics. The interviews were tape-recorded, with field-notes taken, and follow-up interviews were conducted with three interviewees to clarify ambiguous points.

Table 2. Semi-structured Interview Agenda

Examples of questions and prompts used in semi-structured interviews:

1. Recall one or two of the current impressive experiences or events during group participation?
Prompt:
- What did you feel about this experience?
- How importance is it to you? To your family? To the group?
- Any positive or negative impact to you during the group meeting?
- What was the result? What did you learn from it?

Table 2. (Continued)

2.   Recall one or two of the current impressive experiences or events during group participation?

Prompt:

- What did you feel about this experience?
- How importance is it to you? To your family? To the group?
- Any positive or negative impact to you during the group meeting?
- What was the result? What did you learn from it?

3.   Describe the process of your involvement and commitment to the group?

Prompt:

- Please comment on your involvement and commitment during the first and second session. Any changes about this during the next few sessions, also, in the 11th and 12th sessions?
- Any thing/person that facilitated (or inhibited) your involvement/participation in the group?
- When did you feel could trust the members and disclose your personal feelings, caregiving experiences to other group members? What are the key factors causing you such changes?

4.   What are the benefits you obtained from the group participation?

Prompt:

- Please describe any of the events or comments relating to, e.g.,
- Instrumental: practical assistance & material support; emotional or esteem support; information support; problem solving; and social relationship or companionship.

5.   What are the negative aspects of the group?

Prompt:

- Time inflexibility and consuming; inadequate time or number of sessions;
- Negative experiences or feelings; support providing more than receiving;
- Reduced hope for patient recovery; and ineffective coping with caregiving role.

6.   Recall one or two of the current impressive experiences or events during group participation?

Prompt:

- What did you feel about this experience?
- How importance is it to you? To your family? To the group?
- Any positive or negative impact to you during the group meeting?
- What was the result? What did you learn from it?

7.   Describe the process of your involvement and commitment to the group?

Prompt:

- Please comment on your involvement and commitment during the first and second session. Any changes about this during the next few sessions, also, in the 11th and 12th sessions?
- Any thing/person that facilitated (or inhibited) your involvement/participation in the group?

Table 2. (Continued)

8. Recall one or two of the current impressive experiences or events during group participation?

Prompt:
- What did you feel about this experience?
- How importance is it to you? To your family? To the group?
- Any positive or negative impact to you during the group meeting?
- What was the result? What did you learn from it?

9. Describe the process of your involvement and commitment to the group?

Prompt:
- Please comment on your involvement and commitment during the first and second session. Any changes about this during the next few sessions, also, in the 11th and 12th sessions?
- Any thing/person that facilitated (or inhibited) your involvement/participation in the group?
- When did you feel could trust the members and disclose your personal feelings, caregiving experiences to other group members? What are the key factors causing you such changes?

10. What are the benefits you obtained from the group participation?

Prompt:
- Please describe any of the events or comments relating to, e.g.,
- Instrumental: practical assistance & material support; emotional or esteem support; information support; problem solving; and social relationship or companionship.

11. What are the negative aspects of the group?

Prompt:
- Time inflexibility and consuming; inadequate time or number of sessions;
- Negative experiences or feelings; support providing more than receiving;
- Reduced hope for patient recovery; and ineffective coping with caregiving role.

A total of 38 (34 first and 4 follow-up) interviews were conducted with the family caregivers and/or the patients. One research assistant and the first author independently undertook transcription and translation of the first five interviews. One nurse researcher trained in qualitative research methods compared the two sets of transcribed interview scripts and suggested amendments to the research team. Then the research assistant translated and transcribed the remaining interviews. The research assistant and the first author independently identified themes from all of the 38 interview scripts and checked the coding reliability (i.e., > 92% of agreement in coding of the data; Gilstrap, 2004) before categorizing the interview data into themes.

Meaningful entities identified were related to the understanding of the family appraisals of the group process, including the feelings and attitude toward the support group and fellow group members, perceived benefits obtained from and difficulties experienced in group participation, and factors influencing group development and integrity. Preliminary themes were validated and checked with the group sessions data to identify similarities, as well as contradicting evidence. Theme matching and condensation were then performed according to a procedure suggested by Miles and Huberman (1994), who suggested collating in-depth information and accommodating the diversity of experiences and feelings of each informant. This approach consists of six stages of analysis: (a) getting familiar with the diversity of the verbatim data and affixing codes and remarks to each transcript; (b) sorting and sifting through the codes and interview data to identify similarities, differences, and patterns between the codes and noting the recurrent themes emerging from transcripts; (c) elaborating a set of generalizations that cover the consistencies discerned in the interview data and field-notes; (d) isolating patterns and clustering commonalities and differences between the themes and creating a thematic index to transcripts; (e) contrasting and mapping the themes identified, making interpretation and providing explanation; and (f) finalizing the materials, re-examining the data if necessary, and drawing conclusion.

RESULTS

Characteristics of Study Participants

Thirty-four out of the 38 family caregivers (i.e. 89.5% of total number of the support group participants) were interviewed by the researcher. The other four group participants refused to be interviewed, giving as their main reasons: lack of time due to work or being unable to find anyone to take care of the patient; a feeling that talking about their experiences in the group would be of limited value; while those who had exhibited deterioration in their outcomes, felt too embarrassed or guilty about caregiving to discuss family events or their patient's condition with anyone else.

The demographic characteristics of the 34 family caregivers and their 11 patients are similar to the total population of non-participants and participants in the mutual support group conducted within the controlled trial by the research team (Chien et al., 2006). Of the 34 family caregivers (and their patients) selected for interview, 16 reported a marked improvement in the schizophrenia sufferer's condition on three primary outcome measures (i.e., re-hospitalization, patient functioning, and interactions and relationship with family members), a further 10 indicated no or mild improvements, and the final eight indicated deteriorations in all three outcomes. All caregivers reported that this was their first experience of participation in a family mutual support group. The mean ages were 39.1 years (SD = 6.0) for the caregivers and 24.1 years (SD = 5.7) for the patients. There were more female caregivers (n=20; 58.8%) and patients (n=6; 54.5%) than male. Twenty-six of the caregivers were Chinese born in Hong Kong (n=19, 63.3%) or mainland China (n=7, 23.3%), and the remaining 4 were Asian or American Chinese (11.8%). Around 91% of them were a child (n=12), parent (n=10), or spouse (n=9) of the patient. Their average monthly household income was Hong Kong Dollars $12,100.0 (SD=1,940.2) or US$ 1,551.3 (SD=248.7). The mental condition of about 80% of the patients during the previous 3 months was stable or improved. The 34 patients lived with about two family members (M = 2.2, SD = 0.9). Medications taken by the patients were mainly conventional neuroleptics (88.0%), such as haloperidol and chlorpromazine, and of a low or medium dosage (83.3%). The duration of patient illness at data collection was around 2 years (M=2.2, SD=0.9). These patient characteristics were found to be similar between the 11 interviewees and the 23 patients who refused to be interviewed. The major socio-demographic characteristics of the 34 family caregivers (and 11 patients) who were interviewed by the researcher after completion of the support group intervention are presented in Table 3.

Table 3. Socio-demographic characteristics of 34 interviewees and/or their patients

Characteristics	f	%
Family Caregivers (n=34)		
Gender		
Male	14	41.2
Female	20	58.8
Age		
20-29	8	23.5
30-39	12	35.3
40-49	10	29.4
50-62	4	11.8
Education level		
Primary school or below	10	29.4
Secondary school	18	52.9
Tertiary [a]	6	17.6
Relationship with patient		
Spouse	9	26.5
Parent	10	29.4
Child	12	35.3
Sibling & others	3	8.8
Monthly household income (HK dollars)[b]		
10,000 or below	10	29.4
10,001 – 20,000	12	35.3
20,001 – 30,000	7	20.6
30,001 – 40,000	5	14.7
Number of family members living with patient		
One	12	35.3
Two	15	44.1
Three to Five	7	20.6
Characteristics	f	%
Patients (n=11)		
Gender		
Male	5	45.5
Female	6	54.5
Age		
19-24	5	45.5
25-30	5	45.5
31-50	1	9.0
Duration of illness (years)		
Less than 2	4	36.4
2 to 3	5	45.5
4 to 5	2	18.2
Education level		
Primary school or below	2	18.2
Secondary school	7	63.6
Tertiary [a]	2	18.2
Patient's mental condition after intervention [c]		

Table 3. (Continued)

Improved	5	45.5
Staying the same	4	36.3
Worsened/Not stable	2	18.2
Current dosage of antipsychotic medication [d]		
Low	4	36.3
Medium	5	45.5
High	2	18.2

Note: f = frequency, % = percentage.

[a] Tertiary level of education refers to studies completed in university and other postgraduate programs in Hong Kong.

[b] US$1 = 7.8 Hong Kong dollars; UK£ 1 = 15.0 Hong Kong dollars.

[c] Family caregivers' rating of patients' mental condition during the past three months when compared with that before intervention.

[d] Dosage levels of neuroleptic medications were compared with the average dosage of medication taken by patients in haloperidol equivalent mean values in mg/day, as recommended by the American Psychiatric Association (Bezchlibnyk-Butler & Jeffries, 1998).

Going through Different Phases of Group Development

The development of the mutual support group used in this study was designed in terms of the five proposed stages (refer to Table 1), identified by Kimberly (1997) and Wilson (1995) through their experiences in therapeutic groups in a variety of family and patient populations. After about seven to eight group sessions, 25 participants emphasized many times that they had developed a very good interpersonal relationship with other group members, with one to two becoming intimate companions and a source of support. In line with the other 24 caregivers during the interview, one child carer stated:

> I felt I could get adequate help and support from the group from the second group meeting... similar to most of the group members. To gain benefit from and be better involved in the group, it is important to understand and adapt to the group culture. I learned to trust other members and be willing to open ourselves... I still remember that in the first session a few members repeatedly said that we were being 'in the same boat' and that was why we were here for sharing and support. I could express my bad feelings in caregiving with other members because I recognized that they were concerned about me. (Carer 13)

Nevertheless, nine participants including those who showed marked improvements and deteriorations in psychosocial conditions reported some difficulties in getting through the first engagement phase, in particular building trusting relationship with other members and the group facilitator. Reported difficulties pertained to acceptance of roles and responsibilities in mutual learning and support, as well as open discussion of life events and personal feelings in relation to caregiving and the effects of the illness on the entire family. During the second group session, one carer said:

It took time for us to feel comfortable in the group culture and obey the rules, such as open and non-intrusive comments about other members' life events. I think it is better for me to put down my suspicions to all of you. But I am not comfortable to be so open in discussion, because I had been ignored by others such as long period of time and thus I had withdrawn from most social activities with relatives and friends. I have seldom talked about my family with other people because I was afraid of this being the laughing-stock of others. (Carer 4)

From the interview data, the following translated excerpt illustrates the kinds of difficulties that the caregivers perceived:

I can't believe I could be so emotionally involved and time-committed in this group. I felt very uncomfortable in the very beginning of group participation because it is very surprising that some members could discuss their private issues and feelings openly; and they seemed to feel unembarrassed even when they revealed their faults and rudeness to their family members. Also, I did not know what I could do to help others and I just wanted to get something from the group, but it turned out to be 'mutually shared' manner. (Carer 7)

The second phase of the support group (Recognizing their own psychological needs) was not easy for the caregivers to get through, but most of them felt satisfied with the gradual changes that had taken place during this phase. The psychological tensions of group members were indicated from the interview and group session data, together with how the group managed to resolve their issues of power, control and decision-making. Among these issues, perception of control over events and participation in decision-making were the most prominent and explicitly expressed concern within the group. Eighteen caregivers preferred to have some controls to the ways and the extents to which they shared their experiences during group sessions. This caregivers' wish to have control over participation and discussion within the group was a reflection of their wishes, and also a displacement strategy for having better control over the caregiving situation within their families. As one mother carer and her patient stated during the interview:

It is really not difficult for me to follow others' instructions and orders, as our family has always been one where family members met and discuss problems together, before making decisions about family affairs. I would like to play a part in deciding the topics or format of the discussion in some of the sessions, but I felt too insecure and uncomfortable to talk about something that I don't want to share with others. (Carer 20)

Maybe I have already got so many things that my mother and I are worried or concerned about, that I don't want to add any more. At the very least, we need to know what is going to happen during the group meetings so that we can feel confident enough to attend the group. Similarly, it would be wonderful if my mother has the chance and ability to decide on my family activities. (Patient 20)

Such desire for control and decision-making by the members resulted in a more flexible group process and increased team spirit. At the request of some members and the agreement of them all, the group had a short discussion of about 10 minutes at the beginning of each session, about what they were going to do or discuss within the session, and they each took part in choosing some of the activities performed during the session. In the later sessions, half of the caregivers indicated as what one parental carer said:

> I understand that it is very important for each of us to have mutual respect, sharing of information and concerns, and even rooms for expressions of intense emotions and feelings about patient care. If we only focused on concerns and problems of ourselves, we could not listen to others and learn the alternative ways of solving problems from others' experiences. I now really appreciate the fact that the other members could be so patient with me, tolerating my self-centeredness and unreasonable demands on them and listened to what I had said. (Carer 7)

During the third and fourth phases (recognizing self and family needs and adapting to new roles and challenges in caregiving), the support group appeared to be run smoothly and made good progress in dealing with their major concerns about caregiving. Over two-thirds of the participants indicated in the group sessions and interviews that they had gained "more understanding about their relative's illness and its related behavior" (Carer 13). During the sixth group session, five of them admitted that they sometimes had difficulty in applying their newly acquired coping skills to their real caregiving situations. However, on many occasions within the group sessions, the other 15 caregivers (interviewees) emphasized that they had experienced more effective communication and improved relationships with their patients and other relatives, following the fifth sessions. This was reflected in their pleased smiles and their reports of some of the joyful interactions and activities they had had with their patients after the group meetings. Participants also reported that they could establish specific home management strategies, for examples, more effective financial management such as budgeting and better hygiene by maintaining a more tidy and hygienic home environment.

Twenty group participants who had limited social support from their family members and showed deterioration of psychosocial conditions indicated that coping with the caregiving role was found to be very difficult and challenging for them. However, they emphasized that their new learning from group members, such as trying out some positive strategies or activities with patient (e.g., accompanying patient to follow-up consultation), use of problem-solving approach in management of patient's problems and demands, and minimizing conflicts within family, would require more behavior rehearsals and practice in their 'real' family life. Thus, they (and their patients) would like to have extra support and social activities outside the group meetings such as "some practical assistance in caring for their patient or frail family member at home, provided by a few close-linked groupmates" (Carer 29), or "an informal telephone or face-to-face contact every week to meet the others and tackle some immediate problems that have arisen in-between the two sessions" (Carer 18). A few also suggested that continuation of the group, after the six-month period, should be considered.

During the last session (the ending phase), specific time was set aside by agreement of all the group members to evaluate the results of their learning and goal achievement within the group, in preparation for the dissolution of the group, and to discuss related issues such as their emotional reaction towards the forthcoming termination. The importance of independent living and use of problem-solving skills was stressed, especially for the six members who would not be continuing their participation in their self-initiated support group set up for a few close friends among the group members, at the close of the study. Seventeen caregivers during the interviews felt very satisfied with what they had learned about caring for their relative with schizophrenia and with the consistent support they had received from other group members. They expressed satisfaction with the mutual aid and support amongst group members, when working on common goals, agreed tasks and also on some of their own personal concerns. Five of them emphasized that the most important outcome for them was the "true friendship" they felt they had established with other group members. They felt this intimate, personal relationship would be of much value to them in the future.

Assessment of their own problem solving skills and ways of coping with their caregiving role, combined with the support and encouragement of other group members, were found to be effective in reducing their anxiety and in helping them feel more confident about their future independence and caring abilities. Consistent with most group participants, one male carer said in the last group session:

> I was only able to feel secure because I made an agreement with my close friends during the last group session, that we would offer continued support to each other after the intervention. In addition, we knew the facilitator could be contacted for any professional advice if needed. For me, the most important thing is to be able to contact somebody for help whenever there is any great problem within my family in the future. (Carer 6)

These extracts show that the final, closing stage of the intervention was very important for most of the 34 group participants, as it enabled them to review all that they had learned and to prepared, not only for their separation from the other members but also to set up a small peer group for friendship and support with the group members to whom they were closest.

Perceived Benefits and Difficulties Experienced by Family Caregivers for Group Participation

The analysis of the data from the interviews and the audio-taped group sessions elicited some important themes that were seen by the family caregivers as influencing the group process and benefiting individual caregivers, their families and the whole group, as well as benefiting the group development. Three therapeutic mechanisms were then identified by bringing together these themes that had influenced the group development and contributed to the perceived benefits and success of the support group. These four mechanisms were:

M1: Reconstructing a new positive self-image (role identity) in relation to caregiving;
M2: Psychological empowerment of caregivers through acquisition of knowledge and skills in caregiving; and
M3: Extending social support network both within and outside the group.

The three mechanisms and their key elements are depicted in Figure 1. The flow diagram also presents the stages of group development associated with and the potential outcomes achieved by each mechanism. Some of these potential outcomes were demonstrated by the findings of the controlled trial (Chien et al., 2006). These included: decreased family burden might be contributed by reconstructing a new positive self-image for caregiving (M1); increased perceived social support might be resulted from extending social support network both within and outside the mutual support group (M3); and improved family functioning might be contributed by psychological empowerment of caregivers through the acquisition of knowledge and skills for caregiving (M2). The three therapeutic mechanisms are discussed in detail in discussion section at below, along with other research and literature on mutual support groups.

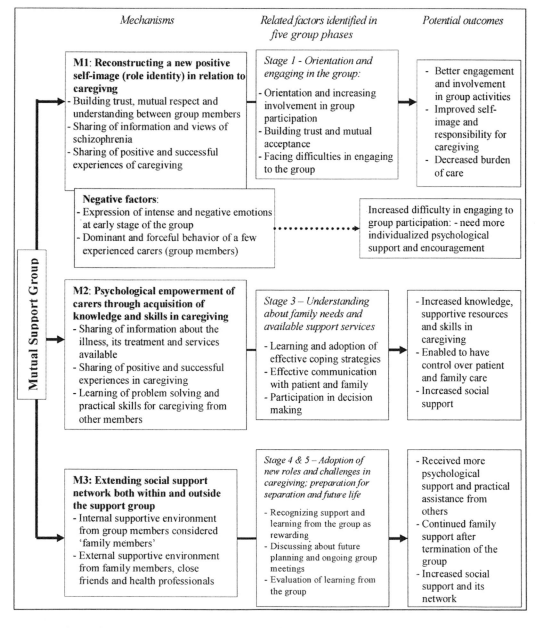

Figure 1. Three Therapeutic Mechanisms of Family Mutual Support Group.

In addition, one major hindrance to the success of the support group was also identified within one of the three mechanisms. The expression of intensive and negative emotions at early group stage and the presence of dominant and forceful behavior of the experienced caregivers might be negatively affected some family caregivers' reconstruction of their positive self-identity (M1), and increased their difficulty in engaging to group participation. These family caregivers might need individualized psychological support and encouragement by peer members and group facilitator to have better engagement in the support group.

DISCUSSION ON FOUR THERAPEUTIC MECHANISMS

This exploratory study is one of the relatively few, in Chinese or Western countries, which have sought to identify the perceived therapeutic mechanisms and limitations of a mutual support group for family caregivers of people with schizophrenia. Brooker (2001) suggested that the hesitation of clinicians to use family intervention might be attributed to the inadequate knowledge of researchers of the particular elements of family intervention that enhance its therapeutic value for family caregivers and patients. Increased understanding of the active components of family intervention, such as are seen in the mutual support group in this study, will facilitate the design of future interventions for family caregivers of the mentally ill and thus produce optimal benefits for patients and their families (Chien & Chan, 2004). Three therapeutic mechanisms of the mutual support group, their related factors in the group phases and their potential outcomes were identified from the main themes that emerged from the interview and group session data, and are discussed in the following sections, in relation to the recent literature.

Mechanism 1: Reconstructing a new Positive Self-Image in RELATION to Caregiving

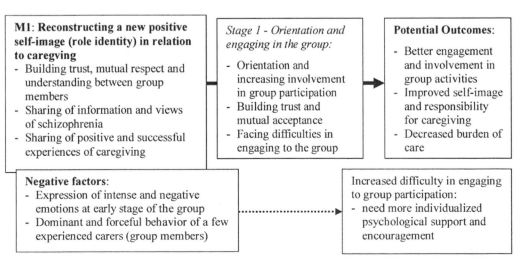

The first therapeutic mechanism mainly refers to changes in the perception of the family caregivers' role in caring for a relative with the mental illness that is induced by participation in a mutual support group. Like their patients, the family caregivers had experienced or felt "being stigmatized or socially isolated by relatives and friends". They emphasized that the major contribution of the support group to those with these perceived negative attitudes, was to enable them to "reconstruct a new positive identity and self-image". Consistent with the findings of Cook et al. (1999) and Yalom (1995) on therapeutic groups for mentally ill patients and their family members, the participants emphasized that interactions with others who were experiencing similar life problems (i.e., the feeling that they were "all in the same boat") was useful in establishing group collectiveness, empathy and a trusting relationship between participants. In other words, the 'universality' of the problems or concerns induced a sense of security and respect between the participants. Willingness to share their experiences and offer help to each other (i.e. the 'altruism' factor) as suggested by Yalom (1995), appears to have been an effective way for the caregivers to maintain their psychosocial health. The caregivers in this study helped each other through the hardships of their stigmatized self-image or 'label' of being a family member of a mentally ill person while supporting each other wholeheartedly in performing their caregiving role.

As a result, the caregivers began to recognize that they, too, could achieve "what the others had attained in caring for their family and patient". During the interviews, they said they felt more positive about self-image and the "importance and responsibility of their role in caring for our patient" (Carer 20), and they acquired an insight into having a more meaningful life, even though some of their difficulties might remain unresolved.

Kurtz (1997) suggested that mutual support is commonly accepted as the process of sharing common experiences, situations and concerns by people within a group, in which participants can learn from one another about how to cope with their own problems, and also about how to care for and be concerned for, other group members. A mutual support group can thus be referred to as a type of mutual helping unit, where participants share and deal with common health needs and concerns and voluntarily offer reciprocal support and satisfy common goals, thereby bringing about desired social and personal changes (Nichols & Jenkinson, 1991; Oka, 2003).

Enthusiastic and autonomous interchange of information and practical skills regarding patient care provision was important for the family caregivers in this study, as it enabled them to adapt to the new role and responsibility of caregiving for their mentally ill relative. Imparting information about the illness and patient management, identifying available community resources, and sharing successful and unsuccessful caring experiences, were important components of the mutual support group in this study. Sharing information and disclosures about their differing perspectives on caring for their relatives with schizophrenia, by the group participants, is important for family caregivers, particularly for those with limited caregiving experience, or inadequate knowledge about the illness. It also helped them make sense of the reality of the illness, as well as giving them plausible explanations about their responsibilities for patient care (Humphreys, 1997). As a result of such interchange, the caregivers gained experiential knowledge from those who had lived through and resolved their own life problems. This was knowledge that would not have been available from health professionals (Chien et al., 2005).

This group behavior helped to change the family caregivers' perceptions of their patient's illness and its management, and facilitated them in reconstructing a new positive personal identity. Prior to their participation in the group, family caregivers in this study had little knowledge about the illness and had found their sense of self being diminished through misunderstandings and distress, caused by their inexpert manner of care delivery. However, their self-image (or identity) changed progressively as they learned about the reality of the illness and gained useful insight into their responsibilities and the difficulties of caring for their patient. These positive changes revealed the effect of the mutual support group in improving the adaptive competence of family caregivers in dealing with short-term crises and life transitions, as well as the long-term challenges, stresses and privations (Gazda, Ginter, & Horneboston, 2001).

Sharing of information about the illness can also be crucial for clarifying misconceptions about the causes of schizophrenia for the family caregivers. For example, participants in this study, confronted with emotions of shame, guilt and anger, also experienced feelings of uncertainty (Barrowclough & Tarrier, 1992; Medvene & Krauss, 1989), because they thought they were required to be responsible for the illness within their family. Through participation in the support group, the group members had the opportunity to think about and share experiences of different ways of doing things and to discuss the pros and cons of their actions. This led to improved psychological well-being and ability to cope with the stigma related to the illness. Mutual support groups are therefore viewed as social worlds, in which the group is a cultural arena with no formal boundaries and whose members were able to attach definitions (and redefinitions) and symbolic meanings to things that are usually unknown or are unfamiliar to outsiders (Humphreys, 1997).

Borkman (1999) suggested that the sharing of caregiving experiences, combined with open discussion about the adverse life situations encountered in caregiving, assists participants in the mutual support group to reframe their life problems and enables them to pinpoint 'what is wrong', or not working, in their management of their relative with schizophrenia. Even though family caregivers recognize that they will have to continue to live with unresolved difficulties, they are able to gain an insight into a more meaningful life and thus gain relief from thinking of themselves as the victim of the illness and begin, instead, to act compassionately towards their sick relative. This reframing of problems and 'letting go' of unsuccessful methods of caregiving is considered crucial by family members for coping effectively with their patients with schizophrenia and other severe mental illnesses (Gazda et al., 2001).

As shown in the first therapeutic mechanism and demonstrated by the interview and group session data, the caregivers' adoption of a new role and more effective coping methods of caregiving, resulted from the group members' sharing their past personal experiences and caregiving difficulties within the supportive group environment. Family caregivers' experiential learning started by listening to the personal stories of other group members from which they learned about communication with their patients and/or other family members. This continued with stories about how support group members had attempted different means of communication and ways of resolving arguments and conflicts with their family members, which had mainly arisen from miscommunication and misunderstandings.

Chou et al. (2002) and Galinsky and Schopler (1995) suggested that, in the experience of their family group, mutual sharing of personal knowledge and experiences among families within a support group is one way of demonstrating their mutual concern and care for each other and, through these social interactions, they are able to practice effective communication with other people. This suggestion is confirmed by similar comments from the interview data of 10 family caregivers in this study. These family caregivers also emphasized that adequate opportunities to practice alternative styles of communication and behavior, enabling them to interact more effectively with their patients and other family members, and deal with problems and conflicts with them, was important in their successful adoption of a new caregiving role.

The findings in this study also suggest a need for continued group participation or a longer period of group development for those few participants who had been less actively involved in the group, or who had made slow progress in accepting the experiences and responsibilities of caregiving. It was sometimes difficult for these participants to build a sufficient level of mutual trust and support to discuss the 'taboo areas' of their family life, within the six-month group intervention. Consistent with the recommendation by Wituk, Shepherd, Warren, and Meissen (2002), a minority (three) of the caregivers in this study indicated that more work was needed to overcome these difficulties, for example, by having more discussion, both within and outside the support group, about the actual scenarios encountered by family caregivers and organizing more outside group contacts and activities. These families might also need more intense individual support from the peer leaders.

This improvement in caregivers' self-image and in their caregiving role occurred mainly during the first stage of group development. This initial stage was perceived by family caregivers as critical and essential to them in building trust and acceptance of each other's role and responsibility in the support group. Once they were successfully orientated towards and involved in participation in the group, they felt comfortable enough to discuss openly their own family issues, and thus to engage actively in the mutual support group and in other social activities outside the group. Yalom (1995) suggested that feelings of mutual understanding and acceptance and subsequent increased empathy with each other's life situation, is the first and most important step towards the successful integration into a therapeutic group.

Two negative factors were identified as having hindered the caregivers' engagement in the support group. They included the expression of intensive and negative emotions by members in the group sessions and the presence of dominant and forceful behavior by a few experienced caregivers within the group. It might have been better if sharing of very intense and negative emotions about family situations had been left to the later stages of the mutual support group, so that the members had more time to establish adequate social support for each other before facing these painful experiences and emotions. The importance of group members and the facilitator being alert to the need to offer positive, concrete support and to demonstrate effective coping methods is highlighted in the literature of family group work (Wilson, 1995). Thus, emotionally weak members become aware that their family situations are not as helpless and hopeless as they previously believed. These patterns of interactions have been highlighted in the literature (Gazda et al., 2001; Yalom, 1998), which offers some guidance on the role of a group facilitator. Yalom (1998) suggests that the group facilitator must be aware that the presence of dominant, forceful and critical group members in such discussions can be discouraging to other members, particularly those who feel more powerless and helpless. Therefore, more positive and balanced views about personal and family situations should be addressed and discussed within the support group as a whole, with appropriate reinforcement from the facilitator and other experienced caregivers, before the weaker group members can start to accept their stigmatized self-image and false beliefs about the illness permanently.

These negative factors were also identified by Mankowski et al. (2001) in self-help groups dealing with alcoholic patients and also by McFarlane (2002) in family psychoeducational groups for patients with severe mental illness. The difficulties of engaging in group participation experienced by a few family caregivers in this study, suggests that individualized psychological support and encouragement should be provided for those members who feel uncomfortable in open self-disclosure within a support group, so as to reduce their tensions and anxieties during the early days of their group participation. Meissen and Volk (1995) suggested that these barriers could be anticipated and reduced, both by group participants and the facilitator if, during the group sessions, they actively encouraged the group's development and individual participants' involvement.

Engaging participants in a support group is the first important, but often difficult, step towards gaining their commitment (Cragan & Wright. 1999). As suggested by the caregivers in this study, group participants themselves perceive this as the most important first step and other factors, such as providing more time and opportunity for each participant to express their own feelings and concerns in the group meetings, are all matters that should be carefully considered by health professionals when designing a mutual support group for family caregivers of patients with schizophrenia.

Family caregivers are confronted with feelings of shame, guilt, and anger because they take the blame personally for the mental illness within their family (Barrowclough & Tarrier, 1992). Cook et al (1994) demonstrated that providing more opportunities for them to vent their feelings and have people in a support group actively listen to their concerns, conveys to them the message that they are of concern to, and are respected by the other members of the support group. This will lessen their feeling of burden of care (Cook et al., 1994). This is also a good place for family caregivers to begin building sufficient trust to be able to disclose their own family issues to other group members.

The second therapeutic mechanism refers to the potency of psychological empowerment that family caregivers would gain in a mutual support group. The essence of empowerment, which is to enable the families to help themselves (Gidron & Chesler, 1995), occurs when the caregivers gain more knowledge about caring for the patient and then practice effectively the skills that they have learned from other group members in their family situation. Similar to patients with schizophrenia in Wong and Chan's (1994) study, most of the support group participants in this study reported gaining a great deal in their ability to reach out to others, despite being shown clearly that they were suffering from difficult life circumstances that were unlikely to be resolved very soon. Nevertheless, this group was able to bring about changes that allowed them to cope with their life situations more positively.

Mechanism 2: Psychological Empowerment of CAREGIVERS through Acquisition of Knowledge and Skills in Caregiving

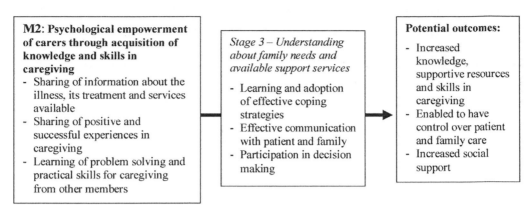

Psychological empowerment at an individual level claims to build on the supportive social context of the group to enable connections with people outside it. Participation in a mutual support group is a social action process, by which individuals learn to gain personal control over issues that concern them, together with a proactive approach to life and a critical understanding of their intrapersonal and social environment (Zimmerman, 1995). This idea has been applied in the USA in an organizational study by Maton & Salem (1995), on a mutual support group program (named GROW) for people with mental illness. They suggested that empowerment in a mutual support group can be enhanced by provision of a peer-based support system, allowing individuals to take on meaningful roles within the group and within their own family, together with the adoption of a belief system that inspires members to strive for better mental health. From the perspective of empowerment, Reissman and Carroll (1995) suggested that mutual support groups enable participants to take control of their life situations and, as a result, cope better with their caregiving role. As indicated in the group session data, members identified what their personal goals were in relation to caregiving and decided what they wanted to learn and obtain through their participation in the group. Participants also gained increased awareness about the availability of external support resources, such as emotional and instrumental support from family members and others in their social network, and expert advice from healthcare professionals. Such resources could thus be used more appropriately by the families and might result in a reduction of their demands for family support services over the 12-month follow-up period.

Although a small-sized mutual support group may not be as developed, for example, as an Alcoholics Anonymous group, Zimmerman (1995) suggested that its members would still be able to benefit from opportunities to form new social relationships that would connect them to new people and ideas. As with most of the family caregivers in this study, most support group participants were able to learn and practice problem-solving skills through actively involving themselves in the group's activities. As an intervention aimed at empowering its participants, mutual support groups provide opportunities for family caregivers to develop, with peer support, new knowledge and caregiving skills for their relative with schizophrenia while, at the same time, helping them to establish a more harmonious family life. Another benefit is that, with this newly found knowledge and confidence, family caregivers also learn to engage with professionals as collaborators, as opposed to engaging with them as authoritative experts (Perkins & Zimmerman, 1995; Wituk et al., 2000).

The families in the mutual support group learned to employ active and interactive coping strategies more frequently, such as exploring in-depth the nature of the problems they encountered in caring for their patients and discussing different ways of coping with their caring role. The development of psychological empowerment in the family caregivers, thanks to the excellent and appropriate ongoing support from other group members, was crucial in strengthening their resistance to feelings of despair and in overcoming their wish to relinquish their caring role. Their confidence increased as their knowledge and caregiving skills grew and, gradually, they became sufficiently confident to take action, both for themselves and on behalf of their family members. The increased social support they received from other group members, whom they came to treat as close family members, continued to encourage them to improve their caregiving skills and, also, to assist them to be more responsible and effective in their caring role.

Despite some minor difficulties such as conflicts between group members, the family caregivers' empowerment grew as they started to better understand their own family needs, and the range of support services available for them. They all acknowledged that it was in the third and fourth phases of the support group investigated in this study, that the most important and rewarding stages in their group participation were achieved, in respect of their caregiving. By that time, most of the caregivers in particular the novice ones, were able to learn and adopt new coping strategies and caregiving skills for their patients, in addition to learning more effective communication with their patients and other family members. Citron et al. (1999) and Chou et al. (2002) suggested in their evaluation studies on mutual support groups for family caregivers that the most frequent and important perceived benefits of group participation included enhanced stress-coping skills in relation to caregiving and the use of a problem solving approach in resolving difficulties in family situations. The family caregivers in this study also learned to undertake positive activities with their ill relatives, such as accompanying them to follow-up outpatient clinics and participating in recreational activities organized by community centres.

As the functional models of mutual support groups prevalent in the United States, Chien et al. (2005) emphasized that the two most important attributes of a mutual support group are: (1) giving and receiving help and (2) the way participants rely on each other's efforts, skills, knowledge, and concerns, as their primary source of help when sharing common life experiences and problems. These models emphasize that inner-focused, supportive groups, comprising families of a relative with severe mental illness, strive to focus on providing personal growth opportunities for caregivers that promote individual change through empowerment and consciousness-raising goals. Such changes would include improvements in knowledge and skills regarding the illness and its care, caregivers being able to deal with their negative emotions concerning patients and own self-care, and improvement in seeking appropriate community services (Heller et al., 1997b). These positive changes were identified as the benefits of group participation in this study.

Mechanism 3: Extending Social Support Network within and outside the Support Group

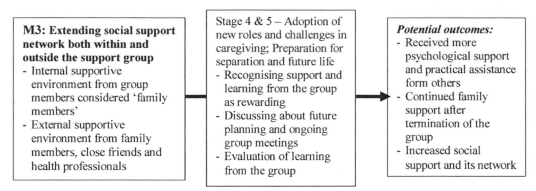

M3: Extending social support
network both within and
outside the support group
- Internal supportive
  environment from group
  members considered 'family
  members'
- External supportive
  environment from family
  members, close friends and
  health professionals

Stage 4 & 5 – Adoption of
new roles and challenges in
caregiving; Preparation for
separation and future life
- Recognising support and
  learning from the group
  as rewarding
- Discussing about future
  planning and ongoing
  group meetings
- Evaluation of learning
  from the group

Potential outcomes:
- Received more
  psychological support
  and practical assistance
  form others
- Continued family
  support after
  termination of the
  group
- Increased social
  support and its network

The final therapeutic mechanism of the mutual support group in this study was the extension of caregivers' social support network both inside and outside the support group. The mutual support group in this study served three functional purposes of social support: (1) instrumental support, providing material aids and practical assistance with daily tasks; (2) information support, providing appropriate information and advice in caregiving; and (3) emotional support, conveying empathy, caring and trust to and from other group members. The importance of these functional dimensions for the family caregivers in the support group was reflected in the interview and group session data. Most caregivers indicated the unity and friendship as being similar to that of a close family member. Some family caregivers also offered to help other group members to manage their family affairs outside the group and, in this way, other members became an additional important part of the family caregivers' social network.

Though this sense of cohesiveness was strong among those family caregivers who had attended the group regularly and participated actively in the group activities, it was also closely linked to their altruistic behavior towards other group members. Conversely, those caregivers who attended the group sessions inconsistently and infrequently, found that the demand to assist and take care of the concerns of others first, sometimes at the sacrifice of their own (i.e. altruism), overwhelmed them and made them question what benefits, if any, they were gaining from the group. This was consistent with recommendations by Yalom (1998), who found that levels of cohesiveness and altruistic behavior are essential factors if the caregivers are to benefit from their group participation.

The results of this study demonstrate the truth of this by finding that the family caregivers who showed high levels of altruism towards, and cohesiveness with, other members in the support group, also reported greater and more substantial positive improvements in their psychosocial health condition over the 12-month follow-up period, compared with those who were not so closely linked with others in the group. It can be seen, therefore, that mutual support groups are able to create strong, cohesive forces while, at the same time, promoting attitudes of unselfishness and concern among participants and helping them to find value in helping resolve each other's problems and concerns before their own. The Chinese family caregivers of patients with schizophrenia in this study, like most Chinese and Asian families, who have already culturally inclined to accept these collective group and cohesive forces (Ma & Yip, 1997), might find no problem in being receptive to the additional social support and practical assistance provided for them.

The findings of high levels of cohesiveness and openness in sharing their own experiences in this mutual support group raise two issues of cultural consideration in the family group work. First, the Chinese family caregivers who actively participated and openly discussed their own family situations in the support group were perceived as obtaining great benefit from their participation. These positive results are in contradiction to previous studies that tended to show that, culturally, Chinese people are passive and reserved when it comes to emotional and personal disclosure (Leung & Lee, 1996), and that a more directive and structured approach to their problems, conducted by the family therapist, was considered more productive (Wong & Chan, 1994). Second, the concept of 'gan qing' (emotional love), which symbolizes mutual good feelings, empathy and friendship among Chinese people and is not easily found in Western people (Sun, 1991), might play an important role in the close supportive relationships of the support group participants in this study. Once this 'gan qing' has been cultivated and affirmed in a relational context by means of mutual aid and care, such as in this study, group members became highly inter-dependent and committed to helping one another.

The supportive environment outside a mutual support group is also an important factor in influencing the effect that such a support group has on its participants. Despite the strong cohesion and support among group members, it is also desirable for the family caregivers to have access to more links and interaction with health professionals and available community support services, thus enabling them to seek professional help and support independently when they need it. The family caregivers in the support group suggested that the group should be run as an adjunct to the local community mental health services, with all their aids, facilities and resources. All the caregivers had welcomed the participation and presentations by the health professionals who had attended at the request of the group.

Ample evidence indicates that the needs of families for professional support partly stems from their experiences of the stigma associated with mental illness (Rose, Mallinson, & Walton-Moss, 2004). This stigma undermines any support that families might otherwise have expected from their social and familial networks. Professional support can reduce these unmet needs of families caring for a mentally ill relative, because some families prefer to share their concerns with professionals as they feel they can rely on the professional conduct and expertise of clinicians, who understand their family situation and concerns, and will not violate their privacy. In spite of acknowledging the importance of professional support for these families, studies have confirmed that families do not receive adequate support from professionals (Solomon, 2000). Therefore, if the mutual support group can run in parallel with adequate support from health professionals, the effect of family intervention may be strengthened and thus the benefits to these families will be optimized.

However, this awareness of the need to obtain external support from health professionals among the families who participated in the support group may not necessarily increase their demands for health services. The findings of this and other studies on family intervention for patients with severe mental illness (Budd et al., 1998; Dyck et al., 2002) indicate that, through their group participation, family caregivers are better able to understand and select the services that they actually need and are most appropriate for them, as similar to that reported in previous family group studies in Western and Chinese countries (Chien & Chan, 2004; Solomon, 2000).

Moreover, more than half of the family caregivers in the support group in this study also indicated that the social support available from their family members and other people within their social networks, such as close friends and relatives, was another important element of support obtainable outside the support group and they considered this help equally important as the help they received from health professionals and the support group. With improved communication and interpersonal relationships with family members, as a result of their support group participation, family members and close friends can become the primary sources of immediate physical and emotional support for caregivers, when they are caring for patients and practicing their newly learned caregiving skills.

The complementary interaction of three different sources of social support (family members, health professionals and support group members) further strengthens group participation and enhances its benefits for family caregivers, in addition to enhancing their ability to cope with the stress of caregiving. Mobilization of adequate family support resources (Langford et al., 1997), such as these, were perceived to be important to the family caregivers in this study, in acting as a protective buffer against the stress experienced by families in providing care for their patient.

The aims of this extended social support network within and outside the mutual support group was clear-cut from the later stage (fourth group stage) when the caregivers were eager to learn and adopt new roles and challenges in caregiving once they had understood their own and family needs. The caregivers felt that this stage of the support group was the most rewarding stage of their group participation. Most of them, in particular the novice caregivers, were able to learn and adopt new coping and caregiving skills, as well as effective communication with their patients and family members. Chou et al. (2002) suggested that these elements are the most important benefits of participation in the group, but the caregivers in this study also learned to undertake constructive activities with their ill relatives, such as participating in recreational activities organized by community centers.

The extension of the caregivers' social support networks was intensified in the final stage of the mutual support group, which, according to Powell (1994), has often been treated as relatively less important by group facilitators and participants, than the earlier phases of the group. The family caregivers also felt that the final meetings provided them with an opportunity to talk about their anxieties about leaving the group and to plan for continued support and make arrangements for further, informal meetings and gatherings with other close group members after the end of the group program. Yalom (1995) suggested that the discussion and psychological preparation for separation from the other members is essential for helping group participants to feel secure about continued support in their future life and thus in relieving their anxieties.

In addition, the final phase was found useful for allowing the family caregivers to evaluate what they had learned during their group participation, as well as facilitating independence in their future family life. Wilson (1995) recommended that, through this evaluation and reflection on their learning in the last session, participants are able to consolidate their knowledge and skills learned in the group and have an opportunity to clarify any unclear concepts and misunderstandings. Before they left the group, arrangements were also made for future referrals to appropriate services, such as respite care, and when needed. Since so much importance was accorded to this period of preparation and evaluation by seven of the group participants in this study, when they requested an additional group session to discuss their learning and concerns, they were allowed to do so in accordance with the usual flexible approach of the support group.

CONCLUSION

The findings of this study indicate that most of the participants (family caregivers and patients) were able to perceive the positive characteristics and effects of the family mutual support group on them. There were three therapeutic mechanisms identified from the interview and group session data. First, consistent with the recommendation by Yalom (1998), the caregivers in the mutual support group emphasized that interactions with others who were experiencing similar life problems was useful in establishing group cohesiveness and a trusting relationship between group members (i.e., "universality" of problems/needs), inducing a sense of security and respect for each other; and willingness to share their life experiences relating to caregiving and offer psychological support and instrumental help to others (i.e., "altruism" factor) appear to have been one way in which the group participants resolved their difficulties in restructuring the self- identity and role of family caregivers of a mentally ill relative.

Second, the essence of empowerment, which is to enable the families to help themselves, can occur when family caregivers in a mutual support group receive more knowledge about caring for their patient and practice the skills learned from other members effectively in family life. Most caregivers would be able to reach out to others and be encouraged to see clearly that they are suffering from difficult life circumstances. As a result, mutual support groups, as such in this study, can definitely bring about family cares' personal changes concerning perceptions of illness and patient recovery and thus they can cope with those difficult life situations more positively. The caregivers can also gain some experiential knowledge from others who had lived through and resolved their life problems, and this knowledge may not be available from health professionals.

The open disclosure and cohesiveness between the group participants are attributed to several important factors established in the early stage of group development, including trusting relationships between group members, feelings of being respected and reciprocal assistance, conflict resolution, and continuous support outside the group. These important elements of therapeutic group establishment are also highlighted in the literature on family mutual support groups (Maton, 1993).

The final therapeutic mechanism highlights the significance of an extension of family caregivers' social support networks both inside and outside the support group. Mutual support groups can serve three functional purposes of social support: providing material aids and practical assistance with daily tasks; sharing of information and advice in caregiving; and conveying empathy, caring and trust to and from other participants. This will establish a supportive environment for the family caregivers and their patients, inside and outside a support group, and thus should be an important factor in influencing the positive effect that such a support group has on its participants.

The findings of this study also indicate that Chinese family caregivers who are considered as passive and reserved in emotional and personal disclosure can actively participate in and openly discuss their family situations in a mutual support group. In addition, the '*gan qing*' (emotional love), which symbolizes mutual good feelings, empathy, and friendship among Chinese people and is not easily found in Western people, can be cultivated and affirmed in a relational context by means of mutual aid and care in the support group. Group members become highly interdependent and committed to helping one another. These issues of cultural consideration should be remembered in future family group work.

It is noteworthy that some inhibitory factors or barriers to the success of the support group were identified from the perceptions of the group participants in this study. These factors include (a) poor group attendance behaviors by some participants, such as low and irregular attendance; (b) dominant and forceful behaviors of a few senior or experienced members; and (c) expression of intense and negative emotions at the early stage. To increase attendance and group cohesiveness, more flexibility in time and venue of group meetings might be useful to encourage family caregivers' group participation, and an increase of informal contacts outside group may increase their group involvement.

A few limitations in this study included: (a) two-thirds of the patients (n=23) refused to be interviewed, and their views and appraisals about the group participation could not have been included; (b) the families were recruited from only two of 15 psychiatric outpatient clinics and thus the results might not be representative of most family caregivers of Chinese patients with schizophrenia in Hong Kong; and (c) the interviews were conducted and analyzed by the researchers, who might have subjective biases to the positive effects of the mutual support group and thus to the responses of the participants. The family caregivers were self-conscious about the purposes of the group intervention and the study; and this might have affected their behavior and responses to the support group program and the interview questions. Methodological triangulation using dissimilar techniques for data collection, such as field notes, participants' personal journals, and group discussion, could have been used to for enhancing the credibility and dependability of the findings. Finally, relationships between family caregivers and other significant people in their social networks such as family members, friends and health professionals, and their views about the changes of support group participants, should be explored to fully reveal the benefits of group participation and the amount of perceived social support outside the mutual support group and its influence on the attendance and thus the benefits of group participation.

This qualitative study provides insights for clinicians and researchers into the therapeutic components of a family group program for people with schizophrenia, which are still relatively unknown in research and practice. These components can be adopted by mental health professionals to produce the most benefits for family caregivers and their patients when they design psychosocial interventions for these families. The therapeutic factors should also be tested further with family support groups from diverse socio-economic and cultural backgrounds.

REFERENCES

American Psychiatric Association. (1997). Practice guidelines for the treatment of patients with schizophrenia. *American Journal of Psychiatry, 154* (suppl.), 8-80.

Anderson, C., Reiss, D., & Hogarty, G. (1986). *Schizophrenia and the family: A practitioner's guide to psychoeducation and management.* New York: Guilford Press.

Asen, E. (2002). Multiple family therapy: An overview. *Journal of Family Therapy, 24,* 3-16.

Barbato, A., & D'Avanzo, B. (2000). Family interventions in schizophrenia and related disorders: a critical review of clinical trials. *Acta Psychiatrica Scandinavica, 102*(2), 81-97.

Barnes, T. R. E., Hutton, S. B., Chapman, M. J., Mutsatsa, S., Puri, B. K., & Joyce, E. M. (2000). West London first episode study of schizophrenia: Clinical correlates of duration of untreated psychosis. *British Journal of Psychiatry, 177,* 207-211.

Barrowclough, C., & Johnston, M. (1996). Distress, expressed emotion and attributions in relatives of schizophrenic patients. *Schizophrenia Bulletin, 22* (4), 691-702.

Barrowclough, C. & Tarrier, N. (1992). *Families of schizophrenic patients: Cognitive behavioural intervention.* London: Chapman & Hall.

Barrowclough, C., & Parle, M. (1997). Appraisal, psychological adjustment and expressed emotion in relatives of patients suffering from schizophrenia. *British Journal of Psychiatry, 171*(1), 26-30.

Bateson, D. H., Jackson, D., Haley, J., & Weakland, J. (1956). Towards a theory of schizophrenia. *Behavioural Science, 1,* 251-264.

Bebbington, P., & Kuipers, L. (1994). The predictive utility of expressed emotion in schizophrenia: An aggregate analysis. *Psychological Medicine, 24* (3), 707-718.

Bellack, A. S., Haas, G. L., Scholloer, N. R., & Flory, J. D. (2000). Effects of behavioural family management on family communication and patient outcomes in schizophrenia. *British Journal of Psychiatry, 177,* 434-439.

Bezchlibnyk-Butler, K. Z., & Jeffries, J. J. (1998). *Clinical handbook of psychotropic drugs.* (8th ed.). Seattle: Hogrefe and Huber.

Bishop, P., Clilverd, A., Cooklin, A., & Hunt, U. (2002). Mental health matters: A multi-family framework for mental health intervention. *Journal of Family Therapy, 24,* 31-45.

Borkman, T. J. (1999). *Understanding self-help/mutual aid: Experiential learning in the commons.* New Brunswick, NJ: Rutgers University Press.

Brooker, C. (2001). Decade of evidence-based training for work with people with serious mental health problems: Progress in the development of psychosocial interventions. *Journal of Mental Health, 10,* 17-31.

Brown, G. W., Monick, E. M., Carstairs, G. M., & Wing, J. K. (1962). Influence of family life on the course of schizophrenia illness. *British Journal of Preventive Social Medicine, 16,* 55-68.

Budd, R. J., & Hughes, I. C. T. (1997). What do relatives of people with schizophrenia find helpful about family intervention? *Schizophrenia Bulletin, 23* (2), 341-347.

Budd, R. J., Oles, G., & Hughes, I. C. T. (1998). The relationship between coping style and burden in the caregivers of relatives with schizophrenia. *Acta Psychiatrica Scandinavica, 98,* 304-309.

Burland, J. (1998). Family-to-family: A trauma-and-recovery model of family education. In H. Lefley (Eds.), *Family coping with mental illness: the cultural context*. San Francisco, CA: Jossey-Boss Publishers.

Butzlaff, R. L., & Hooley, J. M. (1998). Expressed emotion and psychiatric relapse: A meta-analysis. *Archives of General Psychiatry, 55* (6), 547-552.

Canive, J. M., Sanz-Fuentenebro, J., Vazquez, C., Qualls, C., Fuentenebro, F., Perez, I. G., et al. (1996). Family psychoeducational support groups in Spain: Parents' distress and burden at nine-month follow-up. *Annuals of Clinical Psychiatry, 8*(2), 71-79.

Champion, L. A., & Goodall, G. M. (1994). Social support and mental health: Positive and negative aspects. In D. Tantam, & M. J. Birchwood (Eds.), *Seminars in psychology and the social sciences* (pp.238-259). London: Royal College of Psychiatrists.

Champion, L. A. (1990). The relationship between social vulnerability and the occurrence of severely threatening life events. *Psychological Medicine, 20* (suppl. 1), 7-161.

Chien, W. T. (2004). *Report on the controlled trial of mutual support group for Chinese family caregivers of patients with schizophrenia*. Unpublished doctoral report, Florence Nightingale School of Nursing & Midwifery, King's College. London. London: University of London.

Chien, W. T., & Chan, C. W. S. (2004). One-year follow-up of a multiple-family group intervention for Chinese families of patients with schizophrenia. *Psychiatric Services,55* (11), 1276-1284.

Chien, W.T., Chan, C.W.H., Lam, L.W., & Kam, C.W. (2005). Psychiatric inpatients' perceptions of positive and negative aspects of physical restraint. *Patient Education and Counseling, 59* (1), 80-86.

Chien, W. T., Chan, S., Morrissey, J., & Thompson, D. (2005). Effectiveness of a mutual support group for families of patients with schizophrenia. *Journal of Advanced Nursing, 51* (6), 595-608.

Chien, W. T., Norman, I., & Thompson, D. R. (2004). A randomized controlled trial of a mutual support group for family caregivers of patients with schizophrenia. *International Journal of Nursing Studies, 41*(6), 637-649.

Chien, W. T., Norman, I., & Thompson, D. R. (2006). Perceived benefits and difficulties experienced in a mutual support group for family caregivers of people with schizophrenia. *Qualitative Health Research, 16*(7), 962-981.

Chien, W.T., & Chan, C.W.S. (2004). One-year follow-up of a multiple-family-group intervention for Chinese families of patients with schizophrenia. *Psychiatric Services, 55* (11), 1276-1284.

Chou, K. R., LaMontagne, L. L., & Hepworth, J. T. (1999). Burden experienced by caregivers of relatives with dementia in Taiwan. *Nursing Research, 48* (4), 206-214.

Chou, K. R., Liu, S. Y., & Chu, H. (2002). The effects of support groups on caregivers of patients with schizophrenia. *International Journal of Nursing Studies, 39* (7), 713- 722.

Citron, M., Solomon, P., & Draine, J. (1999). Self-help groups for families of persons with mental illness: perceived benefits of helpfulness. *Community Mental Health Journal, 35*(1), 15-30.

Cohen, S., & Wills, T. A. (1985). Stress, social support and the buffering hypothesis. *Psychological Bulletin, 98* (2), 310-357.

Colahan, M., & Robinson, P. H. (2002). Multi-family groups in the treatment of young adults with eating disorders. *Journal of Family Therapy, 24,* 17-30.

Cole, R. E., & Reiss, D. (Eds.). (1993). *How Do Families Cope with Chronic Illness?* Hillsdale, NJ: Lawrence Erlbaum Associates, Inc.

Cook, J. A., Heller, T., & Pickett-Schenk, S. A. (1999). The effects of support group participation on caregiver burden among parents of adult offspring with severe mental illness. *Family Relations, 48* (4), 405-410.

Cook, J. A., Lefley, H. P., Pickett, S. A., & Cohler, B. J. (1994). Age and family burden among parents of offspring with severe mental illness. *American Journal of Orthopsychiatry, 64,* 435-447.

Cragan, J. F., & Wright, D. W. (1999). *Communicating in small groups: theory, process and skills* (5th ed.). Belmont, CA: Wadsworth Publications.

Craig, T. K. J., Garety, P., Power, P., Rahaman, N., Colbert, S., Fornells-Ambrojo, M., et al. (2004). The Lambeth Early Onset (LEO) Team: Randomised controlled trial of the effectiveness of specialised care for early psychosis. *British Medical Journal, 329* (7474), 1067-1071.

Dare, C., & Eisler, I. (2000). A multi-family group day treatment programme for adolescent eating disorder. *European Eating Disorders Review, 8* (1), 4-18.

Dixon, L., Adams, C., & Luckstead, A. (2000). Update on family psycho-education for schizophrenia. *Schizophrenia Bulletin, 26*(1), 5-20.

Dixon, L., Lyles, A., Scott, J., Postrado, L., Goldman, H., & McGlynn, E. (1999). Services to families of adults with schizophrenia: From treatment recommendations to dissemination. *Psychiatric Services, 50* (2), 233-238.

Dixon, L., McFarlane, W. R., Lefley, H., Lucksted, A., Cohen, M., Falloon, I., et al. (2001). Evidence-based practices for services to families of people with psychiatric disabilities. *Psychiatric Services, 52* (7), 903–910.

Doyle, M., Carr, A., Rowen, S., Galvin, P., Lyons, S., & Cooney, G. (2003). Family-oriented treatment for people with alcohol problems in Ireland: A comparison of the effectiveness of residential and community-based programmes. *Journal of Family Therapy, 25,* 15-40.

Drake, R. J., Haley, C. J., Akhar, S., & Lewis, S. (2000). Causes and consequences of duration of untreated psychosis in schizophrenia. *British Journal of Psychiatry, 177* (6), 511-515.

Dyck, D. G., Hendryx, M. S., Short, R. A., Voss, W. D., & McFarlane, W. R. (2002). Service use among patients with schizophrenia in psychoeducational multiple-family group treatment. *Psychiatric Services, 53* (6), 749-754.

Fadden, G. (1997). Implementation of family interventions in routine clinical practice following staff training programmes: a major cause for concern. *Journal of Mental Health, 6,* 599-612.

Fadden, G. (1998). Research update: Psychoeducational family interventions. *Journal of Family Therapy, 20,* 293-309.

Falloon, I. R. H., & Pederson, J. (1985). Family management in the prevention of morbidity of schizophrenia: The adjustment of the family unit. *British Journal of Psychiatry, 147,* 156-163.

Falloon, I. R. H., Boyd, J. L., McGill, C. W., Razani, J., Moss, H. B., & Gilderman, A. M. (1982). Family management in the prevention of exacerbations of schizophrenia: A controlled study. *New England Journal of Medicine, 306* (4), 1437-1440.

Galinsky, M. J., & Schopler, J. H. (Eds.). (1995). *Support groups: Current perspectives on theory and practice.* New York: Harworth Press.

Gazda,G. M., Ginter, E. J., & Horne, A. M. (2001). *Group counselling and group psychotherapy: Theory and application* (pp.33-94). Boston: Allyn and Bacon.

Gidron, B., & Chesler, M. (1995). Universal and particular attributes of self-help: A framework for international and intra-national analysis. In F. Lavoie, T. Borkman, & B. Gidron (Eds.), *Self-help and mutual aid groups: International and multicultural perspectives* (pp.1-44). New York: Haworth.

Gilstrap, L. (2004). A missing link in suggestibility research: What is known about the behavior of field interviewers in unstructured interviews with young children? *Journal of Experimental Psychology: Applied, 10*(1), 13-24.

Goldstein, M., Rodnick, E., Evans, J., May, P., & Steinberg, M. (1978). Drug and family therapy in the aftercare of acute schizophrenics. *Archives of General Psychiatry, 35* (10), 1169-1177.

Greenberg, J. S., Greenley, J. R., & Benedict, P. (1994). Contributions of persons with serious mental illness to their families. *Hospital and Community Psychiatry, 45,* 475-480.

Hazel, N. A., McDonell, M. G., Short, R. A., Berry, C. M., Voss, W. D., Rodgers, M. L., et al. (2004). Impact of multiple-family groups for outpatients with schizophrenia on caregivers' distress and resources. *Psychiatric Services, 55,* 35-41.

Heller, T., Roccoforte, J. A., & Cook, J. A. (1997). Predictors of support group participation among families of persons with mental illness. *Family Relations, 46*(4), 437-442.

Heller, T., Roccoforte, J. A., Hsieh, K., Cook, J. A., & Pickett, S. A. (1997). Benefits of support groups for families of adults with severe mental illness. *American Journal of Orthopsychiatry, 67*(2), 187-198.

Hirsch, S., & Leff, J. (1975). *Abnormalities in parents of schizophrenics.* Maudsley Monograph No. 22. London: Oxford University Press.

Hogarty, G. E., Anderson, C. M., Reiss, D. J., Kornblith, S. J., Greenwald, D. P., Ulrich, R. F., et al. (1991). Family psychoeducation, social skills training, and maintenance chemotherapy in the aftercare treatment of schizophrenia, II: Two-year effects of a controlled study on relapse and adjustment. *Archives of General Psychiatry, 48* (5), 340-347.

Humphreys, K. (1997). Individual and social benefits of mutual and self-help groups. *Social Policy, 27* (3), 12-19.

Ivanović, M., Vuletić, Z., & Bebbington, P. (1994). Expressed emotion in the families of patients with schizophrenia and its influence on the course of illness. *Social Psychiatry and Psychiatric Epidemiology, 29,* 61-65.

Karanci, A. N., & Inandilar, H. (2002). Predictors of components of expressed emotion in major caregivers of Turkish patients with schizophrenia. *Social Psychiatry and Psychiatric Epidemiology, 37,* 80-88.

Katz, L. F. (1997). *Self-help and support groups: A handbook for practitioners.* Thousand Oaks, CA: Sage Publications.

Kavanagh, D. J. (1992). Recent developments in expressed emotion and schizophrenia. *British Journal of Psychiatry, 160*, 601-620.

Kavanagh, D. J., Piatkowska, O., Clarke, D., O'Halloran, P., Manicavasagar, V., Rosen, A., et al. (1993). Application of cognitive-behavioural family intervention for schizophrenia in multi-disciplinary teams: What can the matter be? *Australian Psychologist, 28*, 181-188.

Kimberly, K. C. (1997). *Group processes and structures: A theoretical integration.* Lanham: University Press of America.

Koettgen, C., Soennichsen, I., Mollenhauer, K., & Jurth, R. (1984). Group therapy with the families of schizophrenic patients: results of the Hamburg Camberwell Family Interview study III. *International Journal of Family Psychiatry, 5* (1), 83-94.

Kurtz, L. F. (1997). *Self-help and support groups: A handbook for practitioners.* Thousand Oaks, CA: Sage Publications.

Lakey, B., & Cohen, S. (2000). Support theory and measurement. In S. Cohen, L. Underwood, & B. Gottlieb (Eds.), *Measuring and intervening in social support* (pp.29-52). New York: Oxford University Press.

Langford, C. P. H., Bowsher, J., Maloney, J. P., & Lillis, P. P. (1997). Social support: A conceptual analysis. *Journal of Advanced Nursing, 25* (1), 95-100.

Leff, J., Kuipers, L., Berkowitz, R., & Sturgeon, D. (1985). A controlled trial of social intervention in the families of schizophrenic patients: two year follow-up. *British Journal of Psychiatry, 146* (6), 594-600.

Leff, J., Kuipers, L., Berkowitz, R., Eberlein-Fries, R., & Sturgeon, D. (1982). A controlled trial of intervention in the families of schizophrenic patients. *British Journal of Psychiatry, 141* (2), 121-134.

Lefley, H. P. (1996). *Family caregiving in mental illness.* Thousand Oaks, CA: Sage Publications.

Lehman, A.F., & Steinwachs, D.M. (1998). At issue - Translating research into practice: The Schizophrenia Patient Outcomes Research Team (PORT) treatment recommendations. *Schizophrenia Bulletin, 24* (1), 1–9.

Lehman, A. F., Steinwachs, D. M., & the Survey Co-investigators of the PORT project. (1998). Patterns of usual care for schizophrenia: Initial results from the schizophrenia patient outcomes research team (PORT) client survey. *Schizophrenia Bulletin, 24* (1), 11-20.

Leung, P. W. L., & Lee, P. W. H. (1996). Psychotherapy with the Chinese. In M. H. Bond (Ed.), *The handbook of Chinese psychology* (pp. 441-456). Hong Kong: Oxford University Press.

Linszen, D., Dingemans, P., Van der Does, J.W., Nugter, A., Scholte, P., Lenoir, R., et al. (1996). Treatment, expressed emotion, and relapse in recent onset schizophrenic disorders. *Psychological Medicine, 26*, 333-342.

Loukissa, D. A. (1995). Family burden in chronic mental illness: A review of research studies. *Journal of Advanced Nursing, 21* (2), 248-255.

Ma, K. Y., & Yip, K. S. (1997). The importance of an effective psychiatric community care service for chronic mental patients in Hong Kong. *Hong Kong Journal of Mental Health, 26*,(1), 28-35.

Mankowski, E. S., Humphreys, K., & Moos, R. H. (2001). Individual and contextual predictors of involvement in Twelve-step self-help groups after substance abuse treatment. *American Journal of Community Psychology, 29* (4), 537-563.

Mari, J. J., & Streiner, D. (1996). Family intervention for people with schizophrenia. In Cochrane Library, Issue 1, 1996. Oxford, UK: Cochrane Library Update Software [Electronic database].

Martens, L., & Addington, J. (2001). The psychological well being of family members of individuals with schizophrenia. *Social Psychiatry and Psychiatric Epidemiology, 36,* 128-133.

Maton, K. E., & Salem, D. A. (1995). Organizational characteristics of empowering community settings: A multiple case study approach. *American Journal of Community Psychology, 23* (5), 631-656.

Maton, K. I. (1993). Moving beyond the individual level of analysis in mutual help groups research: An ecological paradigm. *Journal of Applied Behavioural Science, 29* (2), 272-286.

McCallion, P., & Toseland, R. W. (1995). Supportive group interventions with caregivers of frail older adults. *Social Work with Groups, 18* (1), 11-25.

McFarlane, W. R. (2002). *Multifamily groups in the treatment of severe psychiatric disorders.* New York: Guilford Press.

McFarlane, W. R., Dixon, L., Lukens, E., & Lucksted, A. (2003). Family psychoeducation and schizophrenia: A review of the literature. *Journal of Marital & Family Therapy, 29* (2), 223-245.

McFarlane, W. R., Link, B., Dushay, R., Marchal, J., & Crilly, J. (1995a). Psychoeducational multiple family groups: four-year relapse outcome in schizophrenia. *Family Process, 34* (2), 127-144.

McFarlane, W. R., Lukens, E., Link, B., Dushay, R., Deakins, S. A., Newmark, M., et al. (1995b). Multiple-family groups and psychoeducation in the treatment of schizophrenia. *Archives of General Psychiatry, 52* (8), 679-687.

Medvene, L., & Krauss, D. (1989). Causal attributions about psychiatric disability in a self-help group for families of the mentally ill. *Journal of Applied Social Psychology, 19* (17), 1413-1430.

Meissen, G. J., & Volk, F. (1995). Predictors of burnout among self-help leaders. In: F. Lavoie, T. Borkman, & B. Gidron (Eds.), *Self-help and mutual aid groups: International and multicultural perspectives* (pp.241-262). New York: Haworth.

Miles, M. B., & Huberman, A. M. (1994). *An expanded sourcebook: Qualitative data analysis.* (2nd ed.). Thousand Oaks, CA: Sage Publications.

Mueser, K. T., & Gingerich, S. (1994). *Coping with schizophrenia: A guide for families.* Oakland, CA: New Harbinger Publications.

Mueser, K. T., & Glynn, S. M. (1999). *Behavioral family therapy for psychiatric disorders,* (2nd ed.). Oakland, CA: New Harbinger Publications.

Mueser, K.T. (2003). *Mental Health Guidelines - Family services for severe mental illness.* Illinois, USA: Behavioral Health Recovery Management, Fayette Companies & Chestnut Health Systems.

National Collaborating Centre for Mental Health (2002). *Clinical Guideline 1 – Schizophrenia: Core interventions in the treatment and management of schizophrenia in primary and secondary care.* London: National Institute for Clinical Excellence.

Nichols, L., & Jenkinson, J. (1991). *Leading a support group.* New York: Chapman and Hall.

Noh, S., & Turner, R.J. (1987). Living with psychiatric patients: Implications for the mental health and family members. *Social Science and Medicine, 25*(3),263-272

Ohaeri, J.U. (2003). The burden of caregiving in families with a mental illness: A review of 2002. *Current Opinion in Psychiatry, 16*(4), 457-465.

Oka, T. (2003). *Self-help groups for parents of children with intractable diseases: A qualitative study of their organizational problems.* Parkland, FL: Dissertation-com.

Pearson, V., & Ning, S. P. (1997). Family care in schizophrenia: an undervalued resource. In: C.L.W. Chan, & N. Rhind (Eds.), *Social work intervention in health care: The Hong Kong scene* (pp.317-336). Hong Kong: Hong Kong University Press.

Penn, D. L., & Mueser, K. T. (1996). Research update on the psychosocial treatment of schizophrenia. *American Journal of Psychiatry, 153* (5), 607-617.

Perkins, D. D., & Zimmerman, M. A. (1995). Empowerment theory, research, and application: An introduction to a special issue. *American Journal of Community Psychology, 23*, 569-579.

Pharoah, F. M., Mari, J. J., & Streiner, D. (2001). *Family intervention for schizophrenia.* The Cochrane Library Reviews, Issue 3, 2001. Oxford, Cochrane Library Update Software [Electronic database].

Pharoah, F. M., Mari, J. J., & Streiner, D. (2001). *Family intervention for schizophrenia.* In Cochrane Reviews, Issue 3, 2001. Oxford, UK: The Cochrane Library.

Pilling, S., Bebbington, P., Kuipers, E., Garety, P., Geddes, J., Orbach, G., et al. (2002). Psychological treatments in schizophrenia, I: Meta-analysis of family intervention and cognitive behaviour therapy. *Psychological Medicine, 32*, 763-782.

Powell, T. J. (Ed.). (1994). *Understanding the self-help organization: Framework and findings.* Thousand Oaks: CA, Sage Publications.

Reissman, F., & Carroll, D. (1995). *Redefining self-help: Policy and practice.* San Francisco: Jossey-Bass.

Repper, J., & Brooker, C. (1998). Serious mental health problems in the community: The significance of policy, practice and research. In C. Brooker, & J. Repper (Eds.), *Serious mental health problems in the community: Policy, practice and research* (pp.8-30). London: Bailliere-Tindall.

Rose, L. E., Mallinson, R. K., & Walton-Moss, B. (2004). Barriers to family care in psychiatric settings. *Journal of Nursing Scholarship, 36* (1), 39-47.

Saunders, J. C. (1999). Family functioning in families providing care for a family member with schizophrenia. *Issues in Mental Health Nursing, 20*(2), 95-113.

Sellwood, W., Barrowclough, C., Tarrier, N., Quinn, J., Mainwaring, J., & Lewis, S. (2001). Needs-based cognitive-behavioural family intervention for caregivers of patients suffering from schizophrenia: 12-month follow-up. *Acta Psychiatrica Scandinavica, 104* (5), 346-355.

Solomon, P. (2000). Interventions for families of individuals with schizophrenia: Maximising outcomes for their relatives. *Disease Management and Health Outcomes, 8* (4), 211-221.

Steinglass, P. (1998). Multiple family discussion groups for patients with chronic medical illness. *Families, Systems and Health, 16,* 55-70.

Sun, L. K. (1991). Contemporary Chinese culture: Structure and emotionality. *Australian Journal of Chinese Affairs, 26,* 1-42.

Tarrier, N. (1991). Some aspects of family interventions in schizophrenia: I. Adherence to intervention programmes. *British Journal of Psychiatry, 159* (4), 475-480.

Telles, C., Karno, M., Mintz, J., Paz, G., Arias, M., Tucker, D. et al. (1995) Immigrant families coping with schizophrenia: Behavioural family intervention vs. case management with a low-income Spanish-speaking population. *British Journal of Psychiatry, 167* (4), 473-479.

Toseland, R. W., & Rossiter, C. M. (1989). Group interventions to support family caregivers: A review and analysis. *Gerontologist, 29* (4), 438-448.

Wearden, A. J., Tarrier, N., Barrowclough, C., Zastowny, T. R., & Rahill, A. A. (2000). A review of expressed emotion research in health care. *Clinical Psychology Review, 20* (5), 633-666.

Wheelan, S. A. (1994). *Group processes: A developmental perspective.* Boston: Allyn and Bacon.

Wilson, J. (1995). *How to work with self-help groups: Guidelines for health professionals.* Aldershot, UK: Arena.

Winefield, H. R., & Harvey, E. J. (1994). Needs of family caregivers in chronic schizophrenics. *Schizophrenia Bulletin, 20,* 557-566.

Wituk, S., Shepherd, M. D., Slavich, S., Warren, M. L., & Meissen, G. (2000). A topography of self-help groups: An empirical analysis. *Social Work, 45* (2), 157-165.

Wituk, S., Shepherd, M. D., Slavich, S., Warren, M. L., & Meissen, G. (2000). A topography of self-help groups: an empirical analysis. *Social Work, 45* (2), 157-165.

Wong, D., & Chan, C. (1994). Advocacy on self-help for patients with chronic illness: The Hong Kong experience. In: F. Lavoie, T. Borkman, & B. Gidron (Eds.), *Self-help and mutual aid groups: International and multicultural perspectives* (pp.117-140). New York: Haworth.

Xiong, W., Philips, M. R., Hu, X., Wang, R., Dai, Q., Kleinman, J., et al. (1994). Family-based intervention for schizophrenic patients in China. A randomised controlled trial. *British Journal of Psychiatry, 165* (3), 239-247.

Yalom, I. D. (1995). *The theory and practice of group psychotherapy* (4th ed.). New York: Basic Books.

Yalom, I. D. (1998). *The Yalom reader: Selections from the work of a master therapist and storyteller.* New York, NY: BasicBooks.

Zhang, M., Wang, M., Li, J., & Philips, M. R. (1994). A randomized controlled trial of family intervention for 78 first-episode male schizophrenic patients: an 18-month study in Suzhou, Jiangsu. *British Journal of Psychiatry, 165* (suppl. 24), 96-102.

Zimmerman, M. A. (1995). Psychological empowerment: Issues and illustrations. *American Journal of Community Psychology, 23* (5), 581-599.

In: Health Education Research Trends
Editor: P. R. Hong, pp. 95-128

ISBN: 978-1-60021-871-2
© 2007 Nova Science Publishers, Inc.

Chapter II

PERSPECTIVES IN HEALTH EDUCATION FOR INDIVIDUALS WITH INTELLECTUAL/DEVELOPMENTAL DISABILITIES

Margaret E. Williams[1]

[1]Children's Healthcare of Atlanta, Atlanta, GA, USA;
Byrdine F. Lewis School of Nursing, Georgia State University, Atlanta, GA, USA.

ABSTRACT

Individuals with intellectual/developmental disabilities (I/DD) are known to have both health and healthcare disparities. The health disparities are related to the general aging process and to health problems typical of individuals with intellectual/developmental disabilities. Healthcare disparities are experienced by these individuals because historically either these individuals did not survive childhood or they were placed in institutions. Thus, community medical providers, especially adult providers, have had little experience caring for the health of these individuals. As for anyone, healthcare education is important. But, for individuals with I/DD, unique health educational approaches are needed.

As many of the health problems experienced by individuals with I/DD are related to diet, nutrition education is important. One health educational approach is to use a variation of the Plate Method. The Plate Method is a commonly used visual method to show the proportions of a dinner plate that should be used to contain each of the various food groups. This Plate Model could be adapted for use by individuals with I/DD as a way to teach healthy eating.

In addition to a healthy diet, it is important for individuals with I/DD to incorporate into their daily routine activities to promote health. Social stories have been a means of positive behavior supports for children with autism. These social stories could be adapted for use by individuals with I/DD. Each individual would have their own *All About Me Healthy Lifestyle Story* in a book individually tailored to their needs. Pages of the book would cover their day from getting up in the morning to going to bed at night. Various pages would have a picture depicting the desired healthy lifestyle and simple words. Health behaviors that could be promoted include washing hands, brushing teeth, exercising, and taking medications.

In summary, health education for individuals with I/DD presents a unique challenge. Both the Plate Method and the *All About Me Healthy Lifestyle Story* present unique methods of health education for this population.

INTRODUCTION

Health education and promotion of healthy lifestyle choices is important for everyone. However, some individuals need health education geared toward their style of learning such as individuals with intellectual/developmental disabilities (I/DD). This need for health education for individuals with I/DD is highlighted by the disparities that have been noted in both health and healthcare for these individuals. This chapter will discuss the nature of developmental disabilities, the need for health education for individuals with I/DD to help offset their health and healthcare disparities, and will suggest two methods to promote health education and healthy lifestyle choices among individuals with I/DD.

Definition Intellectual/Developmental Disabilities (I/DD)

According to the national Governor's Council on Developmental Disabilities programs and the Federal definition of developmental disabilities, as noted in the Developmental Disabilities Assistance and Bill of Rights Act Amendments of 1994, the term "developmental disabilities" means a severe, chronic disability of an individual five years of age or older that

1. is attributable to a mental or physical impairment or combination of mental and physical impairments;
2. is manifested before the individual attains age 22;
3. is likely to continue indefinitely;
4. results in substantial functional limitations in three or more of the following areas of major life activity: (i) self-care; (ii) receptive and expressive language; (iii) learning; (iv) mobility; (v) self-direction; (vi) capacity for independent living; and (vii) economic self-sufficiency; and
5. reflects the individual's need for a combination and sequence of special, interdisciplinary, or generic services, supports, or other assistance that is of lifelong or extended duration and are individually planned and coordinated..."

(Governor's Council on Developmental Disabilities, 2007)

Demographics

Estimates of the prevalence of I/DD in the United States range from 1.0% to a high of 3.0% with a general prevalence of 1.0%. According to Horowitz, Kerker, Owens, and Zigler (2000), it is estimated that in the United States there are as many as 2.0 to 7.5 million individuals who are mentally retarded. [Note: Historically the term mental retardation (MR) was used. The term now generally used is intellectual/ developmental disability (I/DD). Other terms used are cognitive disabilities, intellectual disabilities, and developmental disabilities. All terms are used in this text depending on the source of the material.] Gaps exist in life expectancy between individuals with I/DD and individuals in the general population. In the United States, the overall life expectancy at birth is currently estimated to be 74.0 to 76.5 years. In contrast, individuals with I/DD have an estimated life expectancy at age 45 of 53.6 years to 66.1 years depending on the severity of the retardation. As individuals with mental retardation age they are prone to the same chronic diseases, including cardiovascular disease, cancer, and diabetes, which confront the general adult population. Yet, disparities in both health and in healthcare have been documented for individuals with intellectual/developmental disabilities (Horowitz et al, 2000).

Health and Healthcare Disparities

Several studies have documented health disparities for individuals with I/DD. The *2006 Disability and Health Chartbook*, from the Centers for Disease Control (CDC), contains information about the health of individuals with disabilities. Profiles of each state show the estimated number of men and women in each state with a disability along with graphs comparing the health of adults with and without a disability. The chartbook data show that, in general, individuals with a disability, compared to individuals without a disability, self-report their health status as much more likely to be fair or poor and much less likely to be very good or excellent. Yet, these same individuals with a disability are more likely to smoke, to be obese, and to be physically inactive (CDC, 2005, 2006).

Havercamp, Scandlin, and Roth (2004) studied health disparities among adults with developmental disabilities, adults with other disabilities, and adults not reporting a disability in North Carolina. The study found that compared to adults without a disability, adults with developmental disabilities were significantly more likely to have fair or poor general health status. Generally, adults with I/DD were at similar or greater risk of having four of five chronic health conditions compared to non-disabled adults.

More specifically, adults with I/DD were much more likely to have diabetes and less likely to have had their teeth cleaned within the previous five years. Compounding the problem, compared to adults without a disability, adults with I/DD were more likely to lead physically inactive sedentary lives. The researchers suggested that health promotion for individuals with I/DD include education regarding the risks associated with various health behaviors as well as education promoting a healthy lifestyle – including information about physical fitness, weight control, smoking cessation, emotional support, and disease prevention (Havercamp, et al., 2004).

Looking at women's health, Parish and Saville (2006) studied 15,831 women, age 18 to 64 years, to determine the extent to which disability-based disparities exist in the healthcare received by working-age women with cognitive disabilities as compared with non-disabled women. These authors found that women with cognitive limitations were less likely to receive breast cancer and cervical cancer screening than non-disabled women. Thus, women with cognitive disabilities may not receive the clinically indicated preventive care.

In recognition of the need to improve the quality of life of individuals with mental retardation, a study was commissioned by Special Olympics, Inc. to examine the health status and needs of children and adults with mental retardation and to identify gaps in service (Horowitz, et al., 2000). A follow-up analysis published in March, 2001, *Promoting Health for Persons with Mental Retardation–A Critical Journey Barely Begun* identified and highlighted the health status and needs of persons with mental retardation and suggested approaches to improve both their length and quality of lives (Corbin, Malina, & Shepherd, 2005, Special Olympics, Inc, 2001a, 2001b).

To determine the health of people with I/DD, more than 3,500 athletes were screened at the 2003 Special Olympics World Summer Games in Dublin, Ireland. According to the data, the athletes with intellectual disabilities had a higher prevalence of serious health problems than the general population. Of these athletes, 30% failed hearings tests (which leads to communication problems), 25% had vision problems, 29% of males and 13% of females had below normal bone mineral density (BMD), 30% were obese, and 23% were overweight (Horowitz, et al., 2000; Special Olympics, Inc, 2001a, 2001b).

Why Are There Disparities?

According to Horowitz et al., 2000, individuals with I/DD are particularly vulnerable to have unmet healthcare needs. Several forces influence the ability of individuals with I/DD to receive appropriate healthcare and health education. With the health and healthcare disparities noted for individuals with I/DD, it is imperative to find ways to provide these individuals with appropriate health education. Yet, factors exist that hinder meeting their health education needs. These factors include deinstitutionalization, an increase in life expectancy for individuals with I/DD, the challenging nature of their healthcare, and a paradigm shift in medicine.

Since the 1970s, there has been a move toward the deinstitutionalization of individuals with I/DD by moving them from the institutions, where they have traditionally lived, back into the community. With deinstitutionalization, all but the most severely disabled individuals are expected to function within the community environment. Along with deinstitutionalization, there has been an increase in life expectancy such that individuals with I/DD who used to die in childhood are now living into adulthood. Consequently, adult primary healthcare providers in the community, who traditionally have had little exposure to the healthcare needs of individuals with I/DD, are now called upon to provide healthcare services for these individuals (Horowitz et al, 2000). To complicate the issue, when individuals have an I/DD, the management of chronic illness becomes more challenging as their medical conditions are more complex and involve multiple disorders (Parish & Saville,

2006). The net effect is that the healthcare needs of individuals with I/DD are not being adequately addressed in the community.

Concurrently to deinstitutionalization and improved life expectancy for individuals with I/DD, there has been a paradigm shift in healthcare and health promotion. In the past, the emphasis in healthcare has been on prevention of disabling conditions with a relative neglect of individual health promotion. The new healthcare paradigm focus is on evaluating and improving the health of individuals along with the prevention of secondary conditions and chronic illness. Health education is an important part of this new paradigm of healthcare (Brown, Watson, & Maloney, 2007c). It is a challenge for us to find ways to communicate health education for individuals with I/DD.

Communication Problems Lead to Disparities

Yet, a challenge to providing adequate care for individuals with I/DD is gaps in communication. These communication gaps takes two forms. There may be a gap in communication between the individual with I/DD and the health care provider. And, the individual with I/DD may not understand the healthcare treatment regimen recommended by the healthcare provider. These communication gaps are often aggravated by severe cognitive disability, hearing problems, autism, mental health disorders, early dementia, or cognitive decline (American Association on Mental Retardation [AAMR], Fact Sheet, 2007).

When individuals with I/DD are non-verbal, healthcare providers find their care to be more challenging and time consuming. Initially, healthcare providers may have difficulty communicating with individuals with I/DD who have difficulty explaining their health problems or symptoms of disease. Then, caregivers need to identify the symptoms and report them to the health providers, who must detect clinical manifestations of disease among individuals who lack the communication skills to describe their symptoms (Horowitz et al., 2000). Thus, the medical problems of these individuals may go unrecognized and untreated. To add to the communication gap, a medical history is often lacking (Brown, et al., 2007c). Compounding the problem, the medical care for individuals with I/DD is often more challenging because of the physical, cognitive, and behavioral difficulties often encountered in treating these individuals (Horowitz, et al., 2000).

Conversely, individuals with I/DD may have difficulty accessing appropriate health services, understanding the risks and benefits of medical treatment, and understanding the effect of their behavior on their health (President's Committee on Mental Retardation, 1999). Because of these problems, the ability of individuals with I/DD to cooperate for healthcare may be limited (Krogman, 2007). For example, treating obesity for an individual with I/DD is compounded if the individual has difficulty understanding the nutritional recommendations (Horowitz, et al., 2000).

Because of the communication challenges, providers must rely on the caregivers to communicate treatment regimens. However, because of staff turnover combined with the movement of individuals with I/DD from one housing location to another, there often is a lack of continuity of care. The result is a lack of the development of a therapeutic relationship with the health provider and a lack of adherence to a treatment regimen. Yet, individuals with

I/DD need to be full partners in promoting their own health, and they have a right to be informed about their health status and healthcare needs (Horowitz et al., 2000.) This need necessitates finding ways to communicate with and to promote health education for individuals with I/DD.

CHRONIC HEALTH CONDITIONS FOR INDIVIDUALS WITH I/DD

Certain chronic health conditions are associated with aging, especially for individuals with developmental disabilities, and the risk of these chronic health conditions increases with age. Chronic health conditions that are common causes of death are cardiovascular disease, cancer, and diabetes. Just as with the general population, chronic age related physical health conditions contribute to the morbidity and mortality of individuals with mental retardation. For individuals with I/DD, the incidence of such chronic conditions occur either with the same frequency (Krogman, 2007) or with a greater frequency than in the general population. The most common causes of death among individuals with mental retardation are cardiovascular diseases, respiratory illness and neoplastic conditions (Horowitz, et al., 2000). Another problem affecting the health of individuals with developmental disabilities is dental health. Encouraging healthy lifestyle behaviors to help prevent these chronic health conditions and dental problems can improve the quality of life for these individuals.

Cardiovascular Disease

Cardiovascular disease is the leading cause of death in the U.S. accounting for 31.4% of deaths in the general population and is a common cause of death among individuals with I/DD (Horowitz et al, 2000). Cardiovascular disease includes such disorders as coronary heart disease, arteriosclerosis, hypertension, peripheral vascular disease, atrial fibrillation, congestive heart failure, angina, and heart attack. There is evidence that most cardiovascular disease is preventable and that lower levels of risk for cardiovascular disease are related to healthy lifestyle behaviors. Components of a healthy lifestyle include maintaining a desirable body weight, eating a healthy diet, exercising regularly, and not smoking. According to Pearson, et al. (2002), "The healthcare professional should create an environment supportive of risk factor change, including long-term reinforcement of adherence to lifestyle and drug interventions" (Pearson, et al. 2002, p. 390-391).

Diabetes

Diabetes mellitus is a disease in which the body has an inadequate supply of the hormone insulin, which is needed to transport glucose into the cells for energy. Diabetes is the seventh leading cause of death in the United States (CDC, 1998) affecting more than 15.7 million people. Obesity is a major risk factor for diabetes and the prevalence of diabetes in the U.S.

has been rising by epidemic proportions along with the increase in obesity and overweight in the population (Klein, et al, 2004). "The prevalence of type 2 diabetes is three to seven times higher in obese than normal weight adults" (Klein et al, 2004, p. 2067). And, individuals with diabetes are at higher risk of heart disease, stroke, high blood pressure, blindness, kidney disease, amputations, and dental disease (CDC, 1998). As with cardiovascular disease, the incidence of diabetes is higher among individuals with I/DD (Horowitz, et al, 2000).

Cancer

According to the World Health Organization (2007), dietary factors account for 30% of all cancers in Western Countries. Being overweight or obese increases the risk for cancers of the esophagus, colorectum, breast, kidney, and endometrium. Eating red meat or preserved meat increases the risk for colorectal and esophageal cancers. As being overweight or obese are both serious risk factors for cancer, dietary modification and physical activity are important in reducing cancer risk. A diet high in fruits and vegetables probably reduces the incidence of oral cavity, stomach, and colorectal cancer. Physical activity also reduces the incidence of colon and breast cancer.

Dental Health

In addition to the above chronic health conditions, dental health is another problem among individuals with I/DD compared to the general population. Poor dental health can have dramatic effects on an individual's quality of life by causing tooth loss and problems with eating, speech, and with self-esteem. Thus, dental health is a national priority under Healthy People, 2010 (US DHHS, 2000). Compared to the general population, individuals with I/DD are more likely to have a higher prevalence of gingivitis and other periodontal diseases. Estimates of gingivitis among individuals with I/DD range from 60 to 97% compared with a prevalence of 28 to 75% in the general population. Gingivitis and periodontitis, which may result in tooth loss, may be related to poor oral hygiene and to the mouth dryness associated with certain medications that may be used by individuals with I/DD (Fenton, Hood, Holder, May, & Mouradian, 2003; Horowitz, et al., 2000)

Oral health is dependent on oral hygiene, yet oral hygiene among individuals with I/DD has been shown to be consistently poor compared with individuals in the general population (Horowitz, et al., 2000). According to Rubin and Crocker (2006), there are many reasons that individuals with I/DD are at risk for dental problems. Tooth decay may occur as a result of offering sweets as rewards for good behavior. Problems with chewing and swallowing may necessitate that the individual eat soft foods, which tend to be higher in carbohydrates and tend to be retained in the oral cavity promoting gingivitis and tooth decay. Many oral medications, especially the commonly used antiseizure medications phenytoin (Dilantin) and valproic acid (Depakene), are mixed in syrups for palatability and ease of administration. Other medications with anticholinergic properties, such as antidepressants and neuroleptic medications, reduce saliva flow making the teeth more prone to decay.

LIFESTYLE CHOICES

Many chronic health conditions, including cardiovascular disease, diabetes and cancer, are related to long-term lifestyle behaviors. Certain lifestyle behaviors, such as poor nutritional habits leading to obesity, decreased physical activity, sedentary lifestyle, and use of tobacco products, are the primary modifiable risk factors for most chronic diseases. These lifestyle behaviors are listed among the leading indicators of health in both Healthy People 2000 and Healthy People 2010 (US DHHS, 2000a). Exercise, proper diet, and weight control need to be promoted in general in order to prevent older age-related health disorders, such as Type 2 diabetes and cardiovascular disease (AAMR Fact Sheet, 2007).

In addition, aging with a disability is impacted by the normal effects of aging, which are compounded by the effects of the disability, the treatment of the disability, and poor lifestyle choices. The negative outcomes of poor lifestyle choices include cardiovascular disease, diabetes, and cancer. The effects of these lifestyle choices are compounded by the individual's lack of understanding of the consequences of these lifestyle choices and a lack of motivation to change behavior. These effects are further compounded as there is limited access to quality healthcare for individuals with I/DD and a lack of knowledge among healthcare providers about aging for people with I/DD (Brown, Watson & Moloney, 2007a; 2007b).

Obesity

Obesity is typically the outcome of poor lifestyle choices. Obesity is associated with cardiovascular disease, diabetes, and breast, prostate and colon cancers. According to one estimate, 23% of adults are obese. Among individuals with I/DD, obesity is more common than in the general population, especially among females. Overall prevalence estimates ranging from 29.5 to 50.5% (AAMR fact sheet, 2007; Rubin, et al., 1998). The risk of obesity is also increased for individuals with I/DD living in a group home (Krogman, 2007).

Sedentary Lifestyle

Regular physical exercise is an important health maintenance activity that is associated with decreased body fat, decreased risk of cardiovascular disease and diabetes, and enhanced psychological well-being (US DHHS, 2000a). The US Surgeon General made regular physical activity a national health priority in Health People 2000 and Healthy People 2010 (US DHHS, 1999; US DHHS, 2000a). Regular physical activity also helps to prevent osteoporosis, which is a problem among individuals with I/DD, especially those who take anticonvulsant medications (Schrager, 2004). To the extent that individuals with I/DD participate in sedentary activities (watching television, listening to the radio or to music) and do not participate in physical activities, their overall health is affected and their cardiovascular fitness is compromised (Horowitz et al, 2000).

Oral Hygiene

Oral hygiene is important for everyone. Yet, oral hygiene for individuals with I/DD is often more difficult because of their disability. Some individuals with I/DD may have impaired coordination and need assistance from caregivers to complete oral hygiene tasks (Horowitz, et al., 2000).

Reinforcing the need for good oral hygiene, there is an association between periodontal disease and cardiovascular disease (Goldfarb, 20005). Dietrick and Garcia (2005) report that brushing and flossing not only maintain healthy gums, they help prevent cardiovascular disease in people with diabetes. Regular visits to the dentist are also important in maintaining dental health.

RECOGNITION OF NEED TO IMPROVE

In recognition of the need to improve health and healthcare for individuals with I/DD, the American Association on Mental Retardation (AAMR, now AAIDD as of January 1, 2007) has issued a *Declaration on Health Parity for Persons with Intellectual and Developmental Disabilities.* According to the AAIDD declaration:

> Health is essential for daily cognitive and physical function and a requisite for full participation in society. Health entails well-being in all facets of life, and all persons, including individuals with I/DD, have a right to achieve and maintain their optimal level of health...Globally there is evidence of market disparity of health between persons with I/DD and the general population. Health services for persons with I/DD often continue to be discriminatory, inappropriate, inefficient, uninformed, and insufficient. Provision of most health services is predicated on treatment of illness (AAMR, 2006).

Correspondingly, the *AAMR/ARC Position Statement: Health Care Issue* states:

> Too many of our constituents have faced numerous challenges, including life-threatening barriers, in accessing timely and appropriate healthcare. Problems in the community include inability to obtain appropriate quality services, lack of access to specialists, and healthcare professionals who refuse to serve or limit the options made available to this population. Many communities in fact lack health professionals overall, but especially those trained to meet the needs of our constituents (AAMR, 2002).

In summary, as with the general population, individuals with I/DD are at risk for the chronic age related medical conditions, such as cardiovascular disease, cancer, and diabetes. Individuals with I/DD are also susceptible to the primary risk factors of chronic diseases including obesity, lack of physical exercise, and smoking. Additionally, although individuals with MR have similar physical health problems as those in the general population, they are less likely to receive adequate medical services, including physical, mental, ocular, or dental care, compared with those in the general population (Horowitz et al, 2000). Therefore, health services must be provided to reduce identified aging and disability-associated health risk.

Horowitz et al. (2000) recommended that individuals with MR should be educated about disease prevention, recognition of symptoms of common health conditions, and health maintenance. Developmentally appropriate teaching material should be utilized with this population to promote self-sufficiency and human dignity. A lifespan approach is needed because many older age-related health disorders have their origin in lifestyle choices made at earlier ages and may result in secondary conditions that can be prevented, or effectively diagnosed and treated, at early stages (AAMR, 2005).

More recently, in 2002, the report of the Surgeon General's Conference on Health Disparities and Mental Retardation was issued. This report was entitled *Closing the Gap: A National Blueprint to Improve the Health of Persons with Mental* Retardation (U.S DHHS, 2002). This report noted that good health is essential to quality of life and that individuals with mental retardation are more likely to receive inappropriate and inadequate treatment. "Compared with other populations, adults, adolescents, and children with mental retardation experience poorer health...." P. xii. Goals and action steps to improve the health of individuals with mental retardation were listed in the report. The first goal was to "Integrate Health Promotion into Community Environments of People with Mental Retardation" (p. 3). As part of the goal, "health promotions programs should accommodate people with MR." Examples of health promotion programs included weight control and fitness programs. To implement this goal, individuals with MR "need to be empowered with adequate and understandable information and reinforcement to avoid health risks and maintain healthy personal habits...Their healthcare providers and the environments where they live, work, learn, and socialize should offer opportunities to inform, support, and reinforce healthy lifestyles" (p. 3).

Closing the Gap listed several action steps to achieve this first goal. Under wellness, an action goal was listed to "educate and support individuals with MR, their families, and other caregivers in self-care and wellness." Self-care and wellness programs designed for general population need to be adapted to the needs of individuals with MR. Models need to be developed and disseminated for health care provider counseling and reinforcement of wellness and healthy behaviors in individuals with MR, their families, and caregivers, especially on the topics of nutrition and weight control, exercise, and oral health. Under caregiver support, it was noted that caregivers need training in healthcare and supporting healthy habits. Areas for assessment of this goal were to "assess the effects of health promotion and wellness activities on individuals with MR: their morbidity, secondary disability, mortality, life satisfaction, independent living, achievement of life goals, and cultural/ethnic identity" (US DHHS, 2002, p. 4).

NEED FOR HEALTH PROMOTION

The consensus is that in order to reduce the incidence of chronic conditions, lifestyle modifications are needed in the areas of diet, physical activity, and exercise (Brown, Watson & Moloney 2007b). To help protect the heart against cardiovascular disease, regular moderate exercise needs to be encouraged along with eating a healthy diet. Diet and exercise are also beneficial in preventing diabetes and cancer and in maintaining musculoskeletal health such as strengthening bones and preventing osteoporosis. The following lifestyle modifications are needed in general, but especially for individuals with I/DD.

Diet

Obesity is a risk factor for high blood pressure, diabetes, high blood triglycerides, cholesterol and lipids, and cardiovascular disease. Conversely, weight loss improves the risk factors for cardiovascular disease by improving blood sugar levels, decreasing blood pressure, improving markers of inflammation related to cardiovascular disease, and improving levels of triglycerides, cholesterol, and other lipids in the blood. Even a moderate weight loss of 5%, combined with exercise, can help prevent or delay the onset of Type 2 diabetes in high risk groups (Klein et al., 2004).

According to Klein et al. (2004), weight loss is recommended for all overweight and obese individuals. The primary approach for achieving weight loss is through lifestyle changes, such as reducing the amount of calories consumed, especially calories from fat, and increasing physical activity. Even a moderate reduction in calories may promote weight loss and improvement in cardiovascular risk factors. To promote weight loss and exercise, behavior therapy is often helpful in helping the individual replace problematic eating and activity patterns with healthy lifestyle behavior patterns.

"A low-fat diet is considered the conventional therapy for treating obesity" (Klein, et al., 2004, p. 2068). Along with reducing fat in the diet, reducing the total amount of dietary carbohydrates, especially sugars, aids in weight loss. Specific recommendations to promote weight loss include portion control and limiting foods that are high in fat by substituting lean meats, meat alternatives, or low-fat dairy foods. The consumption fruits and vegetables, whole grains, and other fiber sources needs to be increased in order to maintain a volume of food for hunger control. A variety of food is also important to promote diet palatability (Brown, Watson & Moloney 2007b; Klein et al., 2004).

Physical Activity and Exercise

Physical activity and exercise are important for weight control and for reduction of risk factors associated with cardiovascular disease such as high blood pressure, high cholesterol, and high triglycerides. Physical activity can make a substantial difference in a person's longevity and quality of life. Benefits of physical activity include controlling obesity, decreasing blood pressure, increasing strength and cardiovascular endurance, improving balance, improving lung and breathing function, improving immune function, decreasing cancer risk, and reducing the depression and anxiety that are common for individuals with I/DD (Brown, Watson & Moloney 2007b). Exercise also assists in protecting the musculoskeletal system by improving muscle strength and decreasing the risk for osteoporosis. Maintaining an optimal weight decreases stress on joints. Additionally, increasing the intake of calcium and vitamin D through supplements is often recommended to promote musculoskeletal health and to help prevent osteoporosis (Brown, Watson & Moloney, 2007a).

Exercise guidelines for individuals with I/DD are generally the same as for the general population (Krogman, 2007). According to the National Center on Physical Activity and Disability (NCPAD) Exercise Guidelines for People with Disabilities Fact Sheet (2007), "Exercise is for EVERY body" as exercise is a key factor in maintaining and improving overall health (p.1). In 1996, the Surgeon General of the United States reported that significant health benefits can be obtained with physical activity, especially daily moderate exercise. These benefits are even more important if an individual has a disability since people with disabilities have a tendency to live a less active lifestyle (NCPAD, 2007, p.1).

The National Heart Lung and Blood Institute (NHLBI) recommends for the general population 30 to 45 minutes of moderate-intensity aerobic physical activity three to five times a week initially and then gradually increasing the duration and frequency of the physical activity. Previously inactive individuals may start with 10 minutes of low-intensity exercise and gradually increase the amount and intensity of exercise as strength and fitness improve. Walking and using the stairs are good ways to start an exercise program, and the amount of time of exercise can be divided into two or more short sessions. The key is to develop an exercise plan that can be maintained without injury so it is important to consult with a physician prior to initiating an exercise program (Klein et al, 2004).

Facilitating Lifestyle Changes

It is acknowledged that making long-term changes in diet and activity are not easy. Often, these lifestyle changes need to be facilitated. According to Heller, Ying, Rimmer, and Marks (2002), the major determinants of exercise in adults with cerebral palsy are caregiver attitude and place of residence. Thus, caregivers can have a major impact on the adoption of healthy lifestyle choices by individuals with I/DD.

To make lifestyle changes, individuals need encouragement, support, and praise of efforts. Self-efficacy is a person's belief in their ability to change their behavior and their belief in their ability to change a behavior strongly predicts their ability to make that change. Strategies that increase self-efficacy are powerful tools to foster behavioral change. It is important to create an atmosphere that is supportive of change and to give the clear message that the person is capable of change. This support helps the individual do the hard work of changing their lifestyle. Other strategies for increasing self-efficacy are encouraging the individual to take small steps, setting goals that can be easily mastered, providing role models, clarifying the meaning of symptoms or conditions, and providing pervasive reasons for change (Brown, Watson & Moloney 2007b). Monitoring an individual's weight can be an important way to promote understanding and to provide feedback as to the individual's progress toward their goals.

The two tools presented in this chapter to promote healthy lifestyle changes for individuals with I/DD focus on providing health education to the individuals along with their caregivers. The tools are *The Plate Method* and *All About Me Healthy Lifestyle Stories*. These tools focus on improving nutrition, by teaching healthy food choices, and on encouraging increased activity and exercise as a part of daily life. Of course, to the extent that caregivers support individual self-efficacy and become healthier role models themselves, individuals with I/DD will be encouraged to make positive lifestyle changes (Brown, Watson & Moloney 2007b).

THE PLATE METHOD

Obesity is a common problem in the United States, but especially among individuals with I/DD. Proper nutrition and a balanced diet are considered to be the main ways to combat obesity (Klein, et al., 2004; Pearson, et. al., 2002). But, it is a challenge to find creative ways to teach proper diet and nutrition. Estimating portion size is hard to do. The Plate Method, which uses a simple visual method for teaching meal planning through the use of pictures, graphs, charts, and food replicas, is commonly used in Europe. As part of the Diabetes Atherosclerosis Intervention Study (DAIS) for persons with diabetes and dyslipidemia, dietitians from Canada, Finland, France, and Sweden explored methods of teaching meal planning and chose the Plate Model. Since 1987, the Plate Model has been promoted as useful dietary education tool by the Swedish Diabetic Association and the Community Nutrition Group of the British Dietetic Association. It is considered by some to be easier to use than the traditional diabetic exchange method (Camelon, et al., 1998). The Plate Model has been adapted by a group of dieticians in Idaho and has been renamed by them as the Idaho Plate Method (Rizor & Richards, 2000).

In both the European and the Idaho Plate Models a dinner plate serves as a visual pie chart to show proportions of the plate that should be covered by certain food groups. According to Rizor and Richards (2000), the Plate Method teaches portion control while helping to increase dietary antioxidant nutrients and fiber, lowering the intake of fat, and keeping a more consistent level of carbohydrate at each meal. Experience with the Plate Method has found it to be a valuable tool in diabetic education (Camelon, et al., 1998; Rizor & Richards, 2000; Rizor, et al., 1996, 1998). The Plate Method is also a simple way to teach proper nutrition for weight loss meal planning. Foods do not need to be weighed or measured so cumbersome scales or measuring cups do not need to be carried around. Also, no special diet foods or meals need to be purchased (Rizor & Richards, 2000; Rizor, et al., 1996, 1998). Benefits of using the Plate Method to teach adult learners about proper diet and nutrition are "the promotion of memory retention and understanding through visual messages and experience of a positive approach to nutrition counseling" (Camelon, et al., 1998, p. 1156). It has been used to teach food portion control in order to achieve tight blood glucose control in diabetics (Rizor & Richards, 2000). Overall, use of the Plate Method can help promote healthy eating, weight loss, and lowering of cholesterol. Information about the Idaho Plate Method is available at www.platemethod.com.

Because of its simplicity and versatility, the Plate Method is being proposed to be used to promote a healthy diet in individuals with I/DD. Since the Plate Method uses a visual format that promotes learning, it promises to be a simple way to present a balanced diet in a format that should be easy to understand by individuals with I/DD and by their caregivers (Dale, 1963).

Using the Plate Method

Over the years, the size of dinner plates has gotten bigger and using a larger plate for meals promotes overeating. So, for the Plate Method, a 9-inch dinner plate, a bowl or small plate, and a glass are used. The part of the plate where the food is placed needs to be 9 inches across. This 9-inch dinner plate is then divided into three sections to indicate the proportions of the plate that should be covered by each of three main food groups: Vegetables, Meat/Protein, and Breads/Starches/Grains. A small plate or bowl and a glass sit off to the side of the dinner plate. The small plate needs to hold about one-half cup and the bowl needs to hold about one cup. The glass should hold 8 ounces. For men, in order to provide the extra calories that men typically need, and for individuals who need to gain weight, another small plate may be placed outside the dinner plate for a starch, grain, or bread. Different depictions of the model are used for lunch/dinner and for breakfast (see figures 1 & 2) (Rizor & Richards, 2000; Rizor, et al., 1996, 1998).

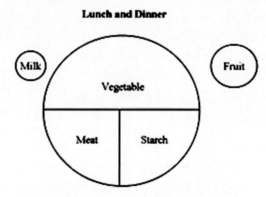

Figure 1. Plate Method for Lunch/Dinner.

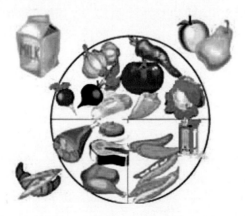

Figure 2. Plate Method: Lunch/Dinner with Sample Foods.

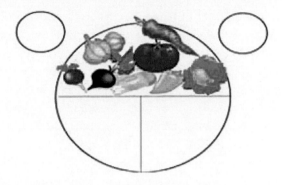

Figure 3. Vegetables.

For the Lunch/Dinner Model, (see figures 1 and 2) the 9-inch dinner plate is divided across the middle into two halves. The top one-half of the plate (see figure 3) is where vegetables are placed. But high carbohydrate vegetables such as corn, peas, potatoes, yams, or winter squash (acorn, butternut, pumpkin, and spaghetti) do not go in this section of the plate. The vegetables provide vitamins, minerals, and fiber. The bulk promotes a feeling of fullness so that less food is eaten. The same vegetable does not need to cover the entire upper half of the plate. A combination of vegetables can be used such as placing both a salad and a cooked vegetable within the Vegetable section of the plate. The vegetables may be cooked or raw. Examples of appropriate vegetables include: green leafy vegetables such as lettuce, tomatoes, onions, cucumber, radishes, broccoli, cauliflower, brussel sprouts, cabbage, beets, carrots, mushrooms, spinach, and summer squash (crook neck and zucchini). The vegetables should be stacked the highest of all the foods on the plate. Also, the foods in each section should not touch each other in order to slightly reduce portion size (Rizor & Richards, 2000; Rizor, et al., 1996; Rizor, et al., 1998).

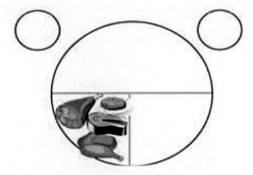

Figure 4. Meat/Protein.

The bottom half of the plate is divided into two-quarter sections. On one of these quarter sections of the plate is placed Meat/Protein (see figure 4). Foods for this section include meat (beef, pork, fish, or poultry) and other high protein foods such as cheese, tofu, eggs, nuts, or soy product substitutes for meat. The basic size of a serving of meat is about the size of a deck of cards. The key is to keep the meat or high protein food totally within the one-quarter Meat/Protein section of the plate. Keeping the amount of the Meat/Protein within this area of the plate will reduce the total amount of fat and cholesterol intake. Moreover, choosing lower fat and cholesterol foods are healthier and will further reduce the fat intake. The method of food preparation can also reduce fat intake. Frying and breading of foods and serving foods with sauces typically add fat. Healthier ways of cooking include removing all visible fat prior to cooking and using cooking sprays instead of oil. Lower fat versions of butter, sour cream, gravies, and other foods are available. Lower fat cooking alternatives to frying include grilling, broiling, baking, boiling, or steaming. Rizor & Richards, 2000; Rizor, et al., 1996, 1998). Another way to reduce fat intake for ground beef recipes is to substitute a ground version of a lower fat protein food such as ground turkey or ground chicken for all or part of the ground beef in the recipe. Even more savings in fat intake can be made if the ground turkey or chicken is the breast portion of the meat, as this portion of poultry is lower in fat than the dark meat. However, some individuals, especially those with I/DD, do not consume enough protein. To add protein to the diet, try adding non-fat dry milk powder to puddings, mashed potatoes, or other similar foods.

In the other one-quarter portion of the plate are placed Breads/Starches/Grains (see figure 5). This group includes starchy foods such as corn, peas, dried beans (garbanzo, pinto, kidney, lima beans), potatoes, yams, or winter squash (acorn, butternut, pumpkin, spaghetti squash) and other breads or grains such as bread, rolls, pasta, rice, cereals, crackers, and tortillas. The serving size of starchy vegetables should be about one cup. A serving of bread is one slice of bread or ½ of a hamburger bun or English muffin. Again, the starchy foods need to remain within this one-quarter section of the plate (Rizor & Richards, 2000; Rizor, et al., 1996, 1998).

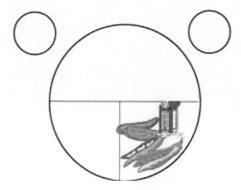

Figure 5. Breads/ Starches/Grains.

On one side of the dinner plate, a small coffee cup for milk is placed (see figure 2). A milk serving is one cup or one small glass. Lower fat forms of milk (skim, 1%. 2%) are healthier. Instead of milk, yogurt or lite ice cream may be substituted. The milk serving provides the needed calcium for strong bones. Calcium also assists in controlling blood pressure and is believed to promote weight loss. Three servings of milk or milk products are recommended daily to obtain the daily requirement of calcium (Rizor & Richards, 2000; Rizor, et al., 1996, 1998).

On the other side of the plate, a small plate or bowl is placed to hold a serving of fruit (see figure 2). A serving of fruit consists of a small piece of fruit such as an apple, orange, or peach that is about the size of a baseball. A small banana may also be used. The small bowl should hold about one-half cup. It may be used for fruits such as applesauce, fruit cocktail, grapes, or berries. Fruit juices may be substituted, but juices are less filling that the whole fruit. The serving size for fruit juice is one-half cup or about one-half of a small coffee cup. It is permissible to substitute a small serving of dessert for the fruit as long as the dessert fits within the small plate or bowl. However, substituting too many desserts for the fruit servings is less healthy and may promote weight gain. Milk, fruit, and starch servings may also be substituted for each other. But, too much substitution is not recommended because a balanced diet includes all of the food groups and skipping a food group on a regular basis may compromise nutrition and not provide the protein, vitamins, and minerals the body needs to stay healthy (Rizor & Richards, 2000; Rizor, et al., 1996, 1998).

For breakfast, the Plate Method can be modified (see figures 6 and 7). The one-half of the plate designated for Vegetables is left empty. One-fourth of the plate may be used for Meat/Protein as desired. The other one-fourth of the plate is still used for a Breads/Starches/Grains. A small bowl can be used to hold cereals instead of using the one-quarter section of the plate reserved for Breads/Starches/Grains (Rizor & Richards, 2000; Rizor, et al., 1996, 1998).

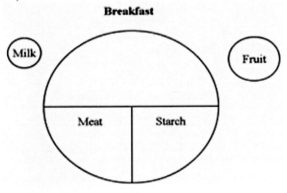

Figure 6. Plate Method Breakfast.

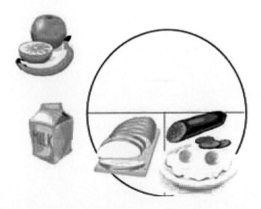

Figure 7. Plate Method Breakfast with Sample Foods.

Serving Sizes

Using the Plate Method will help adjust portions to the proper serving size. There are also several other ways to determine serving size. The nutrition label is a good way to determine the size of a serving. And, the serving size is not always the whole package, so the label must be read carefully. Another way to estimate serving size is to use the hand. The flat part of the hand, excluding the fingers, holds about one-half cup. The whole hand, including the fingers, holds about one cup (Rizor, Thomas, Harker, & Smith, 2002). The serving size of a baked potato is about the size of a fist. For cereals, the serving size can be found on the nutrition label. The serving size of the traditional breakfast cereals, such as corn flakes and puffed wheat, varies from one-half to one cup, or about the size of a fist.

Another way to estimate portion size is to use common everyday objects. The serving size of cooked rice, pasta, or potato is one-half cup or about the size of one-half of a baseball The serving sizes of fresh fruit and ice cream are one-half cup or about the size of one-half of a baseball. A medium whole fruit is about the size of a baseball. The serving size of low-fat or fat-free cheese is one and one-half ounces or about the size of four stacked dice. The serving size of peanut butter is two tablespoons or about the size of a ping-pong ball. For further information on serving size check the following web sites: www.mypyramid.gov or www.medlineplus.gov.

The Plate Method as a Teaching Tool

Various methods may be used to incorporate the plate method as a teaching tool. This is an opportunity for creativity. For the 9-inch plate, a life-size picture of a plate or an actual sectioned plate could be used. Lines could also be drawn on a regular 9" plate. Color pictures or replicas of foods could be given to an individual to place in the appropriate section of the plate. Pictures of foods and beverages could be digital photographs, clip art, sketches, cartoons, or pictures cut out of newspapers or magazines. To teach a nutrition lesson, the plate could be filled according to the plate method in order to show examples of healthful meals consistent with the foods the individuals generally eats. Or, the individual could be shown color photographs of appropriate meals. For non-verbal individuals, finger pointing or eye gaze could be used by the individual to indicate food choices. Various cuisines can be represented by the model (Camelon et al., 1998).

For meals, an actual plate could be used that is sectioned according to the plate method or boundary lines can be drawn on a plate (see figure 8). Then, when the food is being served, the foods could be put into the appropriate section of the plate. The amount of food placed would be guided by the size of the corresponding section of the plate (Camelon et al., 1998). Finally, the Plate Method could be incorporated into the *All About Me Healthy Lifestyle Story.*

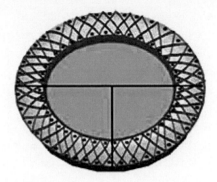

Figure 8. Example of Sectioned Plate.

ALL ABOUT ME HEALTHY LIFESTYLE STORY

An *All About Me Healthy Lifestyle Story* is being proposed as a way to promote a healthy lifestyle for individuals with I/DD. An *All About Me Healthy Lifestyle Story* is based on the behavioral approach of positive behavior support (PBS) and on social stories, which are a commonly used intervention to implement a positive behavioral support plan.

Positive Behavior Support

Currently, "behavior intervention has shifted from the narrow focus of reducing inappropriate behaviors to a more global perspective of improving quality of life" (Carr, 2002). Positive behavior support is used by Lise Fox, Ph.D., University of South Florida, for meeting the needs of young children with challenging behavior and the needs of their families. According to Dr. Fox (2004), positive behavior support is a new applied science of behavior change that is based on humanistic values and research. It is an approach to understand why a child or individual has a problem behavior and to teach a new skill to replace a problem behavior (Fox, Dunlap, & Cushing, 2002; Fox, Dunlap, Power, 2002; Fox, Dunlap, Hemmeter, Joseph, & Strain, 2003; Fox, Lentini, & Hombeck, 2004).

Positive behavior support is based on the recognition that all behaviors are a form of communication and are either a way to obtain something that is desired or to escape something that is not desired. It is different from other approaches as it focuses on the use of positive intervention strategies that are respectful of the child. With positive behavior support, the intervention is proactive rather than a reaction to a problem behavior and the focus is on skill development. Interventions are individualized and based on an understanding of the child, the child's communication abilities, and the unique situations of the child (Fox, Dunlap, & Cushing, 2002; Fox, Dunlap, Power, 2002; Fox, Dunlap, et al., 2003; Fox, et al., 2004).

The process of positive behavior support identifies the problem behaviors, develops an understanding of the purpose and function of the behavior, and develops a behavior support plan to reduce the problem behavior and to help the child develop new skills. Stories can be used as a way of implementing positive behavior support in order to teach expected behaviors. The expectations and the wording of the stories need to be developmentally appropriate to the individual. Positive words are used to tell a child exactly what to do and what not to do. When presenting choices, the options may be communicated by pictures, models, or actual objects. However, choice should involve two desirable alternatives. The behavior support plan helps the child's caregivers teach and interact with the child. For positive behavior support to work, the family/caregivers must "buy in" to the program. Their motivation and enthusiasm are important as the process takes time and resources in order to promote change (Fox, Dunlap, & Cushing, 2002; Fox, Dunlap, Power, 2002; Fox, Dunlap, et al., 2003; Fox, et al., 2004).

Research on positive behavior support has shown its effectiveness for individuals with disabilities from age 2 to 50 years. It has been shown to be effective for individuals with various problems such as mental retardation, autism spectrum disorder[*], oppositional defiant disorder, and other emotional behavioral disorders (Delano & Snell, 2006; Hutchins, 2006; Kuoch & Mirenda, 2003, Reynhout & Carter, 2006).

Social Stories

Social Stories are one way of implementing positive behavior supports. Gray and Garland (1993) introduced the social story as a proactive behavior intervention to teach children with autism how to 'read' social situations and to understand appropriate social behavior. A social story is a short story, written by professionals or caregivers, that describes the subtle cues of a specific social situation that a child may find challenging. Within the social story, the perspectives of the individual and of their caregivers is used to help the individual understand a social situation. With these perspectives, social stories explain the likely reactions of others in a situation and provide information about appropriate social responses (Kuoch & Mirenda, 2003). A social story then becomes a concrete way to improve communication and the links between the individual, caregivers and the external world. As individuals are happier when they fit well within a socially constructed world, social stories can improve quality of life (Moore, 2004).

Social stories are emerging in the research literature as a user-friendly behavioral strategy that is effective in remediating inappropriate behaviors in students with autism. The simplicity and utility of social stories make them functional in both general and special education settings. Social stories have been used as an intervention for children with autism not only to reduce inappropriate behaviors but also to increase prosocial behaviors (Delano & Snell, 2006; Hutchins, 2006; Kuoch & Mirenda, 2003, Reynhout & Carter, 2006). According to Reynhout and Carter (2006), "Social Stories™ stand as a promising intervention, being relatively straightforward and efficient to implement, with application to a wide range of behavior" (abstract). According to Simpson (1993), "Social cognition strategies, such as

---

[*] ASD (Autism Spectrum Disorder) is an umbrella term that includes autism, Asperger's syndrome, atypical autism, pervasive developmental disorder, and childhood disintegrative disorder. Autism is characterized by impairments in social interaction, communication, and behavioral repertoires that occur on a continuum of impairment from mild to severe (American Psychiatric Association, 2000).

social stories effectively guide the social behavior of children and youth with autism by providing social clues and suggestions for appropriate social responses....Social stories have been used successfully to introduce changes and new routines at home and at school, to explain the reasons for another's behaviors, or to teach a new academic or social skill" (para 1).

Positive behavior support, in the form of social stories, works well to communicate with individuals who either do not have the language ability or the social skills for communication. Moore (2004), a behavioral psychologist for the Children's Intensive Psychology Service (ChIPS) uses social stories in a psychology service for children with significant learning disabilities and challenging behaviors. Often these children can not read. Behaviors that are addressed using social stories include: soiling, taking off clothes in inappropriate situations, and problems with eating and sleeping. Typically behavior programs such as ChIPS are "very cost effective as the majority of the behavioral work is implemented by the parents, with support and modification provided by way of regular telephone contact" (p.137).

The effectiveness of a social story is dependent upon its being individualized and personalized to the individual. As social stories are individualized, no two stories are the same. A well-written social story provides information to an individual in a simple, explicit, visually engaging, and personal way. According to Moore (2004), social stories need to be short and written by caregivers or professionals such that the story is individually tailored to the child.

According to Crozier and Sileo (2005), social stories combine the appeal of stories and graphic elements. According to Moore (2004), "visually stimulating and engaging reference pictures are vital to the effectiveness of a social story." Photographs, clip art, or pictures cut out from magazines can be used. Pictures of the child and the people in their environment may be included. Pictures and pages of the story may also be included related to the child's interests. The pages can be laminated or put in page protectors and assembled into a book.

This book can serve as a teaching tool both for the individual and for the people who care for the individual. Moore (2004) has found that the social stories themselves have a reinforcing effect to the child. Pictures give the story personal relevance and provide a sense of routine. Pictures also show a positive outcome–such as child eating vegetables or a child with full plate of food as in the plate model. The time for reading of the book is also time for caregiver individual interaction.

The *All About Me Healthy Lifestyle Story*

To construct a social story, Kuoch and Mirenda (2003), Moore (2004), and Cozier and Sileo (2005) describe specific types of sentences and give guidelines for the use and ratio of these sentences. The *All About Me Healthy Lifestyle Story* is written using some of the basic principles of social stories: individually tailored, giving the perspectives of others, and using age or developmentally appropriate wording in a story format about the individual's daily life. However, the *All About Me Healthy Lifestyle Story* is geared for a purpose other than dealing with a social situation, although teaching about appropriate behavior in a social situation may be part of the *All About Me Healthy Lifestyle Story.*

Soenksen and Alper (2006) suggest the use of social stories to teach functional life skills or leisure skills. As such, the *All About Me Healthy Lifestyle Story* can be used to teach various aspects of a healthy lifestyle: basic hygiene, dental care, proper nutrition, exercise, a positive mental attitude, and getting a good night's sleep. Basic hygiene includes bathing/showering, washing hands, and wearing clean clothes (CDC, 2002). Dental care includes brushing the teeth and going to the dentist. Proper nutrition includes eating a balanced diet as shown in the Plate Method. Drinking water is also important. Exercise can include activities such as walking, dancing, playing ball, or swimming.

First of all, the *All About Me Healthy Lifestyle Story* needs to be geared to the individual and his/her interests. To individualize the *All About Me Healthy Lifestyle Story*, elements of the individual's daily routine, such as going to school or a day rehabilitation program, may be included in the story. Favorite activities can be included as going shopping or going to the park. Pictures of people or places familiar to the individual may also be included. Depending on the individual, a page of the story can deal with encouraging the individual to not smoke. But, the issue of helping an individual quit smoking needs to be part of a behavior plan developed by the individual and their caregivers along with professional assistance.

Next, the story needs to be written within the comprehension of the individual. According to Soenksen and Alper (2006), the story needs to be age-appropriate. With individuals with I/DD the story needs to be developmentally appropriate and geared to the cognitive abilities of the individual such as their reading or comprehension level.

A concept of education involves the use of multisensory teaching modalities. Visual clues reinforce what an individual hears and reads as the cues offer additional information to assist in comprehension. The visual cues need to be simple and easy to understand. Picture cues should be included as they are important for individuals with poor reading skills. The pictures should provide an accurate representation of the concept to be taught. Simple pictures are better than pictures with lots of additional visual clues such as a cluttered background (Dale, 1963).

Assembling the *All About Me Healthy Lifestyle Story*

To assemble the actual *All About Me Healthy Lifestyle Story*, first determine what needs to be included. Either the cover or the first page can be a picture of the individual. Underneath the picture is placed the words, "All About _____ " with the individual's name placed in the blank (see figure 9). The next page could be "I get up in the morning. I am happy." A picture of the sun may be put on the page (see figure 10). This page starts the day with getting up. It also suggests starting the day with a positive mental attitude.

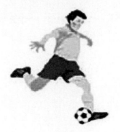

**All
About**

_____

Figure 9. Title Page.

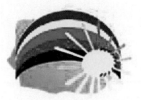

**I get up in the morning.
I am happy.**

Figure 10. Getting Up.

The next pages include the basic morning routine along with basic hygiene. One page could say, "I take a shower." Pictures of soap, shampoo and a towel can be put on the page (see figure 11). The following pages include more basic hygiene. "I brush my teeth" and "I comb my hair" can be put on the page along with pictures of a toothbrush, toothpaste, and a comb (see figure 12). In the page used as an example, brushing the teeth and combing the hair are combined into one page. Depending on the individual's cognitive skills and teaching needs, these two tasks can be separated out into two separate pages.

I take a shower.

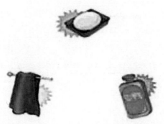

Figure 11. Taking a Shower.

I brush my teeth.

I comb my hair.

Figure 12. Brushing Teeth.

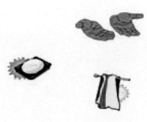

I wash my hands.

Figure 13. Washing Hands.

Another task to include in *All About Me Healthy Lifestyle Story* is washing the hands. Depending on the individual's teaching needs, this page can be very basic as in "I wash my hands" (see figure 13) or more complex as in "I have clean hands. I wash my hands: before eating, after eating, after I go to the bathroom. This makes everyone happy." (see figure 14) Pictures of hands, soap, a towel, and a bathroom sink can be placed on the handwashing page. To finish off the section on basic hygiene, a page can be added such as "I put on clean clothes. I am pretty." Or, "I am handsome" (see figure 15). A picture of the individual all dressed can be placed here or other pictures can be used such as the clip art in Figure 15. Some clip art can be individualized such that the person shown in the clip art picture is wearing the individual's favorite colors.

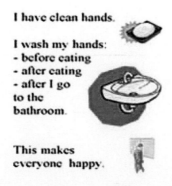

Figure 14. Wash Hands Expanded.

I put on clean clothes.

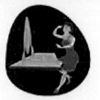

I am pretty.

Figure 15. Clean Clothes.

After morning hygiene typically comes the time for breakfast and medications. Medications are often an important part of being healthy. For the medication page, a clip art picture of medications or a picture of the individual's own morning medications can be used (see figure 16). The medication page can be general as in figure 16, or several pages may be used. A separate page can be devoted to each time of day the individual takes medicine. For each time of day, a clock can be drawn showing the time the individual takes their medicine and placed next to a picture of the medicines that are due at that time. When assembling the story, the medication pages are sorted into the appropriate part of the day.

**I take my medicine in the
morning, at noon, at 4pm
and at bedtime.**

Figure 16. Taking Medicines.

Along with medications, typically comes a meal. So, one page of the *All About Me Healthy Lifestyle Story* can be about mealtimes. A page can say "I eat a healthy breakfast. I like oatmeal. This makes everyone happy" (see figure 17). A picture of cereal or a picture of the plate model format for breakfast can be placed here.

**I eat a healthy breakfast.
I like oatmeal.**

This makes everyone happy.

Figure 17. Eating Breakfast.

The phrase "This makes everyone happy" can be placed at various appropriate places throughout the story as encouragement and positive reinforcement are important for the success of the *All About Me Healthy Lifestyle Story*. Instead of the word "everyone", specific names of individuals or their title such as mom, dad, teacher, etc. can be substituted.

After breakfast, many individuals go to school or to a day program. So, a page can be inserted after the breakfast page to indicate the typical morning routine. "During the week, I go to day rehab" (see Figure 18). A picture of the actual place where the individual goes can be used or a picture of an individual, such as a teacher, may be placed on this page.

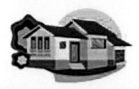

**During the week, I go to
Day Rehab.**

Figure 18. Daily Routine.

The next page can portray other meals generally or pages can be individualized specifically for lunch and dinner. Pictures of a typical healthy meal for the individual can be placed on the page or a picture showing the plate model format for lunch and dinner can be used. Words can be used such as "I eat healthy foods. This keeps me healthy." Or, other words can be used to promote healthy food choices. This is a page for creativity (see figure 19).

Some individuals need special considerations for meals. For example, individuals with dysphagia (difficulty swallowing) may need to consume only thickened liquids. They may also need to sit in a chair or wheelchair to eat. Pages with pictures and words can be included for these special needs (see figures 20 and 21).

I eat healthy foods.

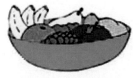

This keeps me healthy.

Figure 19. Eating Healthy.

I eat special foods.
All my drinks are thickened.
I love chocolate milk.

Figure 20. Special Foods.

I sit in my chair to eat.

Figure 21. Sit in Chair to Eat.

I ask permission before
I eat food
or have
anything
to drink.

This keeps me healthy.

This makes everyone happy.

Figure 22. Permission to Eat.

Other individuals may go to the refrigerator or to cabinets to obtain food without first asking. A page may be included for this behavior such as "I ask permission before I eat food or have anything to drink." A reason for changing the lifestyle behavior can be placed on this page such as "This keeps me healthy. This makes everyone happy." On this page, a picture of a refrigerator or of the food cabinet may be included (see figure 22). In this way, the *All About Me Healthy Lifestyle Story* can be used to deal with unhealthy lifestyle behaviors.

Exercise is an important component of a healthy lifestyle. Various pages can be devoted to exercise such as "I walk to keep my legs strong" (see figure 23), "I like to dance" (see figure 24), and "I like to swim and to play basketball" (see figure 25).

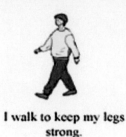

**I walk to keep my legs
strong.**

Figure 23. Walking.

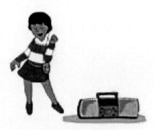

I like to dance and sing.

Figure 24. Dancing.

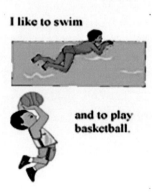

Figure 25. Sports.

As a positive mental attitude is often associated with health, another page can be devoted to being positive. "I am cheerful. I am happy. Everyone loves me." A picture of a smiley face can be put on this page or a picture of someone hugging the individual can be used (see figure 26).

I am cheerful.
I am happy.

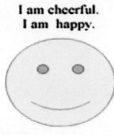

Everyone loves me.

Figure 26. Cheerful.

At the end of the day it is time for bed. Several different types of pages can be used for this time of day. "It has been a busy day. I am tired. I go to bed. I sleep well" can be on a page with a picture of a bed (see figure 27). Another idea is to use a picture of the moon or of an owl with the words "I sleep well. Goodnight" with the individual's name (see figure 28). For some individuals, a picture related to the bedtime routine, such as reading a bedtime story, can be used.

It has been a busy day.

I am tired.

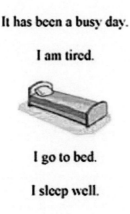

I go to bed.

I sleep well.

Figure 27. Busy Day.

After the *All About Me Healthy Lifestyle Story* individual pages have been created, assemble the pages of the story in chronological order to represent the individual's typical day. Individual pages can be laminated or put into sheet protectors. Then, the pages can be assembled into a notebook or bound into a book. As needed, pages can be revised, added, or removed. It is important to be creative and to keep the *All About Me Healthy Lifestyle Story* relevant to the individual's needs.

To use an *All About Me Healthy Lifestyle Story*, introduce it to the individual. Reading the story should be incorporated into the individual's regular routine. Questions can be asked to determine how well the individual understands the story. After the story has been read, the story may be given to the individual for them to look at as they desire. The story could be read to others or read to oneself (Crozier & Sileo, 2005). But, the story should be accessible for rereading or for just looking at the pictures (Soenksen & Alper, 2006). Other options can also be explored.

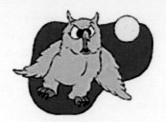

I sleep well.

Good night.

Name

Figure 28. Good Night.

SUMMARY

In summary, health education for individuals with I/DD presents a unique challenge. Health and healthcare disparities for individuals with developmental disabilities contribute to this challenge. Gaps in communication with individuals with I/DD also contribute to the challenge. The Plate Method and the *All About Me Lifestyle Story* use visual images and simple wording as unique methods of health education for individuals with intellectual/developmental disabilities.

REFERENCES

Allen, D. (2005, April). Positive behavioural support: Definition, current status and future directions, *Tizard Learning Disability Review*. Retrieved March 25, 2007, from *http://www.findarticles.com/p/articles/mi qa4141/is_200504/ai_n13635145*.

American Association on Mental Retardation. (2006). Declaration on health parity for persons with intellectual and developmental disabilities. Retrieved March 25, 2007, from *http://www.aaidd.org/Policies/health_declaration.shtml*

American Association on Mental Retardation. (2005). *Fact Sheet: AGING Older Adults and Their Aging Caregivers.* Retrieved March 25, 2007 from *http://www.aamr.org/ Policies/faq_aging.shtml*

American Association on Mental Retardation. (2002). AAMR/ARC Position Statements: Health Care. Retrieved March 25, 2007 from *http://www.aamr.org/Policies/pos_ healthcare.shtml*

American Psychiatric Association. (2000) *Diagnostic and statistical manual of mental disorders (4th ed., text revision.).* Washington, DC: Author.

Brown, S., Watson, K., & Maloney, E. (2005a). Supporting people with developmental disabilities during the aging process. Retrieved February 2, 2007, from *https://depts.washington.edu/aedd/latest_curricula.html*.

Brown, S., Watson, K., & Maloney, E. (2005b). Toward healthy aging: Promoting health through lifestyle changes. Retrieved February 2, 2007, from *https://depts.washington.edu/aedd/latest_curricula.html*

Brown, S., Watson, K., & Maloney, E. (2005c). Getting good health care. Retrieved February 2, 2007a, from *https://depts.washington.edu/aedd/latest_curricula.html*.

Camelon, K. M., Hadell, K., Jamsen, P. T., Ketonen, K. J., Kohtamaki, H. M., Makimatilla, S., et al. (1998). The Plate Model: A visual method of teaching meal planning. Diabetes Atherosclerosis Intervention Study (DAIS) Project Group. Department of Nutrition, Toronto Hospital, Ontario, Canada. *Journal American Dietetic Association, 98*(10), 1155-1158.

Carr, E. G., Dunlap, G., Horner, R. H., Koegel, R. L., Turnbull, A. P., Sailor, W., et al. (2002). Positive behavior support: Evolution of an applied science. *Journal of Positive Behavior Interventions, 4*(1), 4-16.

Centers for Disease Control (2002). Hand hygiene in healthcare settings. Retrieved February 2, 2007 from, *http://www.cdc.gov/handhygiene/*

Centers for Disease Control and Prevention. (n.d.). Disability and health in 2005: Promoting the health and well-being of people with disabilities. Retrieved March 25, 2007 from *http://www.cdc.gov/ncbddd/factsheets/Disability_Health_AtAGlance.pdf*

Centers for Disease Control and Prevention. (2006). Disability and health state chartbook – 2006: Profiles of health for adults with disabilities. Retrieved March 25, 2007 from *www.cdc.gov/ncbddd/dh/chartbook*.

Centers for Disease Control and Prevention. (1998). National diabetes fact sheet: National estimates and general information on diabetes in the United States (Revised Edition). Retrieved March 25, 2007 from *http://www.cdc.gov/dhdsp/CDCynergy_training/Content/activeinformation/resources/Diabetes_Fact_Sheet.pdf*

Corbin, S., Malina, K., & Shepherd, S. (2005, February). 2003 Special Olympics World Summer Games Healthy Athletes Screening Data, Washington, D.C., Special Olympics, Inc. Retrieved March 25, 2007 from *http://www.specialolympics.org/Special+Olympics+Public+Website/English/Initiatives/Research/default.htm*

Crozier, A., & Sileo, N. M. (2005). Encouraging positive behavior with Social Stories: An intervention for children with autism spectrum disorders. *Teaching Exceptional Children, 37*(6), 26-31. Downloaded 1-14-2007 on line version.

Dale, E. (1963). *Audio-Visual Methods in Teaching* (3rd ed.). Austin, TX; Holt, Rinehart, and Winston.

Delano, M, & Snell, M. E. (2006). The effects of social stories on the social engagement of children with Autism. *Journal of Positive Behavior Interventions, 8*(1), 29-42.

Dietrich, T. & Garcia, RI. (2005). Associations between periodontal disease and systemic disease: Evaluating the strength of the evidence. *Journal of Periodontology 76* (11), 2175-2184.

Fenton, S. J., Hood, H., Holder, M., May, P. B., & Mouradian, W. E. (2003). The American Academy of Developmental Medicine and Dentistry: Eliminating health disparities for individuals with mental retardation and other developmental disabilities. *Journal of Dental Education, 67*(12), 1337-1344.

Fox, L., Dunlap, G., & Cushing, L. (2002). Early intervention, positive behavior support, and transition to school. *Journal of Emotional and Behavioral Disorders, 10*(3), 149-157.

Fox, L., Dunlap, G, Hemmeter, M. L., Joseph, G. E., & Strain, P. S. (2003, July). The teaching pyramid: A model for supporting social competence and preventing challenging behavior in young children. *Young Children,* 48-52.

Fox, L., Dunlap, G., Power, D. (2002). Young children with challenging behavior: issues and considerations for behavior support. *Journal of Positive Behavior Interventions, 4* (4), 208-217.

Fox, L., Lentini, R., Hombeck, M. (2004, July). Using Positive Behavioral Support to meet the needs of young children with challenging behavior and their families. Presented at the meeting of the SCEIs Higher Education Research Institute, Helen, GA.

Goldfarb, B. (2005). Periodontal disease linked to mortality in type 2 diabetes. *DOC News,* 2(6). Retrieved February 13, 2007 from *www.docnews.diabetesjournals.org.*

Governor's Council on Developmental Disabilities. *Definition of Developmental Disabilities.* (n.d.). Retrieved February 8, 2007 from *www.GCDD.org.*

Havercamp, S. M., Scandlin, D., & Roth M. (2004). Health disparities among adults with developmental disabilities, adults with other disabilities, and adults not reporting a disability in North Carolina. *Public Health Reports, 119,* 418-426.

Heller, T., Ying, H. S., Rimmer, J.H., & Marks, B. A. (2002). Determinants of exercise in adults with cerebral palsy. *Public Health Nursing, 19*(3), 223-31.

Horowitz, S. M., Kerker, B., Owens, P. L., & Zigler, E. (2000). The health status and needs of individuals with mental retardation. Department of Epidemiology and Public Health, Yale University School of Medicine, Department of Psychology, Yale University, New Haven, Connecticut. September 15, 2000. Revised December 18, 2000. Retrieved February 1, 2007 from *www.specialolympics.org.*

Klein, S., Shear, N. F., Pi-Sunyer, S., Daly, A., Wylie-Rosett, J., Kulkarni, K., et al. (2004). Weight management through lifestyle modification for the prevention and management of type 2 diabetes: Rational and strategies. *Diabetes Care, 27*(8), 2067-2073.

Krogman, L. (2007). The nurse practitioner's role in caring for adults with developmental disabilities. Retrieved February 2, 2007 from *https://depts.washington.edu/aedd.*

Kuoch, H. & Mirenda, P. (2003). Social story interventions for Young children with Autism Spectrum Disorders. *Focus on Autism and other Developmental Disabilities, 18*(4), 219-227.

Moore, P.S. (2004). The use of social stories in a psychology service for children with learning disabilities: A case study of a sleep problem, *British Journal of Learning Disabilities, 32*(3), 133-138.

National Center on Physical Activity and Disability (NCPAD) (2007). Exercise Guidelines for People with Disabilities Fact Sheet (2007). Retrieved March 30, 2007 from *http://www.ncpad.org/exercise/fact_sheet.php?sheet=15.*

National Institutes of Health, National Heart, Lung and Blood Institute, National Institute of Diabetes and Digestive and Kidney Diseases (1998). *Clinical guidelines on the identification, evaluation, and treatment of overweight and obesity in Adults.* Bethesda, MD: Author.

Parish, S. L. & Saville, A. W. (2006). Women with cognitive limitations living in the community: Evidence of disability-based disparities in healthcare. *Mental Retardation, 44*(4), 249-259.

Pearson, T. A., Blair, S. N., Daniels, S. R., Eckel, R. H., Fair, J. M., Fortmann, S. P., et al. (2002). American Heart Association guidelines for primary prevention of cardiovascular disease and stroke: 2002 Update. Consensus Panel Guide to Comprehensive Risk Reduction for Adult Patients without Coronary or other Atherosclerotic Vascular Diseases. *Circulation, 106*, 388-391.

President's Committee on Mental Retardation. (1999). *1999 Report to the President: The forgotten generation.* Washington, DC: Author. Retrieved March 23, 2007 from *http://www.acf.dhhs.gov/programs/pcmr/mission.htm*

Reynhout, G., & Carter, M. (2006). Social Stories™ for children with disabilities. *Journal of Autism & Developmental Disorders, 36*(4), 445-469. [Abstract}

Rizor, H. M., & Richards, S. (2000). All our patient need to know about intensified diabetes management they learned in fourth grade. *Diabetic Education, 26* (3), 392-404.

Rizor, H. M., Thomas, K., Harker, J., & Smith, M. (2002) *Simplified diabetes meal planning includes more than potatoes in Idaho.* Retrieved Janurary 23, 2007 from *http://www.nutritionhawaii.org/newsletter/archive/index5.02.html#2*

Rizor H., Smith M., Thomas K., Harker J., & Rich M. (1996). Have you tried the Idaho Plate Method? American Dietetic Association. Diabetes Care and Education Practice Group. *DCE Newsflash*, 17, 18-20.

Rizor, H., Smith, M., Thomas K., Harker, J., & Rich M. Practical Nutrition: The Idaho Plate Method. *Practical Diabetology.* 1998; 17:42-45.

Rubin, I. L., & Crocker, A. C. (2006). *Medical care for children and adults with developmental disabilities* (2nd ed.) Baltimore: Brookes Publishing Co

Schrager, S. (2004). Osteoporosis in women with disabilities, *Journal of Women's Health,* 13(4), 431-437.

Simpson, R. (1993). Tips for practitioners. *Focus on Autistic Behavior, 8*(3), 15-16.

Soenksen, D., & Alper, S. (2006). Teaching a young child to appropriately gain attention of peers using a social story intervention. *Focus on Autism and Other Developmental Disabilities, 21*(1), 36-44.

Special Olympics, Inc. (2001a, March). *The health and health care of people with intellectual disabilities.* Washington, DC: Author. Retrieved February 1, 2007 from *www.specialolympics.org.*

Special Olympics, Inc. (2001b, March). *Promoting health for persons with mental retardation: A critical journey barely begun.* DC: Washington, DC: Author, Retrieved February 1, 2007 from *www.specialolympics.org.*

U.S. Department of Health and Human Services. (1991). Healthy people 2000, Washington, DC: U.S. Government Printing Office.

U.S. Department of Health and Human Services (2000). Healthy people 2010. (Conference Edition, in Two Volumes). Washington, DC: U.S. Government Printing Office.

U.S. Department of Health and Human Services. (2002). Closing the Gap: A National Blueprint to Improve the Health of Persons with Mental Retardation (Report of the

Surgeon General Conference on Health Disparities and Mental Retardation). Retrieved February 1, 2007 from *www.specialolympics.org*

World Health Organization. (2007) Cancer: Diet and physical activity's impact. (n.d.). Retrieved March 25, 2007 from *www.who.int/dietphysicalactivity/publications/facts/cancer.*

In: Health Education Research Trends
Editor: P. R. Hong, pp. 129-154

ISBN: 978-1-60021-871-2
© 2007 Nova Science Publishers, Inc.

Chapter III

PERSPECTIVES ON HEALTH EDUCATION RESEARCH – VULNERABLE POPULATIONS

Lisa M. Jamieson and Gloria C. Mejía
University of Adelaide, Australia.

ABSTRACT

Health education research is a predominantly Western construct. Problems frequently arise in regards to idea communication and project ownership when investigations are implemented among vulnerable populations, particularly when researchers are from non-vulnerable backgrounds. Participatory Action Research (PAR) is a relevant methodology in health education research involving vulnerable populations because of its fundamental tenets that power be equally shared between the researchers and the researched, that data and information not be removed from their contexts, and that the data collection process be directly influenced by history, culture and local environment. Contemporary health behaviour models, such as the PRECEDE-PROCEED planning model and the Diffusion of Innovation model, suggest that health education interventions among vulnerable populations have much to gain from embracing more holistic, PAR approaches, which in turn are more likely to result in a sustained reduction in harmful health behaviours among vulnerable populations.

INTRODUCTION

This chapter considers perspectives on health education research in relation to vulnerable populations, as separate from health education research perspectives on general populations. The challenges of applying theories for understanding health behaviour change among such groups are addressed, and key concepts to consider when developing sensitive interventions among vulnerable populations defined. PAR as a useful methodology in health education research among vulnerable groups is described, as is the utility of the PRECEDE-PROCEED planning model and the Diffusion of Innovation model. Two case studies are provided by way of example, one in a developing country context and the other in a developed nation.

Definition of "Vulnerable Population"

There is inconsistency in defining "vulnerable" populations (Ruof, 2004). Bio-ethicists such as Kottow (2003) argue that vulnerability is intrinsic to human nature and that at some point all humans are vulnerable. Some argue that labelling certain groups as vulnerable is demeaning (Danis and Patrick, 2002), while others hold that non-vulnerable groups have a special responsibility towards those who are vulnerable (DeBruin, 2001; Goodin, 1985).

Vulnerability is a basic principle in European bioethics and biolaw, along with autonomy, dignity and integrity (Partners in the BIOMED-II Project, 1998). It is thought to express the finitude and frailty of life, and considered to be an object of moral principle. Vulnerable populations may thus be defined as those whose autonomy, dignity or integrity are threatened and for whom assistance should be provided to enable them to realise their potential.

In the health education research context, vulnerable populations may be considered as those groups whose demographic, geographic or economic characteristics impede their health or access to health care services (Blumenthal et al., 1995). The health, and health-related behaviours, of vulnerable populations is unique to that of non-vulnerable groups within a given country or community, with vulnerable groups tending to be less educated, more often living in poverty and less likely to have adequate health care access than their more privileged counterparts. The proportion of persons below the poverty level is higher among vulnerable populations in most developed countries (Australian Institute of Health and Welfare, 2006; New Zealand Ministry of Health, 2006; US Department of Health and Human Services, 2000; Health Canada, 2006).

Many differences in health status and access to health care between vulnerable and non-vulnerable groups can be attributed to socio-economic rather than racial, ethnic or cultural factors. However, as the effects of culture, poverty, racial discrimination and culturally-insensitive health services are usually inter-related, it is often difficult to disentangle the relative contribution of these factors on observed health differences. Other barriers, including language and long travel distances for rural residents, also disadvantage vulnerable populations in relation to access to health care.

The Score of Health Education

Health education is an essential component of health promotion – a social and political process aimed at improving socio-economic and environmental conditions and strengthening community action to improve health (Smith et al., 2006). Simonds (1978) defined health education as "bringing about behaviour changes in individuals, groups and larger populations from behaviours that are presumed to be detrimental to health, to behaviours that are conducive to present and future health". Subsequent definitions of health education emphasised voluntary, informed behaviour changes, for example, in 1980, Green and colleagues defined health education as "any combination of learning experiences designed to facilitate voluntary adaptations of behaviour conducive to health" (Green et al., 1980). The Ottawa Charter for Health Promotion defines health education as "the process by which people are given knowledge, awareness, and the skills needed for them to take greater control of their own health" (WHO, 1986).

Health education includes not only instructional activities and other strategies to influence health behaviour, but organisational efforts, policy directives, economic supports, environmental activities, mass media and community-level programs. It covers the continuum from disease prevention to the detection of illness for treatment, rehabilitation and long-term care. Health education is delivered in almost every conceivable setting – from the most privileged communities in developed nations to the most impoverished areas of third world countries.

APPLYING HEALTH EDUCATION THEORY TO VULNERABLE POPULATIONS

Attention to the unique characteristics of vulnerable populations has been renewed in recent years, as health disparities persist despite advances in modern medicine (US Department of Health and Human Services, 2000; Australian Institute of Health and Welfare, 2006; Morris et al., 2005). The rationale for specific health education research programs among vulnerable populations appears to stem from four observations: (1) the growing diversity among vulnerable groups in many nations; (2) the increase in health disparities between such populations; (3) the differences in behavioural risk factors prevalence across vulnerable groups, and (4) the differences in health behaviour predictors across vulnerable populations.

In order for health education projects among vulnerable populations to be effective, they need to be designed with a deep understanding of the target audience, their health and social characteristics, as well as their beliefs, attitudes, values, skills and past behaviours. As described by Resnicow and colleagues (2002), one of the most fundamental principles in contemporary health education research among vulnerable groups is to "start where the people are". In the same vein, only 200 years earlier, the Danish philosopher Kierkegaard suggested that "in order to truly help someone, I must be able to understand what he/she understands. If I do not do that, then my greater understanding does not help him/her at all. The helper must first humble himself/herself under the person he/she wants to help and thereby understand that to help is not to be the most dominating but the most patient, to have a willingness for the time being to put up with being in the wrong and not understanding what the other understands" (Bloom, 1989).

Some academics contend that conceptual health behaviour models derived from a professionally-centric perspective fail to incorporate the social, psychological, cultural and historical characteristics of vulnerable populations (Sullivan et al., 2006). For example, Social Cognitive Theory emphasises individual-based determinants such as self-efficacy, personal goals, self-evaluative expectations, self-management and assertiveness skills

(Bandura, 2001), which are rooted in what Jones (2004) considers to be Eurocentric, predominantly male values of competitiveness, materialism, personal achievement, impulse control and self-determinism. Such individual-centred models are, some have argued, too mechanistic and fail to adequately account for environmental determinants such as stress, racism, poverty, poor access to health services that for many vulnerable populations may be more influential than individual motivation alone (Crosby, 2006).

In the contrasting approach, it is assumed that the fundamental determinants of behaviour operate similarly among all populations, and that psychological and behavioural models can be successfully adapted across a range of diverse vulnerable groups (Bandura, 2001). However, it has been suggested that successful adaptation requires an integrative understanding of the unique environment of the target population, and that modification of conventional health behaviour change models need to take the unique characteristics of such populations into account.

Health education research among vulnerable populations requires investigators to examine ethno-centric (or professionally-centric) assumptions inherent in their methods and to attempt to incorporate alternative conceptualisations of human experience. This requires a perspective whereby researchers approach a community not from a deficit model, which assumes one way assistance, but with the intention that they will learn and benefit from their experiences as much as the target audience. It means embracing the view that the community has resources, wisdom, solutions and energy that can be mobilised to improve its health status. These are the central tenets underpinning Community-Based Participatory Research (CBPR) and in particular, Participatory Action Research (PAR) approaches, which are increasingly being used in health interventions involving vulnerable populations throughout the world (Baum et al., 2006; Potvin et al., 2003). CBPR and PAR are described in more detail below.

COMMUNITY-BASED PARTICIPATORY RESEARCH (CBPR) AND PARTICIPATORY ACTION RESEARCH (PAR)

CBPR is a collaborative approach to research that aims to produce knowledge that will be translated into positive social change (Israel et al., 2001). It engages the community in all phases of research. CBPR is particularly effective in addressing health and health care disparities, developing culturally sensitive instruments and in providing the means for a deeper understanding of communities and their circumstances. It is an exceptionally useful tool in research involving vulnerable groups.

Although each community-researcher partnership develops its own values in CBPR, pioneers such as Israel and colleagues (Israel et al., 1998; Israel et al., 2001) identify the following set of key principles:

1. Recognise the community as a unit of identity
2. Build on strengths and resources within the community
3. Facilitate collaborative partnerships in all phases of research
4. Integrate knowledge and action for mutual benefit for all partners

5. Promote a co-learning and empowering process that attends to social inequalities
6. Involve a cyclical and iterative process
7. Address health from both positive and ecological perspectives
8. Disseminate findings and knowledge gained to all partners
9. Involve long-term commitment by all partners

CBPR includes several approaches to research that actively involve communities such as PAR, feminist research and community research (Israel et al., 1998; Israel et al., 2001). Among these, PAR is particularly appropriate for research among vulnerable populations; it evolves from critical theories with a focus on oppressed groups and therefore requires an understanding of authority and power relations of all partners (Hagey, 1997). It stems greatly from the work of Freire on critical reflection (action and reflection go together) and his "pedagogy of the oppressed" (Freire, 1970).

At the core of PAR methodology is empowerment through community engagement and capacity building. PAR consequently serves two functions: a research function, to show processes, progress and results, and an action function; a tool for reflection, discussion and decision-making (Baum et al., 2006). In both research and practice, PAR is collective, self-reflective inquiry undertaken by researchers and participants so they can improve health-related practices and situations in which they find themselves. The reflective process is directly linked to action, influenced by understanding of history, culture and local context, and embedded in social relationships.

The researcher is not an external observer in PAR, but is constantly challenged by ideas, events, information and arguments posed by study participants. PAR requires researchers to work in close partnership with the community; requires each player to learn methods of working together to manage potentially conflicting agendas; including differences in priority perceptions, community politics and interpretation of findings. The PAR movement consequently challenges the system of knowledge control established through mainstream research. However, PAR should not necessarily be considered as an alternative to existing scientific processes, but as a way in which theoretical understanding and social progress may be enhanced. PAR expands conventional approaches in three important ways: the focus is on research that aims to enable action; it advocates for power to be equally shared between researchers and the researched; and it does not aim to remove data and information from their contexts. Although in the words of one researcher PAR is "a painful, self-reflective process" (Wallerstein, 1999), it is the ultimate method in health education research among vulnerable populations in regards to ensuring cultural sensitivity.

CULTURAL SENSITIVITY

Cultural sensitivity is one of the most widely accepted principles in health education research, and is particularly pertinent in projects involving vulnerable populations. There is little evidence, however, on how to achieve cultural sensitivity, and how to measure its impact on psychosocial and behavioural outcomes, particularly among vulnerable groups (Patrick et al., 2006). According to Resnicow and colleagues (1999), cultural sensitivity can be conceptualised in terms of two primary dimensions: *surface structure* and *deep structure*. *Surface structure* involves matching intervention messages to observable characteristics of a target population. For print and audiovisual materials, surface structure may involve using people, places, language, music, foods, brand names and locations familiar to the target audience. Surface structure includes identifying the most appropriate settings for program delivery. It also entails understanding characteristics of the behaviour in question, and the context in which the health behaviour occurs. Surface structure refers to the extent to which interventions fit with the culture, experience and behavioural patterns of the target audience (Resnicow et al., 1999).

Deep structure, the second dimension of cultural sensitivity, is less readily visible, especially among vulnerable populations. It reflects how cultural, social, psychological, environmental and historical factors influence health behaviours differently across different populations (Marin et al., 1995). This includes understanding how members of the target population perceive the cause and treatment of illnesses as well as how they perceive specific health behaviour determinants. Deep structure involves appreciation for how religion, family, society, economics and the government, both in perception and influence, target behaviour. For example, many poor farmers in Uganda believe that white workers are covertly encouraging the spread of HIV/AIDS in their communities (Ssali et al., 2005). When implementing health education projects among such groups, including messages that incorporate, though not necessarily condone, such beliefs may enhance program acceptance. Whereas surface structure generally increases message comprehension, deep structure conveys salience. Put another way, surface structure establishes the acceptability of an intervention, whereas deep structure is essential for project impact (Dunn et al., 2006).

Although most vulnerable populations share common values regarding issues such as family, there are differences in some core values that may influence how health behaviour interventions are tailored. For example, core cultural values for vulnerable people of African origin in the United States are often described as including communalism or spiritualism, respect for verbal communication skills, connection to ancestors and history, commitment to family, and intuition and experience versus empiricism (Delva, 2001; Neuliep, 2006). Core cultural values among Australia's Indigenous population include a strong emphasis on oral traditions, with "stories" being an important and time-honoured method in which information has passed between generations (Cass et al., 2002). Indigenous Australians also have a profound connection with their "country", the geographic area in which their ancestors lived and within which strong spiritual connections exist (Burgess and Morrison, 2007). The use of oral communication and stories, religious or spiritual themes, and historical references to convey messages may thus be invaluable when developing health education research programs among vulnerable groups such as these.

DEVELOPING CULTURALLY SENSITIVE INTERVENTIONS

Focus groups are a potentially valuable means for obtaining information to develop culturally sensitive interventions. During the formative phase of intervention planning, members of the target audience can be convened to explore thoughts, feelings, experiences, associations, language, assumptions, and environmentally enabling and constraining factors in regard to the health behaviour of interest (Pope and Mays, 2000). Exploratory focus groups also provide an opportunity in which the role of culturally-based messages, and the unique language that may be used around a particular topic, may be examined. For example, in the ebino-education project described in Case Study I below, rural-dwelling Ugandans revealed the term "slim" to mean AIDS, a term previously unknown to the non-Ugandan researcher, and in the oral health promotion initiative among regional-dwelling Indigenous Australians (Case Study II), the term "sugar" was frequently used to describe diabetes. Incorporating such terminology can increase the surface structure sensitivity of an intervention. It can also be useful to explore how the target population perceives how the determinants of the target health behaviour may differ in their community relative to the population as a whole.

APPLYING HEALTH EDUCATION THEORY AMONG VULNERABLE POPULATIONS

Some models of health behaviour are culturally sensitive by their very foundation. For example, the PRECEDE-PROCEED planning model (Figure 1) relies on the fundamental principle of community participation in defining problems, solutions and programs (Green and Kreuter, 1999). Accordingly, at each step in the PRECEDE-PROCEED assessment, it is essential that input from the program's intended audience is included.

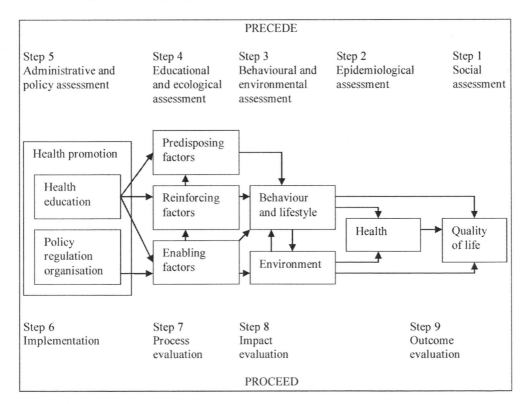

Figure 1. The PRECEDE-PROCEED Planning Model [Green and Kreuter, 1999].

The acronym stands for Predisposing, Reinforcing and Enabling Constructs in Educational/Environmental Diagnosis and Evaluation (Green et al., 1980). PROCEED (Policy, Regulatory and Organisation Constructs in Educational and Environmental Development) was added in 1991, in recognition of the importance of environmental factors as determinants of health and health behaviours. PRECEDE-PROCEED is a nine-step planning process that begins at the end, focusing on the health-related outcomes of interest and working backward to determine which combination of intervention strategies will best achieve the objectives. The planning process begins with the proposition that health behaviours are complex, multidimensional and influenced by a range of factors (Green and Kreuter, 1999).

Step 1: Social Assessment

The purpose of Stage I is to determine a community's perception of their own needs and quality of life (Green and Kreuter, 1999). A social assessment also considers the community's problem-solving capacity, its strengths and resources, and its readiness to change. It is important to establish trusting relationships between researchers and the target audience at this stage, recognising that the building of such trust requires time and consistency (Patrick et al., 2006).

Step 2: Epidemiological Assessment

An epidemiological assessment helps determine what health problems are most important for which groups in the community (Green and Kreuter, 1999). With data on the community's health problems, a researcher is ready to set priorities and write program objectives. Programs that have implemented the PRECEDE-PROCEED model have been successful when decisions were guided by the desires of community members, and when consideration was given to health problems with the greatest impact, those that were previously not a priority, and those for which solutions were realistically available (Patrick et al., 2006).

Step 3: Behavioural and Environmental Assessment

This stage involves examining factors that contribute to the health problem under consideration (Green and Kreuter, 1999). Behavioural factors are individual behaviours or lifestyles that contribute to risk of the health problem, while environmental factors are social or physical factors external to the individual, often beyond an individual's control, but that can be modified to influence the health outcome in question.

Step 4: Educational and Ecological Assessment

This phase involves identifying the antecedent and reinforcing factors necessary for the change process to be initiated and sustained. These factors are classified as *predisposing, reinforcing* and *enabling*. *Predisposing* factors are antecedents that provide the rationale for the behaviour and include individuals' knowledge, attitudes, beliefs, personal preferences, existing skills and self-efficacy beliefs (Green and Kreuter, 1999). *Reinforcing* factors are elements associated with a behaviour that provide continued incentive for behaviour persistence (Green and Kreuter, 1999). Examples include social support, peer influence, significant others and vicarious reinforcement. *Enabling* factors are antecedents to behaviour that allow a motivation to be realised (Green and Kreuter, 1999), and can affect behaviour directly or through environmental factors. They include programs, services and resources and, in some cases, new skills that are required to enable health behaviour change.

Step 5: Administrative and Policy Assessment

Defining the intervention strategies and final planning for their implementation occurs during the administrative and policy assessment stage. Its purpose is to identify the circumstances in a program's organisational context that could facilitate or hinder program implementation. The PRO in PROCEED is defined by Green and Kreuter (1999) as: *Policy;* the set of objectives guiding the organisation's activities, *Regulation;* the act of implementing policies and enforcing rules, and *Organisation*; the bringing together of resources necessary to implement a program.

Steps 6 to 9: Implementation and Evaluation

The program is ready for implementation in this phase (step 6). Data collection plans should be in place for evaluating the process, impact and outcome of the program (steps 7–9). Typically, process evaluation determines the extent to which the program was implemented according to protocol. Impact evaluation assesses change in predisposing, reinforcing and enabling factors, as well as in the behavioural and environmental factors. Finally, outcome evaluation determines the effect of the program on health and quality-of-life indicators.

The following is a case study in which the PRECEDE-PROCEED planning model was used as a framework for a health behaviour change program implemented in a rural district in Uganda. Background of the project is provided, followed by a synopsis on how the specific PRECEDE-PROCEED criteria were met.

CASE STUDY I; THE EBINO EDUCATION PROJECT

Uganda is a landlocked country over 240,000 square kilometres in area in central East Africa. In 2001, the population was estimated to be over 22,780,000, with a density of 94.5

people per square kilometre (Fitzpatrick et al., 2003). Agriculture dominates the economy, contributing 44 percent of the gross domestic product and employing an estimated 80 percent of the working population. The literacy rate is 55 percent for men and 20 percent for women, while current life expectancy is 45.0 years for males and 50.5 years for females (WHO, 2005).

Traditional healers in Uganda are ubiquitous. Because they share the same culture, beliefs and values as their patients, they are often the first point of contact for those seeking health care provision (Accorsi et al., 2003). Traditional healers thus play an important role in the delivery of primary health care, particularly in remote communities (Kubukeli et al., 1999). A common practice undertaken by traditional healers in Uganda is that of ebino ("false teeth" or "maggots") extractions (Accorsi et al., 2003). The custom arose from the belief that unerupted deciduous canine teeth ("maggots") cause fever, diarrhoea, vomiting and other infant illnesses, necessitating their removal. Ebino extractions are usually undertaken with unsterile instruments including bicycle spokes, knitting needles, razor blades, scissors, broken glass or finger nails. The operator uses a tool to make an incision along the top edge of the gum and extracts the suspected cause of child ill health (Stefanini, 1987). In some areas of Uganda, the frequency of ebino extractions is one in every three children (Accorsi et al., 2003; Pindborg, 1969).

Complications often arise from ebino extractions, including septicaemia, anaemia, osteomyletis of the maxilla and mandible, tetanus and haemorrhage (Accorsi et al., 2003). Damage to the developing permanent canines may also occur and cause such teeth to be malpositioned, hypoplastic or missing in adulthood (Holan and Mamber, 1994). Repetition of ebino extractions in multiple infants at the same sitting using the same unsterile instruments may additionally promote transmission of infectious diseases such as HIV/AIDS (Jolles and Jolles, 1998). In some rural areas of Uganda, the frequency of HIV/AIDS is one in three people (Stoneburger and Low-beer, 2004).

Previous initiatives designed to reduce the prevalence of ebino extractions have included health promotion (Kirunda, 1999), cooperation with traditional healers and encouragement to use other traditional customs for ebino symptoms (Accorsi et al., 2003). The Ebino Education Project aimed to explore traditional concepts of ebino through focus group discussion methodology and to develop a context-specific, tailored and targeted community-based ebino education tool that sought to increase knowledge and awareness of ebino extraction alternatives so that the prevalence of such practices, and consequent burden on child ill-health, might lessen. The study framework was based on the PRECEDE-PROCEED planning model.

The project took place at a private-not-for-profit health service in the Rukungiri district, south west Uganda. The hospital services an area of around 200 square kilometres (approximately 10,000 people). The study comprised two components: (1) focus group discussions to identify local perceptions of ebino and (2) development of a culturally-sensitive ebino-education tool based on findings from (1) delivered primarily to women's groups in the community.

The focus group discussions covered five separate themes (what is ebino, what are the causes of ebino, what happens after ebino extractions, what are alternatives to ebino, and what does the group suggest as ways to remove the ebino problem) and were tape-recorded, translated and transcribed. Upon analysis of the focus group discussion findings, and with further dialogue with the hospital and community councils, it was decided to employ three strategies in the ebino education workshops; a role-play, a didactic lecture and a debate/discussion forum. The workshops were conducted by an ebino education team, which consisted of the first author, a local dental assistant and two members of the hospital community outreach team.

The role-play component was aimed at less-literate participants and was designed to be fun, entertaining, informal and visual. Lasting for five minutes, it generally followed the lines of the first author dressing as a local woman with a baby on her back, and consulting with another local woman (dental assistant) about ebino. The dialogue followed several themes: concern that the child was ill and the mother's desire for the child to have ebino extractions; explanation that it was not because of ebino that the child was sick but other factors; distrust of Western medicine and conviction that other children's health had improved following extractions; challenge that some children don't recover after ebino extractions and if they do the children do not develop deciduous canine teeth, suggestion that what was removed was not a "maggot" but a young tooth, that ebino extractions were conducted with unclean instruments that increased the infant's chances of contracting HIV/AIDS; questions as to ways the child's health could be returned without the ebino extractions; information on hygiene, diet and hospital attention; and scientific reasons behind fever, malaise, vomiting and diarrhoea.

The second part of the initiative embraced a didactic approach whereby diagrams, models and posters were used by members of the ebino education team to explain the position of unerupted deciduous canine teeth in the gum, the consequences of their removal with unsterile instruments, the risk of HIV/AIDS transmission when multiple children were treated in one sitting, the importance of deciduous canine teeth in the eruption pattern of permanent canine teeth and scientific explanations for infant symptoms traditionally associated with ebino.

The third component involved a discussion/debate among workshop participants with ebino education team members acting as facilitators. In the debate, those who maintained that ebino extractions were a necessary remedy for infant ailment relief were asked to challenge those who supported the scientific model of ebino symptom aetiology. At the workshops' cessation, attendees were awarded with ebino education certificates and encouraged to discourse with other community members about the program's content.

The program's effectiveness was assessed by follow-up focus group discussions being held with the original focus group participants one and a half years after the program's inception, and by monitoring the prevalence of hospital admissions for ebino extraction complications and other infant illnesses in this period.

The initial focus group discussion findings were grouped into themes that related to the key questions. There were a variety of opinions expressed. The "what is ebino" theme included a range of theories and beliefs that generally involved maggots and poor health. The second theme "what are the causes of ebino" contained a number of responses that illustrated a general lack of awareness of ebino aetiology from a scientific perspective, with some answers revealing a superstitious element. For the "what happens after ebino extractions" theme, responses varied depending on the extent that participants had witnessed children recovering from, or having been traumatised by, ebino extractions. An apparent belief that there were no options to ebino extractions was evident when the question "what are alternatives to ebino" was presented to the groups; an inherent conviction that if the "maggots" were left *in situ*, the infant would become unwell again. For the final theme "what does the group suggest as ways to remove the problem of ebino" a range of solutions were provided, none of which had a scientific basis.

All participants of the pre-intervention focus group discussions took part in an ebino education workshop. There were twenty three workshops held; one in each of the communities serviced by the hospital outreach program and eight to mothers' groups attending the hospital for post-natal care. The number of attendees at each presentation varied from 42 to 112, with a total of 1874 women exposed to the program (mean of 58 women per gathering). There were between 15–20 men who stood around the periphery of each education session but their numbers were not counted as many men were not present for the duration of the intervention. Each session took approximately three hours.

Four follow-up focus-group discussions were held one and a half years after the ebino education program's inception, with the same participants as those in the initial groups. The methodology was the same as that used for the initial focus group discussions, with the same questions being asked by the facilitator. In comparison to the initial answers provided for the "what is ebino" question, the follow-up findings differed markedly, for example, a greater acknowledgement of the scientific reasons behind ebino symptoms was disclosed. Similarly, responses elucidated from the "what are the causes of ebino" question varied considerably from the initial focus group discussion findings, with more scientific causes being understood and discussed. For the "what happens after ebino extractions" item, participants provided a range of responses that differed markedly to those provided in the first instance; again conveying a greater understanding of Western health concepts.

In the initial focus group discussions there appeared to be limited knowledge of alternatives to ebino extractions. However, when this question was repeated in the follow-up discussions, a range of health–promoting options were provided. A number of health-promoting suggestions were similarly offered when the "what does the group suggest as ways to remove the ebino problem" item was asked, which was in direct contrast to responses provided in the initial discussions (direct quotes are available from Jamieson, 2006).

One and a half years following the ebino education program's inception, post-ebino extraction complications fell from being the 5th most common reason for infant admissions in the hospital to the 11th, with the number of admissions for ebino extraction complications falling from 22 to 9 (a decrease of 59.1 percent). Of the nine who were admitted with post-ebino extraction symptoms, seven received the extractions in the previous four hours and presented before gingival swelling commencement, meaning the child's survival prognosis was relatively high. The number of hospital deaths resulting from ebino extraction complications in the same period fell from eight to zero, while the number of in- and out-patient services for infant complaints (predominantly gastro-intestinal) rose from 279 to 498. Four community members were trained as ebino education health workers and employed by the hospital to continue the ebino education series.

After one and a half years of the program's implementation, there appeared to be increased community awareness of the scientific reasons behind infant fever, malaise, diarrhoea and vomiting; and greater acceptance of hospital services for child illnesses historically treated by traditional healers. The program appeared to create a ripple effect whereby the ebino education theme was picked up and incorporated into other areas of hospital services, for example, in AIDS education clinics, ante-natal classes, the rehabilitation clinic, theatre and prayer groups. General hospital staff began discussing the scientific basis of ebino symptoms to patients in many areas of the hospital and it was the topic of discussion in several church services (the ebino education team presented the role play component of the education tool to four church congregations). There was increased dialogue about the ebino tradition and rising acceptance of alternatives to ebino extractions among communities where the ebino education program had occurred. Many people presented at the hospital dental clinic to further discuss the ebino tradition.

The following illustrates more specifically how the PRECEDE-PROCEED framework was helpful in development of the Ebino Education Project.

Step 1: Social Assessment

- Discussions with local councils, church leaders, hospital management, baseline data collection of hospital ebino admissions.
- Ability of community to change with support of key community leaders.
- Local leaders believed it was easier for a person of non-African descent to implement the project in the first instance.

Step 2: Epidemiological Assessment

- Focus group discussions held with a convenience sample of local community members. Ebino considered a problem by all.
- Focus group findings taken back to hospital and community councils. It was decided by these groups that three strategies should be employed in the ebino education workshops; a role-play, a didactic lecture and a debate/discussion forum.
- It was the view of the hospital and community councils that a specific intervention that targeted women was required in order for women to take part; that men in the community would join in as a matter of course.

Step 3: Behavioural and Environmental Assessment

- Individual/lifestyle behaviours considered detrimental in regards to ebino extraction practises included limited education and traditional healers holding substantial power at a community level.
- Social factors included local customs being deeply entrenched, minimal exposure to Western medical/scientific concepts.

- Physical factors included being remotely located (closest town 2 hours drive on a dirt road, minimal car ownership, public transport erratic/non-existent).

Step 4: Educational and Ecological Assessment

- Pre-disposing factors included strong community values, traditional healers, limited education.
- Reinforcing factors were social support, peer influence, scarce knowledge of alternative approaches, limited exposure to Western ideology.
- Enabling factors included increased awareness and education about ebino through the Ebino Education Project – participants in workshops exposed to new ideas, program installed in hospital, women's groups, sustained (1.5 years). Debating skills were enhanced through workshops = empowerment.
- Hospital policy change; at a government level ebino extractions made illegal; hospital role more enforcing.
- Strong role of hospital and church to outrule traditional healers' ebino extraction practises.

Step 5: Administrative and Policy Assessment

- Policy; hospital community outreach, hospital, churches and councils supportive of initiative.
- Regulation; employment of personnel in ebino education capacity (later merged with AIDS awareness).
- Organisation; communication between different sectors; community councils, church councils, hospital councils – often the same people on many committees.
- Barriers to implementation; distance to major centres/large numbers of traditional healers.

Steps 6 to 9: Implementation and Evaluation

- Program successfully implemented.
- Process evaluation; program was implemented according to protocol, but required marked flexibility and last minute changes. Needed to be innovative with ideas.
- Impact evaluation; changes in predisposing (increased education), reinforcing (education at a community level, key community leaders on side), enabling (increased dialogue) factors.
- Outcome by reduction in ebino hospital admissions – marked quality of life changes – no death in period observed.

THEORY OF DIFFUSION OF INNOVATION

Another suitable health behaviour theory useful for health education projects among vulnerable groups is the Theory of Diffusion of Innovation. This theory derives from a body of research that attempts to identify patterns of program diffusion by using a broad range of innovations (Green and Johnson, 1996). It is particularly valuable among vulnerable populations because of its emphasis on creative, novel and innovative approaches. *Innovation* is defined as "an idea, practice or object perceived as new by an individual or other unit of adoption", while *diffusion* is defined as "the process by which an innovation is communicated through certain channels over time among members of a social system" (Rogers, 1995). Rogers (1995) identified characteristics of an innovation that were most likely to affect the diffusion process as:

1. Relative advantage
2. Compatibility
3. Trialability
4. Observability
5. Impact on social relations
6. Reversibility
7. Communicability
8. Time
9. Risk
10. Uncertainty level
11. Commitment
12. Modifiability (Table 1).

Table 1. Characteristics of an innovation most likely to affect the diffusion process [adapted from Oldenburg and Parcel, 2002]

Attribute	Key question
Relative Advantage	Is the innovation better than what it will replace?
Compatibility	Does the innovation fit with the intended audience?
Complexibility	Is the innovation easy to use?
Trialability	Can the innovation be tried before making a decision to adopt?
Observability	Are the results of the innovation observable and easily measured?
Impact on social relations	Does the innovation have a disruptive effect on the social environment?
Reversibility	Can the innovation be reversed or discontinued easily?
Communicability	Can the innovation be understood clearly and easily?
Time	Can the innovation be adopted with minimal investment in time?
Risk and uncertainty level	Can the innovation be adopted with minimal risk and uncertainty?
Commitment	Can the innovation be used effectively with only modest commitment?
Modifiability	Can the innovation be updated and modified over time?

The process of diffusion also typically involves five stages: innovation development, dissemination, adoption, implementation and maintenance. This innovation-development process links together the resource system (professionals, experts, scientists), the diffusion process (activities required to spread the innovation), the linkage system (strategic planning to link the resource and user systems), the implementation process (collaboration to assure diffusion) and the user system (the target audience for adoption) to provide the best opportunities for an innovation to be accepted, adopted and used.

PLANNING FOR DIFFUSION: INNOVATION AND ADOPTER CHARACTERISTICS

Maximising the fit between innovation and user requires consideration of how an innovation is communicated, collaboration between the developers and system users, and characteristics of the environment in which this process takes place. Effective diffusion involves the implementation of strategies through various settings by using a range of communication channels, which can enhance the durability of an innovation and ensure its long-term sustainability. Diffusion theorists view communication as a two-way process rather than one of merely persuading an audience to take action; a central PAR tenet. The *two-step flow of communication* emphasises the value of social networks over and above mass media for adoption decisions (Rogers, 1995).

DIFFUSION AS A MULTI-LEVEL CHANGE PROCESS

Achieving satisfactory diffusion of an innovation involves a complex, multi-level change process (Osganian et al., 2003). The complexity arises from the need to consider change occurring at multiple levels, across many settings, and resulting from the use of numerous change strategies. At the level of the individual, family or small group, uptake of a health behaviour change innovation typically involves changes in lifestyle practices. At the organisational level, successful uptake of an innovation may require the introduction of particular programs, changes in policies, and modification in the roles of particular personnel. This is especially relevant for health behaviour change projects implemented among vulnerable populations, with an enforced need for innovation and creativity.

The following is a case study in which the Theory of Diffusion Innovation model was used as a framework for a health intervention implemented among a regional-dwelling Indigenous population in Australia. Background of the project is provided, followed by a synopsis on how the specific Theory of Diffusion Innovation criteria were met.

CASE STUDY II; THE PIKA WIYA PROJECT

The Pika Wiya study is a community-owned, oral health intervention based on PAR principles that aims to improve behaviours and attitudes affecting oral health and dental service utilisation among the Indigenous population in a regional setting of Australia. Phase I of the study involved implementing focus group methodology to elucidate community perceptions on oral health, and to develop a culturally-sensitive oral health education audiovisual tool to be used in Phase II, the intervention component of the study (in process).

BACKGROUND

Indigenous people in Australia are those who identify as being Aboriginal, Torres Strait Islander or both. In the 2001 Census, Indigenous people represented 2.4 percent of the total Australian population (Australian Bureau of Statistics, 2001a). Indigenous people were believed to have lived in Australia for 100,000 years before European contact (Fullagar et al., 1996). They had a semi-nomadic, hunter/gatherer lifestyle and strong spiritual links with the land (Diamond, 2004). Marked lifestyle changes occurred in the post-colonial era due to the rapid introduction to industrialised society. Traditional lifestyles were discouraged and, up until the late 1960s, children with mixed parents [usually an Indigenous mother and non-Indigenous father] were placed in European homes. The impact of such policies on the social capital of Indigenous groups has been devastating. Rapid dietary changes also occurred in the post-colonial era, with traditional foods being replaced by rations, and more recently, convenience foods, many of which are high in fat and refined carbohydrates (Gracey, 2000). Other Western habits such as smoking cigarettes and alcohol consumption were also introduced (Clough, 2005). Increasingly sedentary lifestyles has meant that diabetes and other chronic conditions have became more prominent among Indigenous groups (Gracey et al., 2006). Such lifestyle changes have also had a marked impact on oral health, which has deteriorated considerably among Indigenous Australian groups in the last 20 years (Jansson et al., 2006).

South Australia is the fourth-largest state in Australia, with the mid-north region having the state's highest population density of Indigenous people (15.2 percent of total population). Such people represent 23 different language groups and mostly reside in the regional centre of Port Augusta and surrounding areas (Australian Bureau of Statistics, 2001b; Spencer Gulf Rural Health School, 2001). Although the overall population in South Australia's mid-north region is decreasing, the Indigenous population increased 6.5 percent from 1996–2000 (Australian Bureau of Statistics, 2001c). At the time of the 2001 Census, over half the Indigenous population in this area were aged 25 years or less, and 15 percent were unemployed (Australian Bureau of Statistics, 2001a). There is an Aboriginal-operated health centre in Port Augusta, which from 2001 has included a dental health service (Parker et al., 2005). Following encouragement by the Aboriginal Health Centre's Board of Management, an oral health promotion initiative that was community-owned and context-specific was developed. The aim of the project was to increase knowledge and awareness of the importance of good oral health to Aboriginal people in the mid-North region of South

Australia, and to increase community capacity in maintaining an oral health promotion program, using PAR methodology under a Theory of Diffusion Innovation health behaviour change model.

Focus group discussions were used to generate data for Phase I of the study, with invitations sent to members of a local Indigenous arts and crafts group (Indigenous adults employed to create arts/crafts products for exhihibition and sale), a chronic disease awareness group (Indigenous elders with chronic diseases who meet at the Aboriginal health service for support and education), and a young mothers Indigenous child care group (Indigenous mothers of children enrolled in an Indigenous preschool programme). Prompt questions were used to help guide discussions in suitable oral-health-related topics. These included: (a) knowledge of oral health; (b) the role of oral health in general health; (c) how the oral health of people known by participants has changed in recent times; (d) the causes of poor oral health; and (e) ways to prevent poor oral health at a community level.

The qualitative approach to data gathering enabled holistic perceptions of Indigenous oral health and well-being to be captured. Participants provided details of the structure of Indigenous knowledge systems and concepts of oral health; the relationships between Indigenous and Western oral health paradigms; and the influence of family, socio-economic status, land ownership and religion on their community's oral health belief systems, behaviours and self-care practices. A core category was identified and labelled "cultural adaptation". Five additional sub-categories also emerged from the data; lifestyle changes, oral health behaviours, barriers to dental care, impact of poor oral health and oral health literacy.

Participants portrayed how ongoing cultural adaptation was required to cope with the social impact of colonialism, living in missions, the stolen generation, loss of land, processes of assimilation and sustained disempowerment. It was explained that such historical legacy impacted on the health, including oral health, of community members, mainly through continued practices of being told what to do, where to live, how/when/if they would receive Government money and what health services were available to them. Participants felt they had little power over their oral health or oral health care decisions.

According to the older study participants, oral self-care behaviours were not a part of traditional lifestyle. This may have translated to contemporary times, with participants commenting that behaviours conducive to oral health were not widely practiced, either by themselves or by other community members. Participants described how regular toothbrushing habits were difficult to instill in children because of the different number of households a child might stay in in any given week. Many barriers to seeking dental care were identified, including dental pain, fear, cost, waiting times and lack of culturally-sensitive dental health services. All participants had experienced negative life impacts resulting from poor oral health, and knew other community members, particularly children, whose poor oral health had similarly affected their life quality. Although some participants were aware of the importance of positive oral health behaviours such as brushing teeth and regular dental appointments, there appeared to be a general lack of understanding at a community level about measures required to achieve good oral health. A sense of powerlessness that good oral health was beyond the control of participants, both at an individual and a community level, pervaded much of the discourse.

Based on the qualitative research findings, an interactive, context-specific oral health promotion audiovisual tool (DVD) was created, using an Indigenous film-maker and using focus group discussion participants as "actors". The DVD was fully endorsed by the Board of Management. Phase II of the project – the intervention – involves a series of four intense, interactive and context-specific oral health education seminars, complete with a range of tools (posters, oral health promotional DVD, toothbrushing and other demonstration models, oral health education pamphlets, toothbrushes, toothpaste, disclosing tablets) being implemented to each of the three community groups involved in Phase I. The tailored messages to each specific group include:

Arts and Crafts group:

- The role of oral health and general health.
- The role of smoking and periodontal disease.
- The role of oral health and diet.
- The importance of regular dental check-ups, with a tour around the Aboriginal Health Centre dental clinic.

Chronic Disease Awareness group:

- The role of oral health and general health.
- The role of diabetes and periodontal disease, the role of medication and dry mouth.
- The role of diet and oral health.
- The importance of regular dental check-ups, with a tour around the Aboriginal Health Centre dental clinic.

Young Mothers group:

- The role of oral health and general health.
- Preventing early childhood caries, simple methods of toothbrushing children's teeth, the role of fluoride and oral health, when to expect teeth to exfoliate, the role of orthodontic work, the "lift the lip" approach to detecting decay.
- The role of diet and oral health.
- The importance of regular dental check-ups, with a tour around the Aboriginal Health Centre dental clinic.

Materials used in the oral health education seminars include the full spectrum of oral health communication tools drawn from a range of everyday contexts; an assortment of written and audiovisual contexts that embrace different components of oral health promotion, oral health protection, dental disease prevention, oral health care and maintenance, and oral health systems navigation. Seminar materials range from the very basic (colour magazine articles advertising toothpaste) to reasonably complex (label on antibiotic container with administration details; how many tablets should be taken at one time; how many times a day should they be administered, when should the next dose should be taken). All seminar materials include images relevant to the Indigenous audience, using words generated in the focus group discussions and local language where possible. Communication strategies include giving meaningful examples, demonstrating procedures, asking participants to demonstrate a given procedure, asking individuals to re-state information in their own words, repeating information several times, presenting the most important information first and last, involving family members or other caregivers, encouraging discussion and involving humour. All participants have been invited to visit the Aboriginal Health Services dental clinic to meet the oral health personnel and to partake in a free dental check-up so that they might become more aware of their current oral health condition, and be less anxious to attend for dental care should it be warranted.

Follow-up focus group discussions for evaluation purposes will be facilitated by the locally-employed Indigenous research assistant and the first author. Discussions will cover the same themes implemented in Phase I so that any changes in oral health knowledge, attitudes, self-care practices and use of services might be captured.

A strong aim of the project is to strengthen the community through allowing participants' ideas and suggestions in the focus group discussions to shape themes/messages in the audiovisual tool (Phase I) and oral health education seminars (Phase II). As with Phase I of the project, communication in the interactive oral health education seminars in Phase II style is being largely driven by the Aboriginal research assistants, with a focus on user-friendly demonstrations, one-on-one tuition when required, discussions and tours through the Aboriginal Health Centre dental clinic. The Aboriginal research assistants and other key community members involved in a leadership capacity in Phase I are driving the oral health education seminars and will do so also for the follow-up focus group discussions. It is hoped this will empower community members through auspices of the Ottawa Charter for Health Promotion, and encourage involvement in other self-determining health promotion initiatives (for example; diabetes control and management; early childhood nutrition).

The following illustrates more specifically how the Theory of Diffusion Innovation is being used as a framework in the Pika Wiya study.

Key innovation attributes were accentuated in the development stage of the Pika Wiya study, as well as in the development of the dissemination strategies (Table 1). *Relative advantage* was shown by emphasising that the program had demonstrated positive effects, such as improved community knowledge of oral health and increased motivation for regular dental care. The demonstrated effectiveness of the Pika Wiya study was presented in dissemination material as an advantage over the previously non-existing oral health promotion programs.

Compatability of the program with current practice is evidenced by four key facts: (1) the National Aboriginal Health Strategy in 1989 identified oral health as a priority for Indigenous communities (National Aboriginal Health Strategy Working Party, 1999); (2) the National Aboriginal Community Controlled Health Organisation recommended that dental health and oral health promotion be incorporated into Indigenous primary health care services (National Aboriginal Community Controlled Health Organisation, 1998); (3) improving Indigenous oral health was listed as one of seven priorities in Australia's National Oral Health Plan (National Advisory Committee on Oral Health, 2004), and (4) a key point that arose from a National Aboriginal and Torres Strait Islander Oral Health Workshop was to "increase oral health promotion activity with the aim of improving health outcomes for Indigenous people" (Commonwealth Department of Health and Aging, 2003). Oral health was also highlighted by the target audience as a priority area requiring action.

Program *complexity* was minimised by developing materials that were informed by, and involve, members of the target audience, are context-specific, simple, colourful and fun. The program is easy to adopt to different settings (outdoor versus indoor use), audience sizes or session length. The oral health education component is formatted for easy use by health workers, with complete instructions and script, copies of powerpoint presentations and videos, and worksheet pages made available.

Good *trialability* is evidenced by the fact that oral health educational materials are available during the dissemination phase as part of the oral health education package, and through the Pika Wiya Health Services Inc. website (in process).

It is possible to show *observability* by illustrating the other attributes—relative advantage, compatibility, and complexity—through demonstration. Aboriginal health workers are able to observe the oral health education activities through professional presentations at the Aboriginal Health Centre, through audiovisual tool guides, and through hands-on training sessions. Innovation and flexibility, as well as PAR tenets such as two-way communication, are essential facets of ensuring the Diffusion of Innovation Theory is followed.

The intervention allows improved social cohesion, indicating that the *impact on social relations* is a positive one, not causing a disruptive effect. Through the intervention the profile of oral health and oral health promotion is raised at a community level, with discourse about oral health-related topics increasing. There are many tangible benefits of the intervention, including but no limited to each participant receiving oral health-related products as part of the initiative.

The project can be easily discontinued, thus emphasising the *reversibility* of the initiative. Much effort is placed on the intervention being articulated simply, thus reinforcing the *communicability* of the innovation. This is particularly achieved through employment of Indigenous research assistants to administer the initiative, who can speak the local language and convey messages in a culturally-sensitive, simple manner.

Considering the aims of the initiative (improve behaviours and attitudes affecting oral health and dental service utilisation patterns), the *time* required to implement the initiative is minimal (two years). However, for the program to be truly sustainable, messages need to be conveyed on a continuous basis, which is why the Board of Management has strongly encouraged the dentist employed by the Aboriginal Health Centre to work on the project one day a week.

There is minimal *risk and uncertainty* in the program, with the opposite occurring in some situations with Indigenous participants who had previously avoided utilising dental services because of fear or other reasons agreeing to have a dental check-up, and in some instances, receiving the necessary care.

Commitment for the initiative was provided from the outset by the Board of Management, and a certain level of trust was consequently in place before the study's commencement. The intervention would have been unsuccessful had this support not been present. The on-going relationship with the Indigenous research assistant and study participants means that commitment from a higher level is not as important following the initial phases of the study, although their support is frequently mentioned in the seminar discourses.

Because the initiative is based on PAR methodology, in which *modifiability* is a central tenet, the agenda items are flexible and able to be adjusted at short notice to better suit the needs of the workshop participants in a given day (for example, Indigenous mothers requiring a distraction for their children at the beginning of the workshops, food required for the chronic disease group when workshops are planned for the afternoon and blood sugar levels are dropping).

MULTI-LEVEL CHANGE PROCESS

Three key levels of the community are targeted for change in the Pika Wiya study; the physical environment, the information environment and the policy environment. Examples of change at the physical environment include the placing of oral health promotion posters at strategic points around the community (arts and crafts centre, Aboriginal Health Centre, pre-school room), and making free drinking water available at places where vending machines are located. Change at the level of the information environment include point-of-food-purchase messages in local stores and tuck shops about health food choices in regards to oral health and take home messages about healthy oral self-care behaviours placed in target audience letterboxes. Change at the policy level to promote positive oral health behaviours involves reviewing existing policies relating to the Aboriginal Health Centre client oral health and then incorporating specific statements about providing access to healthy oral health choices (oral health check-up incorporated as part of general health check-up). There is a strong commitment by the Aboriginal Health Centre Board of Management to allow the employed dentist to spend one day per week working on the project, thus encouraging institutionalisation of the project. Community group leaders play a key role in each of these steps, for example, the arts and crafts leader constantly encourages other members to embrace the project, the diabetes awareness group took part in the audiovisual production, and members of the young mother's group continue dialogue with mothers external to the group.

CONCLUSION

There are many unanswered questions regarding the application of health behaviour theory and health education research among vulnerable populations. However, the evidence suggests that the most debatable questions concern application and not the fundamental utility of health behaviour models (Patrick et al., 2006). Measures of theoretical constructs often need to be altered for vulnerable groups, using a range of innovative diffusion methods such as role plays, debates, videos and interactive websites. Focus group discussions for exploratory purposes, and to allow insight into common language and jargon used, are invaluable as researchers are not often from vulnerable backgrounds themselves. PAR approaches are useful to ensure two-way communication, community ownership and sustainability. Contemporary health behaviour models, such as the PRECEDE-PROCEED planning model and the Diffusion of Innovation model, are useful but often need to be modified to better suit the needs of the vulnerable target audience. Although both are appropriate frameworks, it is essential to appreciate the very real differences between researchers and the researched, and for researchers to avoid adopting professionally-centric views that may alienate the very groups with whom they are hoping to help. Health education researchers interested in working with vulnerable populations would do well to consider not what makes investigations superior in terms of research methods, but what makes them superior in terms of health education outcomes.

REFERENCES

Accorsi S, Fabiani M, Ferrarese N, *et al*. The burden of traditional practices, ebino and tea-tea, on child health in northern Uganda. *Soc Sci Med*. 2003;57:2183–91.

Australian Bureau of Statistics. *Indigenous profile 2001 Census of Population and Housing*. Canberra: Australian Government, 2001a.

Australian Bureau of Statistics. *Census of Population and Housing 2001; Basic Community Profile*. Canberra: Australian Government, 2001b.

Australian Bureau of Statistics. *Basic Community Profile and Snapshot: Port Augusta*. Canberra: Australian Bureau of Statistics, 2001c.

Australian Institute of Health and Welfare. *Australia's Health 2006*. Canberra; Australian Institute of Health and Welfare, AIHW cat.no. AUS 73, 2006.

Bandura A. Social Cognitive Theory: An Agentic Perspective. *Ann Rev Psychol*. 2001;52,1–26.

Baum F, MacDougall C, Smith D. Participatory action research. *J Epidemiol Community Health*. 2006;60:854–857.

Bloom H. *Soren Kierkegaard*. New York: Chelsea House Publishers, 1989.

Blumenthal D, Mort E, Edwards J. The efficacy of primary care for vulnerable population groups. *Health Serv Res*. 1995;30:253–273.

Burgess P, Morrison J. Country. In *Social Determinants of Indigenous Health* Editors Carson B, Dunbar T, Chenhall R, Bailie R. Sydney, Allen and Unwin, 2007.

Cass A, Lowell A, Christie M, Snelling PL, Flack M, Marrnganyin B, Brown I. Sharing the true stories: improving communication between Aboriginal patients and healthcare workers. *Med J Aust*. 2002;176:466–470.

Clough AR. Associations between tobacco and cannabis use in remote indigenous populations in Northern Australia. *Addiction*. 2005;100:346–353.

Commonwealth Department of Health and Aging. *National Aboriginal and Torres Strait Islander Oral Health Workshop: Workshop report and action plan*. Canberra; Commonwealth of Australia, 2003.

Crosby A. Suicidal Behaviors in the African American Community. *J Black Psychol*. 2006;32:1–9.

Danis M, Patrick DL. Health, Policy, Vulnerability and Vulnerable Populations. In *Ethical Dimensions of Health Policy* ed Danis M, Clancy C, Churchill LR. New York: Oxford University Press, 2002. Pp 310–334.

DeBruin D. Reflections of "Vulnerability". *Bioethics Examiner*. 2001;5:1–7.

Delva JD. *Families and Health: Cross-Cultural Perspectives*. New York; The Haworth Social Work Practice Press, 2001.

Diamond J. *Collapse: How Societies Choose to Fail or Succeed*. Los Angeles: Viking Books; 2004; pp12–18.

Dunn AL, Resnicow K, Klesges LM. Improving measurement methods for behavior change interventions: opportunities for innovation. *Health Educ Res*. 2006;21:121–124.

Fitzpatrick M, Parkinson T, Ray N. *East Africa- 6th Edition* Melbourne: Lonely Planet, 2003, 520–521.

Freire P. Pedagogy of the oppressed. New York: Seabury Press, 1970.

Fullagar RLK, Price DM, Head LM. Early human occupation of northern Australia: archeology and thermoluminescence dating of Jinmium rock shelter, Northern Territory. *Antiquity*. 1996;70:751–73.

Goodin RE. *Protecting the Vulnerable: A Reanalysis of Our Social Responsibilities*. Chicago, IL: University of Chicago Press, 1985.

Gracey M. Historical, cultural, political, and social influences on dietary patterns and nutrition in Australian Aboriginal children. *Am J Clin Nutrit*. 2000;72:1361–1367.

Gracey M, Bridge E, Martin D, Jones T, Spargo RM, Shephard M, Davis EA. An Aboriginal-driven program to prevent, control and manage nutrition-related "lifestyle" diseases including diabetes. *Asia Pac J Clin Nutrit*. 2006;15:178–188.

Green LW, Johnson JL. Dissemination and utilization of health promotion and disease prevention knowledge: theory, research and experience. *Can J Public Health*. 1996;87:11–17.

Green LW, Kreuter MW. *Health Promotion Planning: An Educational and Ecological Approach. 3rd Edition*. California; Mayfield, 1999.

Green LW, Kreuter MW, Partridge K, Deeds S. *Health Education Planning: A Diagnostic Approach*. Mountain View, California: Mayfield, 1980.

Hagey RS. The use and abuse of participatory action research. *Chronic Dis Can*. 1997;18:1–4.

Health Canada. *Highlights from the Report of the Royal Commission on Aboriginal Peoples*. Ottawa, Health Canada, 2006.

Holan G, Mamber E. Extraction of primary canine tooth buds: prevalence and associated dental abnormalities in a group of Ethiopian Jewish children. *Int J Paed Dent*. 1994;4:25–30.

Israel BA, Lichtenstein R, Lantz P, McGranaghan R, Allen A, Guzman JR, Softley D, Maciak B. The Detroit Community-Academic Urban Research Center: development, implementation, and evaluation. *J Public Health Manag Pract*. 2001;7:1–19.

Israel BA, Schulz AJ, Parker EA, Becker AB. Review of community-based research: assessing partnership approaches to improve public health. *Annu Rev Public Health*. 1998;19:173–202.

Jamieson LM. Using qualitative methodology to elucidate themes for a traditional tooth gauging education tool for use in a remote Ugandan community. *Health Educ Res*. 2006;21:477–487.

Jansson H, Lindholm E, Lindh C, Groop L, Bratthall G. Type 2 diabetes and risk for periodontal disease: a role for dental health awareness. *J Clin Periodontol.* 2006;33:408–414.

Jolles S, Jolles F. African traditional medicine--potential route for viral transmission? *Lancet.* 1998;352:71.

Jones RL. *Black Psychology. 4th Edition.* New York. Cobb and Henry, 2004.

Kirunda W. "Ebino" (false teeth): how the problem was tackled in Tororo. *Trop Doct.* 1999;29:190.

Kottow MH. The vulnerable and the susceptible. *Bioethics.* 2003;17:460–471.

Kubukeli P. Traditional healing practice using medicinal herbs. *Lancet.* 1999;354:SIV24.

Marin G, Burhansstipanov L, Connell CM, Gielen AC, Helitzer-Allen D, Lorig K, Morisky DE, Tenney M, Thomas S. A research agenda for health education among underserved populations. *Health Educ Q.* 1995;22:346-63.

Morris ZS, Chang LR, Dawson S, Garside P. *Policy Futures for UK Health.* London, Radcliffe Publishing, 2005.

National Aboriginal Community Controlled Health Organisation. *Submission to the Senate Inquiry into Public Dental Services.* Canberra; National Aboriginal Community Controlled Health Organisation, 1998.

National Aboriginal Health Strategy Working Party. *A National Aboriginal Health Strategy.* Department of Health and Ageing, Canberra; Australian Government, 1999.

National Advisory Committee on Oral Health. *Healthy Mouths Healthy Lives. Australia's National Oral Health Plan 2004–2013.* Canberra; Australian Health Ministers' Conference, 2004.

Neuliep JW. *Intercultural Communication: A Contextual Approach. 3rd Edition.* California, Sage Publications, 2006.

New Zealand Ministry of Health. *Whakatātaka Tuarua: Māori Health Action Plan 2006-2011.* Wellington, New Zealand Ministry of Health, 2006.

Osganian SK, Parcel GS, Stone EJ. Institutionalization of a school health promotion program: background and rationale of the CATCH-ON study. *Health Educ Behav.* 2003;30:410–417.

Parker EJ, Misan G, Richards LC, Russell A. Planning and implementing the first stage of an oral health program for the Pika Wiya Health Service Incorporated Aboriginal community in Port Augusta, South Australia. *Rur Rem Health.* 2005;5:254.

Partners in the BIOMED-II Project. *The Barcelona Declaration Policy Proposals to The European Commission.* 1998. Available at http://www.ethiclaw.dk/publication.html

Patrick DL, Lee RS, Nucci M, Grembowski D, Jolles CZ, Milgrom P. Reducing oral health disparities: a focus on social and cultural determinants. *BMC Oral Health.* 2006;6:S4.

Pindborg JJ. Dental mutilation and associated abnormalities in Uganda. *Am J Phys Anthropol.* 1969;31:383–389.

Pope C, Mays N. *Qualitative Research in Health Care* London; BMJ Books, 2000. pp 1–10.

Potvin L, Cargo M, McComber AM, Delormier T, Macaulay AC. Implementing participatory intervention and research in communities: lessons from the Kahnawake Schools Diabetes Prevention Project in Canada. *Soc Sci Med.* 2003;56:1295–1305.

Resnicow K, Baranowski T, Ahluwalia JS, Braithwaite RL. Cultural sensitivity in public health: defined and demystified. *Ethn Dis.* 1999;9:10–21.

Resnicow K, Braithwaite RL, Dilorio C, Glanz K. Applying theory to culturally diverse and unique populations. In *Health Behaviour and Health Education. Theory, Research and Practice.* San Francisco; John Wiley and Sons Inc, 2002. Pp 485–510.

Rogers EM. *Diffusion of Innovations. 4ᵗʰ Edition.* New York. Free Press, 1995.

Ruof MC. Vulnerability, Vulnerable Populations and Policy. *Kennedy Institute of Ethics Journal.* 2004;14:411–425

Simonds SK. Health education: facing issues of policy, ethics, and social justice. *Health Educ Monogr.* 1978;6:18–27.

Smith BJ, Tang KC, Nutbeam D. WHO Health Promotion Glossary: new terms. *Health Promot Int.* 2006;21:340–345.

Spencer Gulf Rural Health School. Working with Aboriginal People in Rural and Remote South Australia; a cultural awareness handbook for people working in the health professions. Whyalla: Spencer Gulf Rural Health School, 2001; 28

Ssali A, Butler LM, Kabatesi D, King R, Namugenyi A, Kamya MR, Mandel J, Chen SY, McFarland W. Traditional healers for HIV/AIDS prevention and family planning, Kiboga District, Uganda: evaluation of a program to improve practices. *AIDS Behav.* 2005;9:485–493.

Stefanini A. Influence of health education on local beliefs. Incomplete success, or partial failure. *Trop Doct.* 1987;17:132–134.

Stoneburner RL, Low-Beer D. Population-level HIV declines and behavioral risk avoidance in Uganda. *Science.* 2004;304:714–718.

Sullivan EA, Abramowitz CS, Lopez M, Kosson DS. Reliability and construct validity of the psychopathy checklist - revised for Latino, European American, and African American male inmates. *Psychol Assess.* 2006;18:382–392.

US Department of Health and Human Services. *Healthy People 2010: Understanding and Improving Health.* Washington DC: US Government Printing Office, 2000.

Wallerstein N. Power between evaluator and community; research relationships with New Mexico's communities. *Soc Sci Med.*1999;49:39-53.

World Health Organisation. *The Ottawa Charter for Health Promotion.* Geneva: World Health Organisation; 1986.

World Health Organisation *Uganda Health Profile http://www.afro.who.int/uganda /overview.html* Accessed 31 March, 2005.

In: Health Education Research Trends
Editor: P. R. Hong, pp. 155-174

ISBN: 978-1-60021-871-2
© 2007 Nova Science Publishers, Inc.

Chapter IV

SEE ONE, DO ONE, TEACH ONE: HIV/AIDS LEARNERS PARTICIPATE IN COMMUNITIES OF PRACTICE

Laura O'Grady

Faculty of Information Studies, University of Toronto, Toronto, Ontario, Canada.

ABSTRACT

Much has been written about consumers using the Internet for health care purposes, including those individuals with HIV/AIDS. Many of those with HIV/AIDS have engaged in self care and are often involved in decisions about their treatment. Yet little is understood about the ways Internet technologies are used to support learning about treatment information or how this resource is used in conjunction with other more traditional sources of information. In this qualitative inquiry twenty three participants attended four focus groups and shared what HIV treatment information sources they used and their means of collaboration. Using Wenger's (1998) Communities of Practice framework as a theoretical lens it was indicated that novice and intermediate learners are apprenticed by those with more experience. Participation is taking place but with little reification, especially within computer mediated communication technologies. Others relying on this technology as a primary source of information may suffer as a result.

INTRODUCTION

Almost since its advent in the late 1980s, the web[1] has been used for health care initiatives. Ranging from uses such as the sharing of genome project data, electronic patient records to telemedicine (Lindberg & Humphreys, 1995), a large percentage of material found

---

[1] A variety of publications related to Internet and web use for health care purposes were cited in this section. In order to be accurate to the source the term used in the cited study was also used in this article.

on the web is health-related. The desire to access this type of information by laypersons or consumers has been a major motivation for many using this technology (Eng, Maxfield, Patrick, Deering, Ratzan, & Gustafson,, 1998). The Internet has provided access to information in volumes not previously experienced (Jadad & Gagliardi, 1998). Interest in obtaining health care information using this technology is on the rise, as more and more people go online to retrieve medical information (Statistics Canada, 2002). Millions are now seeking health care information from the tens of thousands of web sites available (Cline & Haynes, 2001). However, health care web sites for consumer use are not necessarily designed or optimized for learning. Unfortunately many web sites also exhibit problems with usability, which can negatively impact those who are using the site (Badenoch & Tomlin, 2004). Although some research has been conducted in online distance education (Garrison & Anderson, 2003), even less is known about how the general public learns from web-based material presented outside formal educational settings.

A wide variety of health communities use Internet technologies, including web sites, mailing lists, newsgroups, and message boards to share and exchange health information. Web sites have the potential to become an important means of disseminating current HIV treatment information, as well as valued sources of medical information for a community often too stigmatized to seek such information through traditional means (Gomez, Caceres, Lopez, & Del Pozo, 2002). It has also been suggested that people with HIV/AIDS have extensive information needs (Boberg et al., 1995). People with HIV use the web to help cope with their illness (Reeves, 2001). In addition to web resources, many patient advocacy groups provide information to people with HIV (McCoy, 2005). People with HIV/AIDS also learn ways of self care with a variety of sources, including the Internet but also health care professionals, staff at AIDS Service Organizations, and others with HIV (Chou, Holzemer, Portillo, & Slaughter, 2004).

Those with HIV/AIDS want and need information to deal with their illness. Although a variety of sources may be used (Chou et al., 2004) little is yet known about the nature and extent of their application and how working with others facilitates learning. Therefore the research objective in this study was to determine in what ways HIV/AIDS learners are collaborating with others to learn about treatment information and what role the Internet played in achieving this goal.

METHOD

In order to address the research objective a purposive sampling targeting those with a need for HIV/AIDS treatment information was implemented (Morgan, Krueger, & King, 1998). As little is understood about this issue the qualitative method of focus groups was utilized (Morgan, 1997). The research protocol was approved by the HIV/AIDS Research Ethic Board at the University of Toronto. Each of the focus group meetings was audio-recorded and transcribed. The participants in the research study were required to sign an informed consent form at the beginning of the focus group. Four focus groups were conducted, with twelve men and eleven women, for a total of twenty three participants. All participants resided in Toronto, Canada. A survey was used to collect basis demographic information as well as background questions on HIV/AIDS knowledge, Internet skills, and information sources.

RESULTS

Survey: The majority of participants (56.5%) were between the ages of 31 to 40. Four participants (17.4%) were in the age range of 21 to 30. The remaining participants (26%) were over 41 years of age. Most of the participants (73.9%) had incomes less than 30,000 CAD. Most (91.2%) had graduated high school or post secondary. Many (69.6%) of the participants described their knowledge of HIV/AIDS as intermediate. Some (13.0%) declared their knowledge was at expert level, whereas 17.4% choose novice level. The focus group results are presented next.

Theoretical Framework Analysis

In the Lave and Wenger's (1991) ethnographically informed study "Situated Learning" the authors' propose that learning takes place within situations best suited to accomplish the task at hand. They further explain that those with various skill levels, expert, intermediate, and novices all work together to learn this task. Novices initially participated only peripherally. For example, those who are learning to be carpenters may first be involved with ordering supplies, maintaining equipment and tools, and other tasks peripheral to carpentry. These jobs are genuine or legitimate parts of an expert carpenter's task repertoire. This is considered to be legitimate peripheral participation. Once more accomplished, novices take on tasks more closely related to carpentry including measuring, sawing, and installing wood pieces. Over time and with practice the novice moves from intermediate to expert status. When groups of learners of various skill levels learn together it is known as a Community of Practice (CoP) (Lave & Wenger, 1991). This theory was further developed by Wenger in his 1998 publication, "Communities of Practice". Wenger acknowledged these informal learning communities exist in a wide variety of settings including workplaces, schools, and self-help groups (Wenger, 1998). Wenger, along with Lave (1991), first proposed that a self help group, Alcoholics Anonymous (AA), was an example of a CoP. A key component of this theory is the collaborative efforts of individuals to support learning. The findings in this study were examined with Wenger's (1998) "Communities of Practice" (CoP) framework for social learning. The following examination also includes reference to various secondary CoP framework publications by providing an interpretation of those authors' understanding of the framework within the context of this study.

Communities of Practice as a Lens

In the ethnographic study "Communities of Practice" Wenger (1998) observed the work and social habits of claims process workers in a company that prepared medical insurance claims. Similar to the fashion in which office workers do not come to work to participate in a community of practice, HIV/AIDS learners do not seek out treatment information to intentionally participate in a community of practice. These learners seek out information to maintain and improve their health, and ultimately to survive. In reference to workers attending to their jobs while likely wishing they were elsewhere Wenger stated, "It is something they deal with together" (p. 45). This could also describe HIV/AIDS learners, a collection of individuals working together, occasionally with only one thing in common, a desire for HIV-related treatment information. Wenger (1998) reported that the claims processor workers were perceived by management as working in a singular fashion and not collaborating with others to get their work done. It may also have been viewed by many that HIV/AIDS learners were engaged in solitary activity, or at best one, that involves interaction with health care professionals. Many of those not familiar with the AIDS crisis and issues related to the disease are possibly not aware of its impact, including the intensive need for treatment information support.

Social Practice

HIV/AIDS learners engage in a social practice, one that both is certain and explicit and also that which is unspoken or tacit. It is certain that one must attend to health care by accessing the health care system directly. However, accessing other HIV/AIDS learners to find out how to 'work the system' is also an important (and often unspoken) part of this process. For example, in this study one participant shared how his friend informed him of the steps to take when first diagnosed, including which AIDS Service Organization he should contact and what services would be provided. This type of information sharing may be more of a given, something many engage in but may not be overtly discussed. Problems taking medication with certain foods or other tricks of the trade may be readily known amongst HIV/AIDS learners but not necessarily by health care practitioners. Another participant shared an example of this when describing how he learned about a side effect experienced by some while drinking coffee and taking certain HIV/AIDS medications. As Wenger (1998) noted over time this type of information becomes common sense, it is so commonly understood that it may not be intentionally discussed. It is assumed to be known.

Meaning

To exist and participate in a community, one must also share a certain commonality, one that includes meaning. In this context meaning refers to an everyday process by which individuals collectively make sense of the world around them, "Practice is about meaning as an experience of everyday life." (Wenger, 1998, p. 52). This process is attended to in a collaborative fashion, one that is negotiated. Wenger (1998) postulated that to engage in this process there must be an interaction between participation (to take part or share) and reification (to give abstract construct permanence). These are crucial components in the formation of meaning and subsequently, to practice. The negotiation of meaning is a process that involves dealing with individual cases (one's own information), taking that information and generalizing it to others (sharing your information that is similar, but not identical with another learner). It can also involve taking other information that is not identical and making it work in your own circumstances. It is by this process that the meaning is negotiated.

Discussing treatment information, adapting it to suit your circumstances, and engaging with others in this process is how meaning is negotiated. A participant from one of the focus groups shared an example of the formation of meaning:

> So what I do with the information...and it is usually naturopathic stuff that I am accessing...that kind of treatment I am accessing - I try it out. You know I try it out. There's not a lot of people I can ask if they have done it because it's not a popular method of treatment...I try it and ahh what I found with trying it I find other people 'oh you gotta try this vitamin it really gave me my energy'....

Others shared similar ways of finding meaning. When describing how certain everyday things we might eat or drink impact with various HIV medications, one respondent shared the following:

> You can't have caffeine. Like for example, drinking coffee with certain medications, for certain friends. . . is. . . like makes them really kind of wired and . . . so and then I would go to the doctor with that information I would cross reference myself. I mean. . . don't get me wrong I am not writing this stuff down I mean it probably would be a good idea but I take with what I know, I take from the conversation what I can.

Another participant discussed how knowing what had happened to others when taking medication provided meaning for his own understanding. He said, "You learn from their experiences, if they've had, say you're taking the same medication and they're vomiting all the time then you know ok. For example when I started on Sustiva I couldn't even hold food down." Another participant also shared how he found meaning by reading other people's messages and discussing the content with others:

> I try to take a balanced approach to everything. . . like I'll read everything I can find on the Internet and I'll bounce it around as many people I know I can bounce it then I'll sit down there and weigh the options. . . of what I think is right ... somehow it will mush all together to...some sterling answer.

HIV/AIDS learners as members of a community negotiate meaning by sharing their history through their own treatment experiences. One focus group participant mentioned how she shared her information to create meaning:

> So all my information I get, what I do is it's like how we sit here, we have different group every month and we meet and we discuss everything. Like if she doesn't know what's going I have information I share with her. If she has a question she will come and ask. And that's how we use our knowledge and share information with each other. . .

Participation

Wenger (1998) included the concepts of "action" and "connection" in his application of participation in a Community of Practice. Amongst HIV/AIDS learners, "action" is taking the step to engage with others. This is accomplished in many ways, most notably by discussing treatment issues with health care practitioners, ASO staff, and other PHAs. "Connection" is achieved when someone finds a satisfying means to participate. Those who tried to connect with certain information sources and fail, fail to have a connection and end up not participating. One participant described the difficulty he had meeting others while living in another city, "Because I can't talk to people I can't like. . . there is not that much supporting group in Montreal. So I can't go I can't talk to them." Another also shared his frustration with posting messages online that went without an answer, "I've posted to some message boards but nobody responds; people are very shy." It takes the first step of "action" (to seek out the information source) and the second stage of "connection" to find this source useful and applicable. According to Wenger (1998), participation may not be harmonious, as shown by some HIV/AIDS learners who interact with their physicians. One reported that his doctor did not seem to be very organized, stating, "He couldn't find any information in my file if he looked for it." When discussing where he finds information about his own health care, he again mentioned the difficulty the doctor had with his chart, "He never seems to find anything in my files; it's the interns that find more things wrong with me than he does." This participant shared his difficulty finding a connection with his doctor, which in turn affected his ability to participate.

Wenger (1998) stated participation in a community is a two-way exchange, the individual is affected and the individual affects. Many participants in this research shared how they exchange information with others in the community. One participant described how she helped someone on a message board:

> I'm on a message board with the peer outreach project and also last night I was talking to one of the guys on the ...on the Internet, he lived in England and he told me that he was HIV positive and he did not know nothing about it. So I have like so many books at home about it, and I go 'well, I can email you information' and he was 'well, that would be great' and I'm like 'ok'.

Participation in such a community does not cease when the workday is over, Wenger (1998) suggested. Members of HIV/AIDS learning community also exhibit this, many that work or volunteer in this field are also in need of treatment information. This need for health care (and health care information) goes everywhere a person goes; it inhabits your mind, body, and spirit. A participant summed this up when saying, "You know like you know like she [pointing to another focus group member] said before, with HIV if you want to treat ah PHAs successfully you have to treat the whole person you know." Another also shared:

> Some people talk about treatment they think treatment is about taking a bunch of pill. They don't understand treatment can be psychosocial, it can be emotional, it can be physical, it can be mental, it can financial, it can be job, it can be support, it can be companionship, it can be so much that go into treatment. And sometime people don't understand that.

Participation takes on many forms including those of community forums, "As well ACT provides treatment information updates as community forum so PHA have access to those forums as well." noted one focus group member.

Reification

In this context Wenger (1998) intended reification to describe the process of an abstract concept being made real or given permanence. By engaging in reification this concept is expressed. To illustrate the following example is provided. Certain images on recording devices are associated with "stop" (a square box), "play" (a sideways triangle) and "record" (a circle). These symbols have been created to represent actions of the recording device, then agreed upon to have certain meaning. Anyone who understands the meaning can use the device. By engaging in reification we use a short hand form of communication or quick way to ensure understanding. In a work-related environment, establishing a process to handle customer complaints or writing out policies about vacation time could both be examples of reification. It therefore becomes understood that new ways have been established in dealing with these issues. These processes are then applied in the appropriate circumstance. Guidelines about these tasks are often reified or written down. Similar methods are used in our homes and within other communities in which we participate.

Amongst HIV/AIDS learners many reification processes have taken place. For example, vast arrays of acronyms have developed over time to reify certain concepts or as a means of communicating. These include the term ASO (for AIDS Service Organization), PHA (for person with HIV/AIDS), or HAART (highly active anti retroviral therapy). Other processes have been created in one part of the community (health professionals) and used in other parts (disability insurance). The stage of illness to determine when someone is eligible for disability was established by using indicators of health originally devised for medical purposes. Health professionals in the United States first determined the definition of AIDS (as opposed to HIV infection). It comprised of two clinical indications (t-cell count below 200 and diagnosis of at least one opportunistic infection). Insurance companies then began to use these indicators to determine who was eligible for HIV-related disability claims. When doctors reified this definition of AIDS, insurance companies began to apply it in their work.

Within the community of HIV/AIDS learners in this research many examples of reified concepts were demonstrated. Participants readily used a common terminology, referring to various local AIDS Service Organizations such as the AIDS Committee of Toronto by their acronym, namely ACT. Prescription drugs were also referred to by various medical terminologies. For those who read messages posted online by other HIV/AIDS learners, they too were participating with content that had been reified. In this case, one in which the meaning was electronically stored. Some HIV/AIDS learners used the process of seeking out reified content of treatment information. One participant described how he used the written information found in online chat rooms to learn about side effects. He stated:

> Well usually I find out about it on the net, then 'cause I go into a few HIV chat rooms I have the ability to talk with others who are doing it or are considering it. . . its like what are they're concerns or fears?

Another participant also stated he read messages online to find information about HIV. These are examples of how content reified in an online forum was used by study participants.

Duality of Meaning: Participation and Reification

Reification and participation are both individualistic and also dependent upon each other. They are separate entities yet intertwined. Wenger (1998) suggested they must coexist or neither will survive. A group may participate together to create a set of rules in order to self-govern, but these rules must be reified (written down or recorded in some fashion) so they can be remembered and followed. However, the process of creating the rules must be done within the group context, with everyone participating or the process will fail in the same way that creating policy in a vacuum fails. It is difficult to create rules or guidelines for a new committee before meetings begin, as issues that will affect its operation are not yet known. It is also difficult to create laws in advance around new concepts, for example privacy and the Internet.

There must be an implicit understanding of reified requirements amongst participants or the rules will not make sense. Participation addresses this issue. Many groups have similar collective processes, workers establish together an understanding of new rules required to do their jobs and teachers work with others to interpret new curriculum for providing instruction. In this research study respondents provided instances in which they participated with others using reified content. In one focus group a participant shared an example in which a friend helped her understand information:

> ...so he went on the Internet and downloaded all kinds of stuff, he came over to my apartment and he sat down with me and said, 'Ok we are going to go through this'. I was privileged that I had a friend like this right and he took me through it, he was explaining everything and translating it...

One "old timer" in this study recalled his memory of how meaning was negotiated in the early days:

> ...people found out and they like traveled, they went down to New York City and talked to other gay men there and they brought the information back up to Toronto because New York and San Francisco were being hit the hardest and that's where people were more getting information. And there was no information up in Montreal or Toronto, hardly anything, you know...

Wenger (1998) stated that when participation takes places in the form of spoken word, the process of writing it down reifies it for future clarification and use. Many organizations use this technique. Writing down rules and regulations, recording bylaws, and creating FAQs (frequently asked questions) online are a few examples. One participant mentioned that he felt as though he must look up any HIV information he desires, as no one will do it for him. In this instance he is accessing a reified collection of knowledge, shared by others, to learn. There were some instances in which participants wanted mainly to access information from their doctor. One shared her preference of "experts" (health care professionals) as her main information source. This content was not reified or written down, but rather took the form spoken word in a conversation. Others stated they will not use messages posted in online forums, dismissing them as not being credible. For example, one participant shared this opinion:

Not in my experience. Because I just...I can't see it being credible. I really can't. There's too much out there that's just...like anyone can post a web site. Anybody can put like you know little letters behind their name to say that there are such and such anybody can do it. Like I am sorry to be negative but that's the truth.

This would be considered an example in which reified content was rejected. Other examples include participants who shared comments about feeling overwhelmed with the amount of content found online. One participant articulated this as follows, "Look I know this and this and this and I'm concerned with this and I'm freaking out, this is an overload. I mean I have friends telling me this I have the Internet telling me this." Another added, "It's an information overload." Yet another participant stated, "...they didn't want to go to the web site like aidsmed.com to look up their information 'cause there's the...there's all the proof in the pudding in the name in the URL." Stigma can also be an issue in accessing information online. In summary, a variety of reasons were shared by the participants as to why online-based reified content was not utilized including credibility, information overload, negative issues using computer mediated communication (CMC), and stigma related to accessing HIV services online.

Community and Practice

According to Wenger (1998) the process by which we negotiate meaning is considered practice. A community of practice therefore constitutes a collection of individuals negotiating meaning and understanding about a practice. The two terms, community and practice, mean different things on their own. As Wenger (1998) noted the concept of community may refer to a group of individuals such as students who attend a university. But many of these students may have no interaction with each other. They are members of the university community but they do not all participate together.

An example of the process by which one engages in an activity habitually could be someone whose practice is to attend to her garden on Sundays. However, the context by which Wenger (1998) associated community and practice was intended to distinguish from these singular interpretations of the gardener and university student. Wenger (1998) stipulated three components (mutual engagement, joint enterprise, shared repertoire) by which practice indicated connectivity in the community. These three dimensions are used to bind community and practice (Wenger, 1998) and are further explored in the next section.

Mutual Engagement

Simply put, people must interact to learn. Interaction is required to negotiate meaning. Learning is not a solitary process. In formal education most either ask the teacher or other students questions at one point during learning. To engage with others in such a fashion indicates membership in a CoP. Proximity is not required but the process must be facilitated by some mechanism. Office workers need to speak to each other, in the same way individuals in a health-related support group need mechanisms to both find and communicate with each other (Wenger, 1998). For many HIV/AIDS learners, including the participants in this research, this process entailed engagement with health care professionals, staff at ASOs, and also with others affected by HIV/AIDS. While online, some participants reported using web sites and computer mediated communication (mailing lists, newsgroups, and message boards) as a means to find and understand treatment information about HIV/AIDS.

Rogers (2000) further expands on Wenger's (1998) concept of mutual engagement by stating there must be a mechanism for the group to share this common activity in a meaningful manner. Examples of this mechanism amongst participants in this research were both formal and informal. One participant described a casual relationship he had with an acquaintance to discuss HIV treatment information:

> I have a friend, I mean not a very good friend, just more of an acquaintance. But every now and again we'll bump into each other. Its like, he's really informed. Like he's seen everything, right from the like get go. Going to him just talk. . . chatting he up for an hour for coffee is amazing; you know it's inspiring. And I think it really helps.

One participant shared how he went to community forums whereas another mentioned attending conferences. More formal means of mutual engagement included discussing treatment information with health care professionals as a means to engage with others. One participant described how she would ask her physician to explain something she did not understand:

> ...Like I can't get clarification from the medical journals but if like my doctor gives me weird information, uses words I don't understand which has happened a few times using clinical language and I'm like 'What? That's like ten syllables in that word' and then I say 'What like what does it mean?', and break it down and get it familiar in my head 'cause there is no way I'm consenting to anything that I don't understand the language to it so ahh, so that's what I do. . .

Others included his pharmacist as one means of obtaining clarification about treatment issues related to medications.

Rogers (2000) also suggested that group members maintain their identity while mutually engaging in order to negotiate meaning. When researching an online workshop for English as Second Language (ESL) teachers he found that a connection to identity was often illustrated as participants reflected on their experiences in different teacher roles (teaching elementary school before they taught ESL, as an example). Participants used their previous experiences in other roles to help illustrate their points while participating in the workshop.

Similarly, those participants in this research with health care backgrounds shared often about how this affected their health care treatment. This occurred frequently in one focus group, as three of six participants were health care professionals. One stated his nursing background helped him, especially in understanding the language used by the medical professionals that he interacts with when seeking HIV/AIDS information. Another, also a nurse, discussed how his work experience impacted when he decides to contact his doctor:

> … I have a nursing background so usually I treat myself so he knows usually when I call I've done everything I can do. And he's quite quick at picking up on things and going from there. And I know how to navigate through the system fine...

One participant mentioned his medical background and how this impacted meeting his HIV/AIDS information needs:

> I was a paramedic for fourteen years and I have one year of nursing. But...I guess essentially I can't shake this. . . I hope it's a healthy skepticism. I don't take things at face value too often. So I . . . second, third, fourth opinions.

Other identities also have an impact. One participant described her use of a specific web site that is tailored to her cultural origins. In another focus group some participants shared how different their information needs were as women. One described how HIV/AIDS treatment research is mostly done on men:

> . . . there is still a lot of areas in the HIV community like with treatment access right. . . there is that ongoing that women are not a big part of clinical trials. Is it because we don't. . . we don't participate or is it because we are not given access to participate? And then you know so lets say that there's treatment study done or a clinical trial done and five. . . five men are studied and they're all you know 210 pounds, and very well built and very healthy.

Other issues for HIV positive women include dealing with children. One participant provided this example:

> I can't tell you how many mothers I know who - and it's predominately mothers - and I'm sure there's fathers too who experience it - but predominately mothers who don't want to send their kids to daycare, which means they can't go to work, which means they have to stay maybe stuck in a place they don't want to be stuck in. Maybe there's other things they could be doing or rather be doing like they want to go back to work or they want to whatever. But then they have to explain to the daycare workers about the medication and then they have to explain to the grade one teacher about the medication.

These identities affected how the participants interacted with other HIV/AIDS learners. Those with health care backgrounds are affected in their interactions with those health care workers from whom they are seeking care. Women who are HIV/AIDS learners may have less treatment information to choose from as much research is conducted with men. Those who are parents must deal with issues in relation to their HIV positive children.

Through this process of mutual engagement Rogers (2000) observed that members participating together began to form relationships. Participants in all four focus groups in this study discussed how they interacted with others in the course of meeting their information needs. Mentioned earlier were comments from one regarding how he learned about side effects of medications from others. Another participant described how the process of discussing HIV information was at first awkward, and eventually snowballed beyond a core group of friends:

> I think that is an uncomfortable situation for me. . . going up to people and trying to ask for that kind of information because for one usually its within your group of friends. . . initially and then from there you sort of network, and you spread out and then. . .

Another participant shared her example of mutual engagement. She said:

> Sometimes it is just bumping into somebody on the street. I work in a building that's commonly known to people as a place where people accessed services and programs where HIV is concerned. So I bump into a lot of people so maybe I have that advantage. I do a lot of emailing with people, phone calls. We have. . . . there is a women's' retreat that I go to every year and there's forty women from all over the province who get together...

Another participant described how she engaged with others to find out about an online message board:

> 'Cause a lot of people in my building were using it. They were going to get their information there and they said they got a lot of current stuff; they were downloading a lot of good stuff. So I just went there I was just thinking, I was just reading stuff and I saw the opportunity, the possibility of message boards, whatever like leaving a message, asking a question and a real doctor writing back to you ...

Relationships were formed with others in social and work situations in order to access information.

Shared Repertoire

A repertoire is a set of tasks or skills associated with an activity or job. A chef must be able to both prepare and cook food; these are skills within her repertoire. Likewise, a manager must both lead her staff as well as complete other non-managerial tasks required in her own job. For example, the head of an accounting department may manage a number of accountants as well as maintain accounts for clients. Accomplishing both of these assignments requires a set of skills that constitute part of a manager's job repertoire. Wenger (1998) suggested that the repertoire of a CoP includes a variety of written and spoken dialogues, ways of accomplishing tasks, and equipment used to complete these tasks. Application of the repertoire is what is considered to join participation with reification (Wenger, 1998).

Many of the participants in this research engaged in the repertoire required to be an HIV/AIDS learner. Most described examples of how they accessed information from a variety of sources, how they used this information, and who they ask others for help in understanding this material. These are examples of the skill set in the repertoire of an HIV/AIDS learner. In fact, many of the participants in this study engaged in very similar repertoires. Most used the same sources of information and collaborated with the same types of people to learn this information. One example included when a participant explained how she first finds a way to learn HIV/AIDS information and then how one PHA teaches it to another. Describing the latter part of how other are taught, she stated: "You go to another PHA and they'll be able to explain to you ok, 'oh don't pay that no mind, this is what it means' and then in words that we with both can understand."

Learning

The Apprenticeship: CoPs and Shared Histories of Learning

Wenger (1998) observed that members facilitate the ongoing process of participation and reification in a CoP. These members come in to the CoP with varying degrees of expertise and skill levels. As a result, those with more experience often instruct the new members on the practices and procedures of the group. In a work place a new employee is trained by a current staff member with more experience (Wenger, 1998). They may be instructed about procedures related to their job and they may also be taught about culture practices of the office.

Other more informal CoPs such as support or hobby groups have the same process. New participants to a bridge club are instructed about the particular rules this group practices. Over time, the new members move towards more of an intermediate status, once they have gained more knowledge about the workings of the CoP. Eventually they become the experts (Wenger, 1998). Results from this research provide examples of this process. In the survey administered in this research participants self-identified as novice, intermediate, or expert in terms of their knowledge of HIV information, demonstrating a mix of skill levels.

Participants leave and new ones enter the fold as time passes (Wenger, 1998). Although the participants of this study were purposive sampled and thus not a random selection of the population, they exhibited an extensive range in the length of involvement as HIV/AIDS learners from two months to fifteen years. One-fifth of the participants in this study ranked themselves as novices on the subject. Some described the process by which they were educated by those with more expert experience. One participant who identified as novice discussed how those who have been HIV positive longer know more and often help those new to the issue learn. Another, who rated herself as intermediate, described how one of her information sources, her doctor, had been HIV positive for a long period time and therefore,"He's doing something right." Another who also self-ranked as intermediate described how he asked his cousin for help in learning HIV information. He said his cousin had been positive longer than he and therefore knew more. Also mentioned earlier, another with intermediate knowledge shared how she preferred information from expert health care professionals.

Some participants had in the past or were currently working or volunteering at an AIDS Service Organization. These experiences changed their level of involvement as HIV/AIDS learners by providing them with more access to information and other learners. Some would volunteer for a period of time, stop, and then volunteer again. This is an example of what Wenger (1998) referred to as generational discontinuities. Wenger (1998) argued that these discontinuities are an essential aspect of a CoP. Individual participants in this research shared many reflections of how their commitment has changed over time. One focus group member discussed volunteering in the community and how her participation with this activity had fluctuated over the years. Another shared how he had dropped out of various support groups. One participant described how she used to follow HIV issues more closely. She stated, " I've been feeling kinda of like tired about HIV already. And like too much information too much HIV. Ok I am sick of it. It's been so many years."

In reference to legitimate peripheral participation, Wenger (1998) wrote, "No matter how the peripherality of the initial participation is achieved, it must engage newcomers and provide a sense of how the community operates." (p. 100). A participant suggested that those who are more experienced should help others new to the issue learn:

> I mean anyone that's HIV positive and on medication or HIV positive and they've been positive for a couple of years. . . and you know... will have more information maybe than you'd have and. . . . I'm sure anybody in that situation would be more than happy to help. It's sort of a given in a way. . . I am sure that if someone came up to me I wouldn't turn them away."

Another described how a friend provided instruction on accessing services related to HIV, "...he ran me through the whole PWA routine just like an expert. And I couldn't be. . . I couldn't have coped. Because at that point certainly I wasn't coping well."

Wenger (1998) also stated that the apprenticeship process must be welcoming to the newly initiated. In this study examples of both how this did and did not happen were provided. One participant discussed how she did not see herself in any of the posters advertising services at the AIDS Committee of Toronto. She stated:

> ...and I didn't feel like I was. . . . it was the place for me I didn't feel very comfortable there. I looked around and I didn't see myself. So I saw all kinds of treatment posters and all kinds of things about how to live with HIV but they were all you know men predominately...

Alternatively, many of the participants in one group, who were women, discussed how they felt comfortable with one AIDS Service Organization whose mandate is to treat women.

DISCUSSION

Implications

Little of the anecdotal information used by participants in this research appeared to be reified in a written format, or by using CMC. Most participants shared examples of conversations used to learn about HIV that had taken place in-person. Some stated they had read or currently do read online messages. Yet few contributed to these exchanges by either posting questions or answers. Therefore although some participation in online forums is apparent by respondents in this study, the process of reification is not. HIV/AIDS learners appeared to be engaged in participation and reification in-person but not online. This may be happening for a variety of reasons. Some expressed that they are overwhelmed or overloaded with the amount of HIV-related information available. Another issue is stigma in relation to HIV infection. A few participants expressed concerns with using the Internet to find credible treatment information about HIV. This may also impact their use of CMC in collaborating with other HIV/AIDS learners. Some shared negative comments about CMC use in general.

Another issue not shared explicitly by the participants in this research but one that may be inferred is the location in which this study took place in. With the largest population of HIV positive persons in Canada (McCoy, 2005) Toronto has over forty different ASOs serving these individuals, three hospital clinics (Toronto General, St. Michael's, Mount Sinai), and many health care practitioners specializing in HIV/AIDS. There may be little motivation to use CMC to learn about treatment issues. Why read or post online when there are so many available to ask in-person? Using in-person contacts means the HIV/AIDS learner does not have to concern themselves with the stigma of posting a message online that could be tracked back to them. This contradicts the notion prpposed by Gomez et al. (2002) that using online environments would help avoid stigma. Further, in-person contacts known to the HIV/AIDS learner are not likely to require credibility assessments.

Other HIV/AIDS learners who are geographically disadvantaged (living in remote or under-serviced areas) may rely heavily on online postings as a source of information for learning. Those who have access to a rich source of information such as in Toronto should be sharing their information with these other HIV/AIDS learners by means of CMC. HIV/AIDS learners are considered members of this community of practice, including people across Canada and also the world. If this CoP is intended to be a combination of in-person and online mechanisms for communication then the participants of this research study would not be considered full members as they are not engaging in online reification. In turn this implies that the online CMC component of this CoP is not an effective mechanism to aid learning.

Reification in a written format does take place in other forms in HIV/AIDS but seemingly rarely with any anecdotal information. There is documentation that includes information about various treatments and side effects available from local AIDS Service Organizations, both in-print and online. However, the content of these materials is mainly generated from peer reviewed research. It still may be necessary for HIV/AIDS learners to speak with others, especially regarding side effects as they search for anecdotal information. Many participants in this study shared that they had access to written or online information associated with AIDS Service Organizations. Yet they also stated that anecdotal information was still important. Examples of this include comments shared by one participant about learning about drug side effects from others:

> ...but the real personal experience with the drug... they can texturize it like when a person is speaking about the side effects they can provide more texture and say 'not only do you get diarrhea, you get diarrhea like this - ten times a day'...

While discussing online message boards one participant shared that he would like to learn more from other people with HIV. He describes this as hearing from others in their own voice and said, "...but I would like to have a little bit more of conversation with other PHAs in the same forum as well with that particular moderator, that doctor, or that specialist at the time." As described earlier one participant stated how he would have liked access to a support group while living in Montreal.

According to Wenger (1998) lack of reification may lead to the eventual demise of a CoP. Problems will be experienced if these participation and reification are not in balance. For example, cases in which participation continues but reification does not, understandings may be lost or misinterpreted in the future because they have not been written down. Conversely, if reification occurs and concepts are recorded but this is done without participation, there will be no collective interpretation and understanding of this knowledge. Recording content does not always make understanding self-evident. One is likely to need engagement with others to make sense of the material. Wenger (1998) elaborated on the relationship between participation and reification. He stated that there is a symbiotic relationship between the two, one that is mutually beneficial. Both participation and reification are necessary in order to negotiate meaning. Temporal contiguity is required between these two processes in order for meaning to be established. One process feeds off the other. There is little point in participating collectively to create a set of rules to govern an organization without making an effort to document the outcome. Otherwise this new set of rules may later be forgotten, misunderstood, or misinterpreted. However, re-reading any such documentation at a later date can still lead to misunderstanding and misinterpretation. Therefore, collective participation is required to interpret what was originally decided upon, especially by including experts or old timers who were involved in the process. Attending to this activity is paramount in health care, especially when a body of knowledge (anecdotal information) is being derived informally, outside institutional efforts. HIV/AIDS learners are unlikely to write up insights about treatment or what they are learning from others in any formal format such as a journal article or publication. This process is taking place informally by means of in-person communications, primarily with other HIV/AIDS learners. CMC would provide a means to engage in such a process.

Legitimate Peripheral Participation

In a publication on online communities of practice Johnson (2001) contrasts the mix of expert, novice, and intermediate in online environments with what occurs in traditional classroom education. In the school system students are deliberately grouped together based on age, which also means they tend to have similar skill levels. He argued that a mix of novice, intermediate, and expert is necessary to facilitate learning as skill development requires exposure to others with these various skill levels (Johnson, 2001). Mechanisms to ensure that legitimate peripheral participation is supported and old timers are able to instruct intermediates and novices are clearly important. But it also should be recognized that old timers or experts can learn from intermediates and novices as well. There must be methods for sharing information that encourages participation from all levels. The respondents in this study had the advantage of being located in an area with many resources and HIV/AIDS learners to connect with. As previously stated Toronto has a large HIV population, providing a mix of experts, novices, and intermediates with many resources for in-person communication. For those in a small community where the population of HIV/AIDS learners may be small, CMC may be one means to achieve this goal.

Issues such as stigma in relation to accessing both in-person and online services and credibility in content must be addressed if these environments are to be successful. Johnson (2001) noted that knowledge derived from collaboration is superior to any knowledge an individual may have. If HIV/AIDS learners cannot collaborate they cannot learn. With the shift towards consumerism in health care and as one participant stated, "nobody is going to do the work for you", the development and growth of mechanisms for HIV/AIDS learners must be supported and maintained. It has also been suggested that participation in CoPs provides a means for collaborative decision-making (Collier & Esteban, 1999). Participants in this research study demonstrated many mechanisms of collaboration for learning about HIV/AIDS information. A large part of learning for those who are HIV positive is done in order to make decisions about treatment. Participants expressed a strong desire to have anecdotal information in order to help make these decisions. Therefore the means to aid collaboration should also be supported for HIV/AIDS learners to help with treatment decisions.

Limitations and Future Research

This research study was conducted in a large metropolitan city (Toronto, Canada) where there is a wide variety of resources available to HIV/AIDS learners. Similar research conducted in places with fewer resources may have yielded different results. For example, another investigation may have found that more were participating in online forums to exchange information as in-person resources were not available. More research in smaller communities is therefore necessary. Alternatively other illness communities without the resources available in HIV/AIDS may have an entirely different experience. More research could also provide insights into how collaboration around treatment issues occurs.

This study required that participants have access to the Internet as use of computer mediated communication was part of the research objective. Other research should include those who do not have access or have chosen not to use the Internet to learn about HIV treatment issues. Some participants in this research provided examples of why they did not like to use online message forums or newsgroups. Observational research examining how participants use this aspect of Internet may provide insights into issues related to using these environments.

CONCLUSION

The research objective in this study was to determine in what ways HIV/AIDS learners are collaborating with others to learn about treatment information and what role the Internet played in achieving this goal. Despite much research indicating Internet use by consumers for health care education few participants in this study were using it as a source of communication to discuss HIV/AIDS treatment issues. Many preferred in-person contacts. Both off and online information sources and mechanisms for collaboration to aid learning were found. Framework analysis suggested participants in this study were engaged learners involved in much participation but little reification. Lack of reification may lead to the eventual demise of the CoP. When information is not written down or saved it can be forgotten. This includes online formats as well (unless electronic or hard copies are created).

HIV/AIDS learners are very knowledgeable about this disease. Indeed, evidence for this was shared in the focus groups conducted in this study. But little of this content has been reified or stored in any formal means. HIV/AIDS learners in this research were apparently not recording anecdotal or other information by using CMC, which in turn could be shared and used by others. Instead this valuable knowledge remains in many cases only within the mind of the learner or shared within a small, local circle of other HIV/AIDS learners. Although this community of practice is failing to reify by using CMC, it appears at this point that knowledge is still surviving and circulating. One means for this may be the rapid mechanisms for sharing amongst this group of participants. Many were located in downtown Toronto and see each other socially. Others have connected through local ASOs. Only over the long term will any effects of the lack of reification on the community of practice be fully understood.

The large populations of HIV/AIDS learners who reside in urban areas such as Toronto, Canada have accumulated much anecdotal information, which needs to be shared with those HIV/AIDS learners who live in rural areas. Similarly, Canadians with knowledge of HIV/AIDS have a responsibility to distribute this material to other countries. Valuable and insightful anecdotal information can come only from those taking the HIV/AIDS treatments. Government decision makers supporting e-health applications should be made aware that these technologies may not be well utilized amongst HIV/AIDS learners and perhaps amongst other illnesses as well. There needs to be more awareness that HIV/AIDS learners, one of the first groups to use this technology, strongly value anecdotal information. Such content must be presented online in a credible way that is not overwhelming. Efforts must be made to educate about privacy and protection in the use of Internet so that people can learn about HIV/AIDS issues safely. Information overload must be reduced by ensuring proper supports that help discern what content is relevant. Providing experts who monitor online resources will aid in this process. Consumers may end up resisting the responsibility of their own care. Government agencies need to be aware that not everyone will want to take responsibility for their health care, nor should they be expected to because technological advances have made it possible.

ACKNOWLEDGEMENTS

Assistance for this study was provided by Jim Hewitt, Clare Brett, Rosemary Waterston, Wendy Freeman, and Nobuko Fujita (Ontario Institute of Studies in Education of the University of Toronto), Kevin Leonard, Peter Coyte, and Andrée Mitchell (Health Policy, Management and Evaluation, University of Toronto). Thanks also to the anonymous participants.

The research reported herein was supported by a Canadian Institutes of Health Research (CIHR)/Ontario Women's Health Council (OWHC) post doctoral training award. Funding was also provided by the CIHR training program Health Care, Technology, and Place (HCTP).

REFERENCES

Badenoch, D., & Tomlin, A. (2004). How electronic communication is changing health care: Usability is main barrier to effective electronic information systems. *British Medical Journal, 328*(7449), 1564.

Boberg, E. W., Gustafson, D. H., Hawkins, R. P., Chan, C., Bricker, E., Pingree, S., et al. (1995). Development, acceptance, and use patterns of a computer-based education and social support system for people living with AIDS/HIV infection. *Computers in Human Behavior, 11*(2), 289-311.

Chou, F. Y., Holzemer, W. L., Portillo, C. J., & Slaughter, R. (2004). Self-care strategies and sources of information for HIV/AIDS symptom management. *Nursing Research, 53*(5), 332-339.

Cline, R. J., & Haynes, K. M. (2001). Consumer health information seeking on the Internet: the state of the art. *Health Education Research, 16*(6), 671-692.

Collier, J., & Esteban, R. (1999). Governance in the participative organization: freedom, creativity and ethics. *Journal of Business Ethics, 21*, 173-188.

Eng, T. R., Maxfield, A., Patrick, K., Deering, M. J., Ratzan, S. C., & Gustafson, D. H. (1998). Access to health information and support: a public highway or a private road? *Journal of the American Medical Association, 280*(15), 1371-1375.

Garrison, D. R., & Anderson, T. (2003). *E-learning in the 21st century: a framework for research and practice*. London; New York: RoutledgeFalmer.

Gomez, E. J., Caceres, C., Lopez, D., & Del Pozo, F. (2002). A web-based self-monitoring system for people living with HIV/AIDS. *Computer Methods and Programs in Biomedicine, 69*(1), 75-86.

Jadad, A. R., & Gagliardi, A. (1998). Rating health information on the Internet: navigating to knowledge or to Babel? *Journal of the American Medical Association, 279*(8), 611-614.

Johnson, C. M. (2001). A survey of current research on online communities of practice. *Internet and Higher Education, 2*, 45-60.

Lave, J., & Wenger, E. (1991). *Situated learning: legitimate peripheral participation*. Cambridge [England]; New York: Cambridge University Press.

Lindberg, D. A. B., & Humphreys, B. L. (1995). The high performance computing and communication program, the National information Infrastructure and health care. *Journal of the American Medical Informatics Association., 2*(3), 156-159.

McCoy, L. (2005). HIV-positive patients and the doctor-patient relationship: perspectives from the margins. *Qualitative Health Research, 15*(6), 791-806.

Morgan, D. L. (1997). *Focus groups as qualitative research* (2nd ed.). Thousand Oaks, Calif.: Sage Publications.

Morgan, D. L., Krueger, R. A., & King, J. A. (1998). *Focus group kit*. Thousand Oaks, Calif.: SAGE Publications.

Reeves, P. M. (2001). How individuals coping with HIV/AIDS use the Internet. *Health Education Research, 16*(6), 709-719.

Rogers, J. (2000). Communities of practice: a framework for fostering coherence in virtual learning communities. *Educational Technology & Society, 3*(3), 384-392.

Statistics Canada. (2002). Households using the Internet from home, by purpose of use.
    Retrieved November 7th, 2002, from http://www.statcan.ca/english/Pgdb/arts52a.htm
Wenger, E. (1998). *Communities of practice: learning, meaning, and identity.* Cambridge,
    U.K.; New York, N.Y.: Cambridge University Press.

In: Health Education Research Trends
Editor: P. R. Hong, pp. 175-193

ISBN: 978-1-60021-871-2
© 2007 Nova Science Publishers, Inc.

Chapter V

SHIFTING SANDS- EVALUATING EFFECTIVENESS IN COMMUNITY-BASED HEALTH PROMOTION INITIATIVES

Katja Mikhailovich[*]

Healthpact Research Centre for Health Promotion and Wellbeing;
University of Canberra; Bruce, Canberra

ABSTRACT

Interest in exploring what is effective in health education and promotion   initiatives has increased over the last decade leading to more evaluative   research in the health promotion field. This article outlines some of the   contemporary debates about measuring effectiveness in health promotion and   examines the unique characteristics and features of community-based health   promotion programs and what makes them challenging to evaluators. The paper   then discusses the emergence and value of mixed method approaches in health   promotion research and outlines some of the potential benefits and barriers   in using mixed method approaches including opportunities for innovation,   time, cost, expertise and strength of evidence. The paper presents a framework for conducting mixed method research in health promotion and   discusses the lessons learned from two evaluation studies utilising a mixed   method approach: the evaluation of a youth suicide intervention project and the evaluation of a smoking cessation program for marginalised and   disadvantaged groups.

[*] Katja Mikhailovich; Bruce. Canberra; ACT, 2601; Australia; Ph: 61 02 6202446; Fax: 61 02 62016623; Email: Katja.Mikhailovich@canberra.edu.au

INTRODUCTION

Health promotion and education can be described as both a science and an art. As a science the theory and practice of health promotion strives to bring control and predictability to our efforts to improve and enhance the health of individuals, communities and populations as well as certainty about how we might prevent illness, disease or suffering. As an art it requires creativity, intuition, vision and a recognition that the landscape in which we work is constantly shifting.

Increasingly questions of efficacy and how best to draw conclusions about what might be good practice in health promotion are at the for-front of policy makers, researchers and practitioners minds. Experts and scholars from across the globe conduct heated debates at scientific and technical meetings about how best to gain quality evidence of efficacy. Practitioners want to convince funding agencies that their programs work. Funding bodies want to know whether they should spend more money on a program and want evidence to support their purchasing decisions. Finally consumers want to know which interventions are going to bring about most benefit for improved health. Providing answers to these questions is not so simple.

Evaluators and researchers lead the way in providing evidence of effectiveness in health promotion and tacking the challenges of evaluation, particularly in a community-based context. This chapter outlines some of the contemporary debates about measuring effectiveness in health promotion and examines the unique characteristics and features of community-based health promotion and what makes them challenging to evaluators. The chapter then discusses the emergence and value of mixed method approaches in health promotion research and outlines some of the potential benefits and barriers in using a mixed method approach including opportunities for innovation, time, cost, expertise and strength of evidence. This is followed by a framework for conducting mixed method research in health promotion and a discussion of the lessons learned from two evaluation studies utilizing a mixed method approach: the evaluation of a youth suicide intervention project and the evaluation of a smoking cessation program for marginalised and disadvantaged groups.

HEALTH EDUCATION AND PROMOTION: CONTESTED TERRITORY

Health promotion is an emerging cross-disciplinary field with a growing knowledge base, theories and strategies for practice (Cottrell, Girvan and McKenzie, 2006). It can be thought of as an umbrella term for a range of activities seeking to improve the health of populations or as a specific set of actions to improve the health of individuals or groups. Tones and Green (2004) claim that it is well known that the concept of health promotion is essentially contested: the philosophical basis and principles governing the definition and practice of health promotion is open to multiple interpretations. In this sense, health promotion is a complex and multifaceted endeavour characterised by diverse opinions. These diverse opinions about health promotion also extend to the practice of evaluation.

Here we begin to see that health promotion is not only an art or science but inherently political and ideological. It is political because it overtly seeks to bring about change in the conditions that create disease and poor health by challenging existing structures and relationships of power. It is ideological in that it enshrines particular beliefs or ideas as fundamental to health promotion practice such as, doing good, avoiding harm, respecting autonomy, pursing social justice and valuing community involvement, empowerment and participation. (Tones and Green, 2004)

Internationally, contemporary health promotion practice emerged in the context of modern industrialized nations spurred by the World Health Organisation and the primary health care movement, marked by the Declaration of Alma-Ata in 1978. In 1986, the World Health Organization made a second declaration, the Ottawa Charter for Health Promotion (WHO, 1986). This charter has since provided an international framework for health promotion action.

The Ottawa Charter described health promotion as a process for enabling people to increase control over the determinants of health. Health was conceptualized as a positive concept emphasizing social and personal resources as well as physical capabilities. (WHO, 1986) The Charter promoted the idea that health promotion was not only the responsibility of health services but required action from other sectors. It promoted advocacy and equity in health and identified five main action areas that have become central to health promotion practice:

- Building healthy public policy;
- Creating supporting environments;
- Strengthening community action;
- Developing personal skills;
- Reorienting health services. (WHO, 1986).

Specific strategies for promoting health within these action areas include:

- Screening and immunization;
- Social marketing and the provision of health information;
- Health education and skill development;
- Community action and community development. (Victorian Government, 2005).

While the Ottawa Charter definition remains widely accepted internationally, variations in what constitutes health education and health promotion are common and will continue to change and transform as different cultural, social and political interests engage with the field. For example in the United States of America, the American Journal of Health Promotion (1998) describes health promotion as the science and art of helping people change their lifestyle to move toward a state of optimal health. Optimal health being defined as a balance of physical, emotional, social, spiritual, and intellectual health. While lifestyle change is paramount in the definition, the social determinants of health are identified as having great impact in producing lasting change. So too are advocates of Indigenous health forging their own models of health promotion that are culturally appropriate, community controlled, self-determining and based on the goals of Indigenous communities (Durie, 2004; McLennan and Khavarpour , 2004). Health promotion for Indigenous people needs to take into account culture, diversity within populations; socio-economic circumstances; languages and dialects, geographic location, and the consequences of colonisation.

In practice, a range of different initiatives and interventions are called health education or promotion and they occur in a wide variety of settings such as schools, health care services or the community. They are implemented across different disciplines including, education, health, housing, transport or public health. Examples of health promotion and the strategies that are utilized are given in table 1. Some of these initiatives will target individuals, groups or whole populations across the lifespan or target different age groups, genders or cultures. Some will be planned, implemented and initiated by governments and others by non-government or small community groups. All of them are usually motivated by good intention and with hope of improving health or preventing illness. This however is not always enough to bring about results or effective change.

Table 1. Examples of health promotion initiatives

Issue	HP Initiative	Strategies and actions used
Diabetes education	Teaching people skills in self management and self care of their illness	Health education and skill development
Mental health	An arts program to promote better mental health for people living with mental illness	Skill development, community action, creating supportive environments
Social health	Social support networks for newly arrived migrant groups including refugees	Creating supportive environments
Cultural diversity	Developing culturally appropriate health education resources for Indigenous people in primary care settings	Social marketing, health education, reorienting health services
Domestic violence	Program to increase parental awareness of the effects of domestic violence on children	Social marketing, health education
Smoking	Smokers cessation programs	Developing personal skills
Sun protection	Spot clinics for the early detection of cancers	Screening
Depression	Community run awareness and support program for people experiencing depression in rural communities	Strengthening community action, creating supportive environments
Healthy weight	A national campaign to raise awareness about healthy weight and eating.	Social marketing, health education
Alcohol and other drugs	Legislation restricting blood alcohol levels for drivers	Building healthy public policy

* Table adapted from Hawe, P., Degeling, D. and Hall, J. *Evaluating Health Promotion*, 1990 p4.

Community-Based Programs: Characteristics and Special Features

A 'community' may be identified by geography, place or as a community of interest unified by culture, health issues, age, ethnicity, sexuality or class. When health promotion occurs in the community setting rather than within health care services, workplaces, schools or Government agencies, they are generally conducted by not-for-profit agencies or non-government organisations (NGOs) that are philosophically committed to the community or population they serve (Kenny, 1994; Baum, 2002). They can operate at an international, national or local level. Some utilize volunteers while some have paid staff. The resource base of these or groups can vary enormously. A regional organization might employ 8 designated health promotion officers while another organization or group will have a single person working from a home office for two half days a week on a voluntary basis. Some of these may not necessarily identify their core business as health promotion, but apply for health promotion funding for special projects, such as a domestic violence refuge conducting parenting programs.

Community-based health promotion is designed to promote health in a manner consistent with the principles of the Ottawa Charter and aims to encourage empowerment amongst the community. It is based on a model of professional practice that stresses partnership rather than professional dominance (Baum, 1998: 69). Understanding some of the features and characteristics of community-based health promotion initiatives can be helpful to evaluators working in this context.

Many community-based health promotion programs are complex and multi-faceted in that they:

- Have multiple program goals, objectives and strategies;
- Seek to address multiple health issues, risk factors or health determinants in a single program;
- Vary in how rigorously the programs are planned prior to implementation;
- Are dynamic and opportunistic in that the program may be adapted during the implementation in response to consumer needs or new opportunities; and
- Use multiple strategies to achieve their objectives.

It is these types of characteristics that can make them particularly challenging for evaluators.

Across the health promotion and planning literature there is a consensus that systematic planning is critical for achieving program success and that evaluation should be an integral part of the program planning. From the perspective of the community-based practitioners some argue that in a perfect world they would design their health promotion program and evaluation before beginning the program. However, for some this is still seen as a luxury.

> "Even when we design our evaluation beforehand it can sometimes be easier, more economical and less intrusive for participants if we use the information readily available and collected as part of our everyday health promotion practice and use it for evaluation purposes" (Macdonald and Druitt, 2006).

Communities face a range of practical challenges when seeking to undertake planning and evaluation of programs, not the least of which are time and resources. Other challenges may include:

- Limited knowledge of existing research or evaluation in their area;
- Insufficient funding for the level of evaluation they desire;
- A lack of research infrastructure within their organization;
- Limited knowledge and skills in evaluation practice;
- Difficulties in conducting health promotion research in accordance with evidence based requirements.

In response to these challenges communities frequently seek the services of external consultants to conduct evaluations of their health promotion initiatives or programs. Over the last decade increasing numbers of community-based initiatives have been funded and the requirements for evaluation of these initiatives has changed. As funding for the evaluation of health promotion has increased, so too has the need for accountability. There are now greater expectations that initiatives or programs are able to demonstrate the delivery of outcomes. In contrast, at the community level, practitioner interest in evaluation has focused not only on meeting the demands of funding bodies but primarily upon using evaluation for ongoing program improvement.

In many cases there are divergent views between stakeholders over what the purpose of an evaluation ought to or how the evaluation should be conducted. Frequently, insufficient time and attention is given to the type of evaluation that might be appropriate, achievable, meaningful and affordable. Despite the fact that evaluability assessments have been identified as good practice since the early 1980s these are infrequently requested or funded as a precursor to formal evaluation. An evaluability assessment refers to a process undertaken to make sure that the program is ready for evaluation according to a number of critical preconditions such whether a logical fit exists between clearly defined program activities, objectives and goals and if the program has been properly implemented. (Hawe, Degeling and Hall, 1990)

EVALUATIVE RESEARCH

There are now a plethora of evaluation resources and publications outlining why we should evaluate, what evaluation is, how to do it, how to plan, design and implement evaluations, what to measure and the merits and limitations of different evaluation designs and methods. Some excellent resources in program evaluation include: Dignan, 1986; Hawe, Degeling, and Hall, 1990; McKenzie and Jurs, 1993; Pawson and Tilley, 1997; Wadsworth, 1997; Overtveit, 1998; Owen and Rogers, 1999; McDavid and Hawthorn, 2006. Definitions of evaluation, like definitions of health promotion, vary considerably as shown below. Evaluation is described as:

"...an assessment of the extent to which health promotion actions achieve a 'valued' outcome (WHO, 1998);

"The critical and objective assessment of the degree to which services or interventions fulfil stated goals. The achievement must be compared with predetermined standards of expectations" (Rootman et al, 2001);

"A process that attempts to determine as systematically and objectively as possible the relevance, effectiveness, and impact of activities in the light of their objectives". (Last, 2001)

Inherent to all these definitions is the notion of assessment or judgment. Regardless of variations across definitions, evaluative research is characterized by two features: observation and data collection and comparison of what is observed with some criterion or standard. (Hawe, Degeling and Hall, 1990). Although evaluation is defined to be objective, it is, like much of health promotion, political. This is because it is not value free and there are often vested or competing interests at play, such as who the evaluation is for, what the purpose of the evaluation is, or how the results are to be used.

The American Evaluation Association recognizes over 100 types of evaluation (Tones and Green (2004) some of which include:

- *Process evaluation* – assessing the strategies or activities used in a program, including resources, participant satisfaction and program reach;
- *Impact evaluation:* assessing the achievement of program objectives and immediate and intermediate effects on the targets of change such as policy, attitudes, and behavior;
- *Outcome evaluation:* assessing the achievement of program goals and the consequent effect of a program in terms of longer term health and social outcomes;
- *Formative evaluation:* referring to information collected throughout the program and used during the program to make changes designed to maximize the achievement of program outcomes;
- *Summative evaluation:* referring to an end assessment of the extent to which the program goals and objectives are achieved.

Health practitioners and educators, managers and researchers all need to have a basic understanding of evaluation terms, types of evaluation and different designs. This understanding helps to clarify and resolve different stakeholder expectations about what can be achieved through evaluation, the limits of various evaluation types and the evidence they can provide. (Overtveit, 1998)

The Evaluation, Effectiveness, Evidence Nexus

There is an inexorable nexus between evaluation, effectiveness and evidence-based health promotion. In order to have an evidence-base for health promotion we first need to establish the effectiveness of a health promotion initiative, intervention or program. In order to determine effectiveness we need to have evaluative research to inform our understanding of effectiveness. (See figure 1)

Wiggers and Sanson-Fisher, (1998: 141) offer the following definition of evidence based health promotion:

> "the systematic integration of research evidence into planning and implementation of health promotion activities".

This definition is premised on the idea that the best evidence of effectiveness derives from research and advocates for the utilization of hierarchies of research evidence. In such a hierarchy, the randomized control trial (RCT) is at the top of that hierarchy and stands as the gold standard for producing quality evidence. This hierarchy tends to disregard other forms of evidence as gained through clinician expertise, professional judgment, expert working groups, systematic reviews or qualitative research.

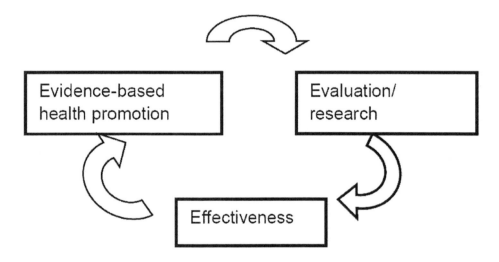

Figure 1. Evaluation, evidence, effectiveness nexus.

The notion of the RCT as the gold standard of quality research evidence for health promotion has been argued and debated thoroughly over the last decade and continues to be vigorously supported by some (see Rosen, Manor, Engelhard, Zucker: 2006 and opposed by others. Opposition to this notion is demonstrated in the WHO European Working Groups statement:

> The use of randomized control trials to evaluate health promotion is, in most cases, inappropriate, misleading and unnecessarily expensive. For a better understanding of the impact of health promotion initiatives, evaluators need to use a wide range of qualitative and quantitative methods that extend beyond the narrow parameters of randomized controlled trails (Rootman et al, 2001: 3).

Subsequently, Tones and Green (2004: 331) proposed that we begin to think about evidence-based health promotion differently: as *systematic planning requiring a series of decisions to be made and that these decisions should be informed by a thorough appraisal of available evidence.* They claim that the growing consensus is that the best evidence in relation to health promotion interventions includes both quantitative and qualitative research and addresses process and context, as well as outcomes (2004: 331).

Categorising types evidence generated through research and evaluation is useful for understanding how they contribute to an evidence base for health promotion. *Type 1* evidence is derived from research that describes risk relations, identifying the magnitude, the severity and preventability of public health problems; *type 2* evidence identifies the relative effectiveness of specific interventions aimed at addressing the problem; and *type 3* evidence is concerned with information on the design and implementation of the intervention, the contextual circumstances in which the intervention was implemented and information on how the intervention was received (Rychetnic et al. 2004:538). Under this type of classification most evaluations of health promotion fall within *type 2 and 3* evidence.

DEBATES ABOUT EFFECTIVENESS

According the World Health Organization (WHO) Global Program on Health Promotion Effectiveness (WHO, n.d.) we need evidence of effectiveness to:

- Identify the best possible ways to promote health;
- Make decisions for policy development and funding allocation;
- Demonstrate to decision makers that health promotion works and is an effective strategy;
- Support practitioners in project development and evaluation;
- Show the wider community the benefits of health promotion actions; and
- Advocate for health promotion development.

Although there may be a good understanding of why evidence of effectiveness is needed in health promotion the concept of effectiveness is not always well understood by community practitioners. Amongst researchers, the question of how best to gain evidence of effectiveness continues to be contested in the evaluation research literature (Rychetnik, Frommer, Hawe and Shiell, 2002).

The terms efficacy and effectiveness are long established concepts originating in epidemiology. Rawson (2001) suggests that efficacy and effectiveness are complementary but non-interchangeable concepts that require different methods in evaluation. Efficacy is more suited to experimental studies and the RCT, whereas effectiveness requires the use of a broader range of methods and is more open to being affected by external influences and differing interpretations. A useful definition of efficacy for health promotion is the extent to which an intervention produces a beneficial result under ideal conditions, whereas effectiveness is the extent to which an intervention when deployed in the field does what it is intended to do for a specified population. (Last, 2001)

Positivist experimental approaches have traditionally served the domains of public health and health promotion by providing research evidence of efficacy. Fundamental to quality evidence within the positivist experimental paradigm are the concepts of reliability and validity. Validity being the extent to which instruments measure what they intend to measure, the degree to which the results are correct for the sample being studied, or the degree to which the results can be generalized. Reliability refers to the extent to which methods and techniques produce consistent results. Within such a paradigm evaluators seek to utilize methodologies with strong reliability and validity and hence a high level evidence or *proof,* where *proof* is the evidence that produces a belief in the 'truth' of an argument (Rychetnik, Hawe, Waters et al. 2004).

If however we are interested in exploring effectiveness in health promotion we might turn to a broader range of research approaches and draw upon constructionist or interpretive paradigms of research where a diverse range of approaches to evaluation are available (Eakin, Robertson, Poland, Coburn, Edwards, 1996; Simpson and Freeman, 2004). In such paradigms validity and reliability remain paramount but *proof* of effectiveness lies with the party responsible for providing the evidence of their proposition. This idea has been adopted from the judicio-legal tradition (Rychetnik et al 2004). Rather than seeking an ultimate truth, we seek to prove 'beyond a reasonable doubt' or we take into account the 'balance of probabilities'[2]. Applying such an argument to evaluation one would seek to gain sufficient evidence of effectiveness to show 'beyond reasonable doubt' that a program was effective in achieving certain specified ends under particular circumstances. The burden of proof then determines how evidence-based practice is interpreted and applied. For example, should a program be considered useful until proven ineffective or assumed to be useless until proven effective? *"If the burden of proof rests on demonstrating ineffectiveness, the default is to do everything: if it rests on demonstrating efficacy, the default is to do nothing"* (Rychtnik et al 2004:540)

Mixed Method Approaches to Studies of Effectiveness in Health Promotion

According to Nutbeam (1999) the most compelling evidence of effectiveness comes from studies that combine different research methodologies—quantitative with qualitative and use a diverse range of data sources. They will provide more relevant and sensitive evidence of the effects of multi-dimensional health promotion interventions than a single 'definitive' study.

Despite the fact that mixed methods approaches to research have been discussed in the literature for over half a century, the approach is still evolving particularly in its application to the evaluation of health promotion initiatives. Mixed methods research involves the investigator collecting and analyzing data, integrating the findings, and drawing inferences using both qualitative and quantitative approaches or methods in a single study (Tahakkori and Creswell, 2007: 4). Most typically the concept encompasses the notion that both qualitative and quantitative approaches are used and that a triangulation of methods is involved or seeking convergence of results from different methods and data sources. (Johnson and Onwuegbuzie, 2004).

The underlying logic of this form of research is that neither qualitative nor quantitative methods alone are sufficient to capture the trends and details of a situation but used in combination they yield a more complete analysis and they complement each other (Creswell,

---

[2] See Tones and Green (2004) for a further discussion of the judicial principle in assessing the validity of evidence.

Fetters and Ivankova, 2004). There are a number of benefits that have been attributed to mixed methods approaches including:

- A reduction in the potential for bias in combining data sources, investigators or methods;
- Adding scope and breadth to a study;
- Providing a more complex range of research questions; and
- Stronger evidence for conclusions. (Creswell, 1994; Johnson and Onwuegbuzie, 2004)

Some of the barriers and weaknesses identified in the literature about mixed method approaches include the difficulty for a single researcher to carry out both qualitative and quantitative research, hence the approach being better suited to suitably qualified research teams. For these reasons, the research may more expensive and time consuming.

Models for Mixed Method Research

Johnson and Onwuegbuzie, (2004) provide an eight step process for conducting mixed method research involving: (1) the determination of research questions; (2) determining whether a mixed design is appropriate; (3) selecting the mixed method model or framework; (4) collection of data; (5) analysis of data; (6) interpretation of the data; (7) legitimating the data; and (8) drawing conclusions.

Having decided that a mixed method approach is appropriate, it is necessary to determine the degree of mix and the stage of the research at which mixing of methods will occur. Ultimately, there are a number of possible ways in which mixing can occur. Three common models for mixed method research include: *a two-phase design* in which the qualitative and quantitative are presented and discussed in two distinct phases; *the dominant-less dominant design*, in which one approach dominates the study; and one that combine both qualitative and quantitative approaches in an integrated way throughout the study (Creswell, 1994). Which framework should be used is dependent on the research or evaluation questions, objectives and the context and scope of the study.

CASE STUDIES OF HEALTH PROMOTION EVALUATIONS USING MIXED METHOD APPROACHES

Two case studies will be used to illustrate the use of mixed method approaches in evaluations of health promotion initiatives. A brief description of each of the health promotion initiatives will be provided incorporating details of the evaluation methodology and a summary of evaluation findings. This is followed by a discussion of the benefits and challenges of using mixed method approach in each of the evaluations. Table 2 provides a summary of the two evaluations with their respective study characteristics.

**Table 2. Mixed Method Investigations of Two
Community-Based Health Promotion Initiatives**

Study characteristic	Suicide Intervention Project	Smoking Cessation for Disadvantaged Groups
Content area	An evaluation of a 2 year suicide intervention pilot program utilising a collaborative participatory research strategy on a University campus.	An evaluation of a smoking cessation program for hard-to-treat smokers across three population groups (drug and alcohol addicted, living with mental illness, Indigenous)
Rationale for Mixing	To allowed for data source triangulation of multiple data sets in a collaborative research project.	To collect data from difficult to access groups.
Forms of data collection *Qualitative*	Document analysis of meetings, progress reports and health education materials produced by students. Focus groups with participating students. Face to face interviews with key personnel and stakeholders.	Document analysis, narrative group interview, key informant face to face interviews
Quantitative	Surveys: student participants and staff	Audit of pre-existing records Clinical monitoring using new instrument
Analytical procedure *Qualitative*	Thematic analysis of focus groups and interview data. Content analysis of education materials and documents	Thematic analysis of narrative group interviews and key stakeholder interviews
Quantitative	Descriptive statistics	Descriptive Statistics
Model	Two phase model: Qualitative and quantitative data collection collected by separate teams of researchers followed by integration of all results by single researcher at completion of research.	Qualitative dominant- quantitative less dominant model

Suicide Intervention Project (SIP)

The Suicide Intervention Project was conducted at the University of Canberra in Australia, funded by the Commonwealth Government and implemented in partnership between the YMCA and the University. The program was an ambitious two-year pilot project commencing in 2002, aiming to increase young peoples' connectedness, resilience and mental health literacy utilising a peer based education strategy to identify, support and refer students at risk of suicide.

The program objectives included:

- Increasing awareness of support services available on campus;
- Providing information and raising awareness of suicide and its contributing factors;
- Identifying barriers to young people accessing support services;

- Training peer leaders to provide information and raise awareness of suicide and contributing social factors among young people.

The project utilized a complex multi-faceted peer education strategy that consisted of:

- Two types of suicide awareness training program (3.5 day peer educator training vs a single 2 hour peer educator training program;
- A range of mental health promotion activities across the University campus designed and implemented by students for students.

The project provided training to 335 students and 11 staff between 2002 and 2003. One hundred and twenty five students received the 3.5 day training and 210 students received a short 1-2 hour training session. The majority of students receiving training were between 17-25 years. The initiative also targeted students who were male, Indigenous or from culturally diverse backgrounds and achieved some success in attracting and training participants from these groups, however the majority of training participants continued to be younger women and students studying in the helping or human service professions.

SIP Evaluation Methodology

The evaluation adopted a participatory and collaborative approach to evaluation by utilising staff and students from within the University as well as external evaluators, working in collaboration with the SIP project manager and student peer educators. Nine researchers worked collaboratively to conduct the evaluation over a 2 year period in two stages. An evaluability assessment was not conducted prior to the evaluation.

A two phase mixed method approach was adopted for the collection of evaluation data with separate teams working independently on specific subsets of research questions that were then integrated into overall evaluation findings. The evaluation was designed to collect both formative and summative information. A mix of qualitative and quantitative methods was used in the evaluation. Initially only a quantitative evaluation was planned by the project team. Twelve months into the program implementation the funding body requested an external independent evaluation be undertaken. This required the incorporation of the existing quantitative data and adding qualitative data collection retrospectively and prospectively. Quantitative data included attendance records, demographic data and survey data related to effectiveness of training programs for participants on measures of attitudes, subjective norms, social distance, perceived behavioural control, intentions, mental health literacy and social connectedness. (Pearce, Rickwood and Beaton, 2003). Qualitative data was provided from questionnaires, focus groups and interviews. In summary, the following methods were used.

- Document analysis: previous evaluation documents, records of participation, publicity records, progress reports, minutes, health promotion materials;
- Observation at specific events including the SIP training and health promotion events;
- Focus groups with SIP participants;

- Interviews with SIP participants and key informants;
- Questionnaires for University staff and student participants; and
- Pre and post self-report surveys for students participating in training programs.

This data was then triangulated to make judgements about effectiveness and outcomes. Over the course of the pilot project the SIP initiative underwent considerable change and development. This is not uncommon in community health promotion interventions where change in the objectives and strategies of an initiative are made in response to community demand or need.

SIP Key findings

The most significant demonstrable impacts of the SIP program were for the 335 students who received peer education suicide awareness training. Although the training outcomes for both groups were similar, as would be expected, the evaluation indicated that the participants who received the longer training program made greater improvements and changes on more measures than the participants receiving the shorter training program.

The results demonstrated partial support for the achievement of the aims and objectives of the project including:

- Changes in participant connectedness and mental health literacy identified from both qualitative and quantitative data analysis;
- Improvements in participant perceptions of control, confidence and attitudes about talking with others about mental health identified through quantitative analysis of surveys;
- Positive life value in the training expressed through qualitative data;
- Capacity building and social capital within the campus community identified through qualitative data analysis; and
- Lessons about the training program structure identified through qualitative analysis.

Smoking Cessation Programs for Special Populations

Between 2004 and 2006 the Cancer Council (a local NGO) delivered smoking cessation programs for hard-to-treat smokers in for three populations. The goal of this initiative was to reduce the prevalence of smoking in hard-to-treat groups within the community. Over a number of years the Cancer Council had developed partnerships with other local agencies such as an Aboriginal health service, a mental health service and a therapeutic drug and alcohol rehabilitation service to deliver smoking cessation programs to clients utilizing these services. The Cancer Council trialed a smoking cessation program for clients of each of the above services using a complex intervention incorporating individually tailored free nicotine replacement therapy within a group context.

Smoking Cessation Program Evaluation Methodology

An external evaluation of the program was commissioned by the funding body one year into the implementation of the program and a team of three researchers worked with the Cancer Council to establish a retrospective (2004-2005) and prospective (2006) evaluation of the program. The aims of the evaluation were to:

- Examine the effect that NRT had made in the trial program;
- Identify changes to participants' subjective feelings of wellbeing and subsequent changes to factors impacting upon health and wellbeing;
- Identify strategies and factors utilized in the program that supported behavior change and program success.

The development of the evaluation involved stakeholder consultation to clarify objectives and agree on the methodology. No evaluability assessment was conducted. Prior to the commencement of the evaluation, the intention had been to combine qualitative and quantitative approaches equally throughout the study. This was not possible due to difficulties in locating past program participants and a lack of retrospective quantitative data from the organisation. This resulted in a model in which the qualitative data collection become dominant and the quantitative became secondary. The following data collection methods were used:

- Document analysis: of program records including funding applications, progress reports, data collection instruments and program documentation.
- Pre- and post-intervention physiological and clinical records: records of attendance, weekly expired CO levels, type of NRT used, previous cessation attempts, age started smoking, number of cigarettes smoked daily and time of first cigarette in the morning, cessation at program completion and at six months post-intervention.
- Semi-structured interviews: with key staff from the organizations whose clients were participants in the smoking cessation programs.
- Narrative interviews with program participants: utilising storytelling to understand lived experience and to use these stories to help make meaning of and judgements about, the worth of the program. (McClintock, 2003; Morgan, 2000)

Smoking Cessation Program Key Findings

Difficulties in accessing program participants retrospectively and a lack of quantitative data from the organization impacted significantly on the findings that could be drawn from this evaluation. The qualitative document analysis of the evaluation revealed:

- Discrepancies in the implementation of the program across services and over time;
- The provision of free NRT was highly valued by program participants and services and contributed to smokers attempts to quit;
- The narrative interviews revealed complex motivations for wanting to quit, and the role that other people (partners, children and others on the program) played in helping to support them to stop smoking.

The quantitative data demonstrated that a total of 80 participants received the smoking cessation program. Of the total 80 participants, 26 had ceased smoking at the completion of the program. Of these 26 people, 6 people remained abstinent at six months post-intervention (7.5%). This rate is markedly less than that achieved within the general population, typically around 22%, however the pattern was comparable with other studies using NRT with hard-to-treat populations in smoking cessation programs (Mallin, 2002; Ivers, 2003).

BENEFITS AND CHALLENGES OF USING MIXED METHODOLOGY APPROACHES

A number of issues emerge on reflection of the two case studies above. They include the impact of unexpected changes to programs and the resulting effects on evaluation plans and methods, the quality of the evidence available to evaluators and considerations for reporting on effectiveness.

Any changes to a health promotion program at any stage of the implementation will impact upon an evaluation. In the two case studies provided, both evaluations underwent significant unexpected change, impacting on timeframes, budgets, the evaluation design and potentially the quality of the data.

In the Suicide Intervention Project (SIP) the scope of the program and the types of activities that were implemented increased during the life of the initiative. This meant more people were engaged, new interventions were introduced and in effect new program objectives were added. This required the evaluation team to make strategic decisions about evaluating the original component of the program as planned, or to attempt to assess the process and impact of the initiative as it emerged and evolved dynamically. In this case the second alternative was selected. The collaborative and participatory methodology combined with a mixed method approach was advantageous as it was possible to expand the size of the evaluation team and use both qualitative and quantitative methods to incorporate a range of data sets to make evaluative judgements about the original aims and objectives of the program as well as tell the story of the changing program that emerged.

In the evaluation of the smoking cessation program the opposite was the case. That is, the program itself was not fully implemented and their was a considerable amount of data that was not available to the evaluators as initially expected. Again a mixed method approach enabled the evaluation team to triangulate the available data to provide developmental feedback on the program and assess the extent to which the program had succeeded against its original objectives. Useful information was also generated about new methods that had been trailed in the smoking cessation program (algorithm for tailoring NRT) and new evaluation techniques (narrative evaluation methodology).

In each case it is the role of the evaluator to draw conclusions from the evaluation data on the basis of the strength of evidence available. It is the evaluator who has the obligation to provide the *proof* for those conclusions - 'beyond a reasonable doubt'. In both of the case studies described, the evaluation data was of variable quality. In the SIP data new instruments were being developed and validated. In the smoking cessation evaluation the data itself proved to be extremely limited. In both cases the evaluators could not predict accurately which data sets would yield the strongest evidence from which to draw conclusions and make recommendations. For example in the SIP evaluation it was anticipated that the quantitative survey data would play a significant part in being able to address to what extent the program had been able to reach its aim of "increasing young peoples' connectedness, resilience and mental health literacy to support and refer students at risk of suicide". However the quantitative data was only partially able to establish changes in participant connectedness and mental health literacy. It was the qualitative data that provided robust supplementary evidence about student's ability to support and refer students at risk of suicide that gave confidence and strength to the conclusions. It was the combination of the qualitative and quantitative results that enabled the evaluators to conclude that the program had only partially met its aims and objectives and how improvements could be made.

Neither of the two evaluations provided evaluation data of sufficient strength to conclude 'beyond a reasonable doubt' that the project was effective against their stated aims and objectives. However because of the multiple data sets available, the extent to which they were effective and the conditions that contributed to that level of effectiveness were more clearly understood and described. It is the illumination of these conditions and contextual issues that may be of greatest use to others when examining whether an intervention or program might be useful to another population group or setting.

CONCLUSION

As health promotion matures as a field, so too will our capacity to provide evidence of effectiveness using evaluative research. Good science demands that evaluations show rigor in research design, methods and analysis in order to draw credible conclusions (*beyond a reasonable doubt*) and make useful evaluative judgements about a program or intervention. There should be no reason to move away from such an approach. On the other hand, the art of health promotion evaluation might seek compelling stories about an initiative, rich in detail, perhaps provocative and 'meaning-full'. Such a combination of art and science could be more actively explored through the use of mixed method approaches to evaluation. In this way there may be opportunities to explore a wider range methods that could enhance our ability to build an evidence base for health education and promotion practice.

REFERENCES

American Journal of Health Promotion (1998) Definition of health promotion. [Accessed 24 April, 2007) *http://www.healthpromotionjournal.com/*

Baum, F. (1998) Measuring effectiveness in community-based health promotion. In J.K. Davies and G. MacDonald Eds. *Quality, Evidence and Effectiveness in Health Promotion: Striving for certainties*. Routledge: London.

Baum, F. (2002) *The New Public Health: An Australian Perspective*. South Oxford University Press: Melbourne.

Cottrell, R.R. Girvan, J.T. and McKenzie, J.F. (2006) *Principles and Foundations of Health Promotion and Education.* Pearson: San Francisco.

Creswell, J.W. (1994) *Research Design: Qualitative and Quantitative Approaches.* Sage: Thousand Oakes.

Creswell, J.W. Fetters, M.D. and Ivankova, N.V. (2004) Designing a mixed method study in primary care. *Annals of Family Medicine.* 2 (1) 7-12.

Dignan, M. (1986) *Measurement and Evaluation of Health Education.* C.C. Thomas, Springfield.

Durie M. (2004) An Indigenous model of health promotion. *IUHEP 18th World Conference on Health Promotion and Health Education,* Melbourne, Australia.

Eakin, J. Robertson, A. Poland, B. Coburn, D. and Edwards, R. (1996) Towards a critical social science perspective on health promotion research. *Health Promotion International.* 11 (2) 157-164.

Hawe, P. Degeling, D. and Hall, J. (1990) *Evaluating Health Promotion.* MacLennan and Petty: Sydney.

Ivers, R.G. (2003) A review of tobacco interventions for Indigenous Australians. 27 (3) 294-9

Johnson, R.B. and Onwuegbuzie, J. (2004) Mixed method research: A research paradigm whose time has come. *Educational Researcher.* 33 (7) 14-26

Kenny, S. (1994) *Developing Communities for the Future: Community Development in Australia.* Nelson: Melbourne.

Last, J.M. Ed. (2001) *A Dictionary of Epidemiology.* 4th Edn. Oxford University Press: New York.

Macdonald, E. and Druitt, S. (2006) The contribution of program data mining to health promotion Evaluation. *Healthlink: The health promotion journal of the Canberra community.* Spring.

Mallin, R. (2002) Smoking cessation: Integration of behavioural and drug therapies. *American Family Physician.* 65 (6) 1107-1114

McDavid, J.C and Hawthorn, L.R.L. (2006) *Program Evaluation and Performance Measurement.* Sage:Thousand Oaks.

Mckenzie, J.F. and Jurs, L.J. (1993) *Planning, Implementing and Evaluating Health Promotion Programs.* MacMillan: New York.

McLennan, V. and Khavarpour, F. (2004) Culturally appropriate health promotion: its meaning and application in Aboriginal communities. *Health Promotion Journal of Australia.* 15(3) 237-239.

Nutbeam, D. (1999) The Challenge to provide 'evidence' in health promotion. *Health Promotion International.* 14 (2) 99-101.

Overtveit, J. (1998) *Evaluating Health Interventions.* Open University Press: Buckingham.

Owen, J.M. and Rogers, P.J. (1999) *Program evaluation: Forms and approaches.* Sage: London

Pawson, R and Tilley, N. (1997) *Realistic Evaluation.* Sage: London.

Pearce, K. Rickwood, D. and Beaton, S. (2003) Preliminary evaluation of a university-based suicide intervention project: Impact on participants. *Australian e-Journal for the Advancement of Mental Health.* 2 (1) 1-11.

Rawson, N. (2001) 'Effectiveness' in the evaluation of new drugs: A misunderstood concept? *The Canadian Journal of Clinical Pharmocology.* 8 (2) 61-62.

Rootman, I. Goodstadt, M. Potvin, L. and Springett, J. (2001) A framework for health promotion evaluation, In I. Rootman, M. Goodstadt, B. Hyndman, D.V. McQueen, L. Potvin, J. Springett and E. Ziglio, Eds. *Evaluation in Health Promotion: Principles and Perspectives.* WHO: Copenhagen.

Rosen. L, Manor. O, Engelhard. D, and Zucker, D. (2006) In defense of the randomized controlled trial for health promotion research. *American Journal of Public Health.* 96 (7) 1181-1186.

Rychetnik. L, Frommer. M, Hawe. P, and Shiell, A. (2002) Criteria for evaluating evidence on public health interventions. *Journal of Epidemiology and Community Health.* 56. 119-127.

Rychetnik, L. Hawe, P. Waters, E. Barratt, A. and Frommer, M. (2004) A glossary for evidence based public health. *Journal of Epidemiology and Community Health.* 54. 538-545.

Simpson, K. and Freeman, R. (2004) Critical health promotion and education- a new research challenge. *Health Education Research: Theory and Practice.* 19 (3) 340-348.

Tahakkori, A. and Creswell, J.W. (2007) The new era of mixed methods. *Journal of Mixed Methods Research.* 1 (1) 3-7.

Tones, K. and Green, J. (2004) *Health Promotion: Planning and Strategies.* Sage: London.

Victorian Government, Department of Human Services (2005) *Health Promotion Interventions and Capacity Building.* [Accessed 24 November, 2005]. *http://www.health.vic.gov.au/healthpromotion/hp_practice/interventions.htm.*

Wadsworth, Y. *Everyday Evaluation on the Run.* 2nd Edn. Allen and Unwin: Sydney.

World Health Organisation Global Program for Health Promotion Effectiveness. (n.d.) [Accessed 20 February, 2007] *http://www.who.int/healthpromotion/areas/gphpe/en/index.html*

World Health Organisation. (1986) *Ottawa Charter for Health Promotion.* [Accessed 20 February, 2007]. *http:www.who.int/hpr/NPH/docs/OttawaCharterforHealthPromotion.pdf*

In: Health Education Research Trends
Editor: P. R. Hong, pp. 195-210

ISBN: 978-1-60021-871-2
© 2007 Nova Science Publishers, Inc.

Chapter VI

A PEER LEADER INTERVENTION TO INCREASE PARTICIPATION IN ORGANIZED SCHOOL SPORTS AMONG LATINA GIRLS: THE *LIDERES LATINA* DEMONSTRATION STUDY

Guadalupe X. Ayala[1,*], Kelley DeLeeuw[2] and Victoria Gonzalez[3]

[1]Division of Health Promotion, Graduate School of Public Health, San Diego State University, USA;
[2]University of Puerto Rico, Ponce School of Medicine, Ponce, PR 00732, 858-35306644;
[3]Psychology Department, University of North Carolina at Chapel Hill, Chapel Hill, NC 27599-7440, USA.

ABSTRACT

The study was designed to increase organized school sports participation among middle school Latina girls. Two schools in a rural community were matched on important characteristics and recruited to serve as an intervention or control school. Thirteen Latina girls were identified by school personnel and nine were trained as peer leaders. Following training, the peer leaders implemented intervention strategies involving material development and distribution, and interpersonal communication with school personnel, peers, and parents. The primary outcome was sports participation among Latina girls. Data on participation were obtained from the school athletic directors and verified by observation. Secondary outcomes included peer leader knowledge, confidence and self-esteem measured at pre-training, post-training, and post-intervention activities using self-administered questionnaires and interviews. At the intervention school, the percentage of spring athletes who were Latina rose from 15% in 2004 to 27% in 2005 versus a drop in participation in the comparison school (10% in 2004 to 0% in

* Correspondence concerning this article should be addressed to: Guadalupe X. Ayala, PhD, MPH, San Diego State University, Center for Behavioral and Community Health Studies, 9245 Sky Park Court, Suite 221, San Diego, CA 92123. E-mail: ayala@mail.sdsu.edu; Tel.: 619-594-6686.

2005). Significant changes in peer leader knowledge and confidence were observed after training. This study reveals that peer leaders are able to implement an intervention to change sports participation patterns. Increasing participation in organized school sports may be an underutilized area for increasing adolescent physical activity levels.

Keywords: Latinas, organized school sports, peer leader.

INTRODUCTION

Adolescent risk for overweight has steadily climbed since 1980; currently 31% of children aged 6 to 19 are considered at risk for overweight (BMI between 85th and 95th percentile) and 16% are considered overweight (BMI $\geq 95^{th}$ percentile; Hedley, Ogden, Johnson, et al., 2004). Twenty percent of Mexican-American girls aged 12 to 19 are overweight compared with 13% of non-Hispanic white girls (Hedley et al, 2004). One risk factor for overweight is insufficient physical activity. Adolescent girls are significantly more at risk for physical inactivity than boys (CDC, 2003), and Latina adolescent girls are more likely than Caucasian girls to report insufficient levels of physical activity (35% versus 29%, respectively). Parents of Latino youth report more barriers for their children being physically active than parents of other racially/ethnically diverse families (CDC, 2003).

Given the high rates of childhood overweight and physical inactivity, it is important to identify methods for raising activity levels. One outlet for encouraging youth physical activity are organized school sports programs which exist for both boys and girls in 99% of U.S. middle and high schools (CDC, 2004a). Participation in school sports involves high levels of physical activity and thus increases the amount of physical activity in an adolescent's day (Pate, Trost, Levin, & Dowda, 2000). Children who participate in sports are much more likely to have a lower BMI and less likely to be overweight (Forshee, Anderson & Story, 2004). This association is stronger than the correlation between television viewing and BMI, race/ethnicity and BMI, and consumption of soft drinks and BMI (Forshee et al., 2004).

In addition to the health benefits of participating in organized sports, participation also offers many other positive benefits to girls, including increased self confidence and self esteem (Ference & Muth, 2004; Richman & Shaffer, 2000), higher academic achievement (Melnick, Sabo, & Vanfossen, 1992), less hopelessness (Baumert, Henderson, & Thompson, 1998) and fewer risk behaviors such as drug use (Pate et al., 2000), teen pregnancy (Sabo, Miller, Farrell, Melnick, & Barnes, 1999), and school dropout (Yin & Moore, 2004). Yet, despite all of these benefits, disparities in organized sports participation have been noted with 26% of Latina girls age 9 to 13 reporting participation in an organized physical activity during the preceding 7 days compared with 47% of Caucasian girls (CDC, 2003).

Increasing Participation

Girls report being influenced to participate in organized school sports for social reasons such as wanting to be with friends or be part of a team (Allen, 2003). Participation is also positively associated with parental and peer support, as well as with positive parental attitudes about physical activity (Brustad, 1996; Prochaska, Rodgers, & Sallis, 2002). This information provides a framework for understanding influences on sports participation.

School-based interventions designed to increase physical activity or reduce overweight among adolescents target improvements in physical education classes or new programs (Gortmaker, Peterson, Wiecha, et al., 1999; McKenzie, Sallis, Prochaska, et al, 2004, Stevens, Murray, Catellier, et al., 2005; Story, 1999; Veugelers & Fitzgerald, 2005). A review of 11 controlled experimental school-based studies for preventing and treating obesity found that relatively few primary prevention research studies exist. Eight interacting components were identified as playing a key role in intervention success: health instruction; health services; school environment; food service; school-site health promotion for faculty and staff; social support services; physical education classes; and integrated and linked family and community health promotion efforts (Story, 1999). The review suggests that schools are in a unique position to play a pivotal role in promoting healthy lifestyles and preventing obesity.To our knowledge, however, no study exists which seeks to increase girls' participation in organized school sports.

Peer Leader Interventions

Peer leader programs are a popular approach to adolescent health promotion (Mellanby, Rees, & Tripp, 2000; Story, Lytle, & Birnbaum, 2002). Peer leadership involves training selected adolescents on specific health topics so that they, in turn, may educate and influence their peers in formal or informal settings. The underlying concepts are that peer leaders may be viewed as more credible sources of information than adults and know how to communicate sensitive health information in a linguistically and socially appropriate level (Mellanby et al., 2000). Peer leader programs are also based on evidence that teens most often seek advice from friends before adults and are influenced by the expectations, attitudes, and behaviors of the peer groups to which they belong (Lindsey, 1997).

Several reviews have shown peer-led interventions to be as or more efficacious than adult or "expert" led health intervention programs (Cuijpers, 2002; Mellanby et al., 2000). The peer leader model has been used to intervene on sensitive topics such as drug and alcohol use (Cuijpers, 2002), HIV/AIDS and sexual education (Milburn, 1995; Zibalese-Crawford, 1997), and youth violence (Wiist, Jackson, & Jackson, 1996). Less sensitive health issues have also been targeted such as poolside skin cancer prevention (Lombard, Neubauer, Canfield, & Winett, 1991), bicycle helmet use (Hall, Cross, Howat, Stevenson, & Shaw, 2004), dental health (Laiho, Honkala, Nyyssonen, & Milen, 1993), and nutrition (Story et al., 2002). One health behavior theory underlying the peer leader model is Social Support theory (Heaney & Israel, 2002). Social support can be defined as the functional content of relationships as it relates to emotional, appraisal, informational and instrumental support

(Heaney & Israel, 2002). Peer leaders may be able to provide more support than adults, or their support may be of higher value, given that peers may be able to communicate feelings and information at a more age- and socially-appropriate level than adults (Mellanby et al., 2000).

Purpose

The present study sought to increase middle school Latina girls' involvement in organized school sports. The peer leader model was chosen as the primary intervention strategy given the cultural divide that exists between new immigrants and the systems they must learn to navigate. A unique aspect of this study was the participatory nature of intervention development with the peer leaders. The peer leaders chose and implemented intervention strategies that were most appropriate for the target audiences they were trying to reach. The outcome of the intervention, participation in spring school sports, was compared with a control school.

METHODS

Study Design

This study comprises a two-group quasi-experimental design involving implementation of a peer leader intervention at one middle school to increase Latina girls' participation in organized school sports. A no-treatment comparison middle school was identified in the same school district with similar student characteristics. In addition to the primary outcome of school sports participation, impact of the program on the Latina peer leaders was examined using quantitative and qualitative methods. All study protocols were approved by the Public Health Institutional Review Board at the University of North Carolina at Chapel Hill.

Setting

The two schools selected for this study are located in a semi-rural county in central North Carolina. North Carolina in general, and this county in particular, experienced a substantial growth in the size of the Latino population between 1990 and 2000 (1% [n=736] to 7% [n=8,835] respectively; U.S. Census Bureau, 2000). This growth was also observed in the schools selected for participation. For example, during the 2001-2002 school year, 20% (n=161) of the student body in the intervention school was Latino, compared with 30% (n=212) in 2004-2005 (National Center for Educational Statistics, 2005). Not surprisingly, changes were also observed in the number of students eligible for the free or reduced-price lunch program, from 68% to 75% in same three years.

Selection of this setting and methods used were informed by a qualitative research study conducted with Latino families in the county (Ayala, Maty, Cravey, & Webb, 2005). The goals of the previous study were to identify family and community influences on obesity. Adolescent Latina girls who participated in the in-depth interviews and community mapping project cited the lack of available resources for being physically active. A school-based project was identified as a feasible and appropriate method for promoting physical activity. After securing permission from the school principal and cooperation from the girls' soccer coach and the English-as-a-Second-Language [ESL] teacher, we began the process of identifying, selecting, and training peer leaders. Our decision to partner with the girls' soccer coach was due, in part, to the popularity of soccer among Latina girls at the intervention school.

Identification and Selection of Peer Leaders

The methods used to identify and select peer leaders for this study were consistent with previous research with peer leaders (Cuijpers, 2002) and lay health advisors in general (Elder, Ayala, Campbell, et al., 2005). In this study, the girls' soccer coach first prepared a list of Latina girls who had participated in organized sports the previous year, and who were still enrolled in the school. These girls would have some familiarity with the requirements for participating in organized school sports. The second and third characteristics used to identify peer leaders were leadership potential and involvement in extracurricular activities (e.g., school club participation). Identification of girls using these criteria was based on teacher reports made to the girls' soccer coach. The coach then confirmed Latino/Hispanic ethnicity using information from school enrollment forms. All identified girls were invited to an informational session, and received a letter that contained a parent consent form and an adolescent assent form. All girls were required to return a signed parental consent form and to sign the adolescent assent form.

Development and Implementation of the Peer Leader Training

A review of other peer leader and lay health advisor programs informed the development of a six-session bilingual curriculum and accompanying peer leader manual. Table 1 provides an overview of the six sessions, the content and goals of each session, and teaching methods employed. Training of peer leaders occurred over a four-week period during the months of November and December, 2004. The training sessions were held during the 30-minute lunch period and in the girls soccer coach's classroom. Free lunch was provided during the training as a small incentive for participation and to minimize time spent in the cafeteria line. Following the training, peer leaders participated in a graduation ceremony, during which the peer leaders described the purpose of the program and lessons learned to family and friends present, and received a certificate of completion and a small gift.

Peer Leader Intervention Activities

Between January and February 2005, immediately prior to the spring sports season, the peer leaders met to brainstorm and implement intervention activities appropriate for the target audience. Each meeting included creating an agenda and action steps to be completed before the following meeting. All meetings were held after school and lasted approximately 1.5 hours. This necessitated providing transportation home for at least half of the peer leaders.

Implementation of this phase of the project used principles consistent with community based participatory research (CBPR; Minkler & Wallerstein, 1996) and those endorsed by adolescent medicine professionals (Litt, 2003; Society for Adolescent Medicine, 2003). One of the benefits of community participation in the research process is leadership development, a goal CBPR shares with the peer leader model (Minkler & Wallerstein, 1996). Backett-Milburn and Wilson (2000) also stress that peer leaders often lack power to influence intervention activities which is a significant limitation of most peer leader programs.

Over the course of six meetings, the peer leaders identified the various audiences, the primary messages to communicate, and intervention strategies to reach these audiences with targeted messages. The peer leaders, with help from the researchers, considered the feasibility, potential efficacy, and the cost of each strategy. The identified audiences included peers, school personnel, and parents. The two most important messages they wanted to send to peers and parents were the requirements necessary to participate in school sports, and the benefits of exercise and sports in the lives of young girls. School personnel (i.e., teachers, administrators, and coaches) needed to know that Latina girls were interested in sports and wanted support for pursuing extracurricular opportunities.

The intervention strategies agreed upon by the peer leaders through consensus gathering included: t-shirts; bracelets (similar to the "Livestrong" campaign); posters; interpersonal communication between peer leaders and peers, and between peer leaders and school personnel; and, support for getting required physicals. The t-shirts and bracelets were designed by the peer leaders and included the school colors. The t-shirts were to be worn by the peer leaders to solidify their identity as leaders and to prompt discussion about school sports among peers. The t-shirts were also given to key school personnel who were in a position to demonstrate support for the peer leaders' efforts (e.g., coaches, principal, counselors, and selected teachers). The bracelets, initially identified as a potential fundraiser, were also used by the peer leaders to start a conversation with an unfamiliar peer in the school and for talking about the program with parents. Across both strategies, the materials were given away free and contained a consistent logo written in Spanish and English: "Believe in yourself, *Cree en ti*". During the intervention development meetings, the peer leaders practiced communication skills acquired in the training and role played ways of distributing the materials and encouraging participation in school sports.

The third and fourth intervention strategies were targeted at the school and included interpersonal communication and bilingual posters. The peer leaders scheduled, prepared for, and held several meetings with the school principal to discuss methods for supporting sports other than football. They also talked about limitations on the type of font that could be used on all materials (the principal prohibited use of Old English font because of its association with gangs). The posters were designed by the peer leaders and displayed in the school one week prior to tryouts. Information on the posters included: requirements to participate and dates of tryouts. The final intervention strategy involved obtaining support for acquiring a sports physical. One of the researchers scheduled a visit with a clinic and provided transportation for a group of girls interested in trying out for sports. Formal intervention activities ceased once tryouts were completed; however, the peer leaders requested the opportunity to continue meeting to discuss fundraising ideas for both the girls and boys soccer teams. They wrote a letter to distribute to local businesses and met with the school principal and vice principal to better understand school fundraising policies, and began soliciting local businesses to become team sponsors.

The peer leaders also considered the following intervention strategies but decided against them because of cost or logistical challenges: short video on the requirements for participating in sports (cost barrier and peer leaders not comfortable appearing in a video); parent night to inform parents of the requirements (logistical challenge given parent work schedules); parent letters sent home on the requirements (challenge due to low literacy among many new immigrants); and a girls' sports day (cost, logistical challenge, and not enough time to organize).

Table 1. Peer leader training content, goals, and teaching methods

Session	Content and Goals of session	Teaching methods
1. Welcome	• Become acquainted with each other • Develop a group identity • Review goals of the program	• Warm-up activity • Group name • Interactive lecture
2. Importance of exercise	• Understand relationship between exercise and health • Identify developmental exercise needs • Describe safety issues in exercise	• Stretching activity • Interactive lecture • Role model letters[1]
3. Athletics at your school	• Learn requirements to participate in school sports • Identify with whom to interface to participate • Describe barriers to participation	• Guest lecture and discussion with coach • Small group discussion
4. Peer communication	• Learn methods for communicating with peers • Identify personal communication style • Discuss importance of confidentiality	• Interactive lecture • In-class assignment • Role playing
5. Creating understanding	• Develop listening and problem-solving skills • Describe the steps in conflict resolution	• Interactive lecture • Role playing
6. Advocacy	• Identify a support network • Understand the role of an advocate • Challenges of working with parents and schools	• Group discussion • Problem solving • Role playing

[1]We partnered with *Latina* magazine to advertise the program and solicit letters from readers about the influence of school sports participation on later success, self-esteem, and health. We shared letters received from the readers with the girls.

Measures

Our primary outcome of interest was participation in organized school sports during the spring season among 7th and 8th graders. Sixth graders are restricted from trying out for organized school sports. Data from the intervention and comparison schools were obtained from the athletic director of each school. These data were confirmed using observational methods during sports practice sessions and games. Secondary outcomes of interest included changes in knowledge, confidence and self-esteem among the peer leaders. Peer leaders completed a 15-minute self-administered survey at baseline (pre training), at post training (before graduation) and at post intervention. In addition, six of the peer leaders also participated in an interview at post intervention to determine their satisfaction with the program and generalization of skills and knowledge acquired as peer leaders. The contents of the survey and interview are outlined below.

Demographics

Information on the peer leaders' age, race/ethnicity, country of origin and parent's country of origin, years living in the U.S., and self-rated health were collected on the survey.

Knowledge

Twelve true/false questions were developed based on content contained in the training manual. Sample topics included the recommended amount of daily physical activity and the requirements necessary to participate in school sports. Each correct response received a score of one for a maximum score of 12.

Confidence to be a Peer Leader

Five items measured confidence in competencies required of a peer leader. The scale included the following statements: I am sure I have the skills to be a good peer leader; I am sure I can make presentations in front of school administrators; I am sure I can clearly express myself to peers; I know what it takes for someone to get involved in school activities; and I am sure I can help people solve a problem. Responses were made on a four-point Likert-type scale from 1=not at all confident to 4=very confident, with respondents receiving an overall mean confidence score.

Self-Esteem

Self esteem was measured using Rosenberg's (1965) 10-item scale which is easily administered and has high face validity and test-retest reliability. Response options range from 1=strongly disagree to 4=strongly agree, with five items requiring reverse scoring before computing a final mean self-esteem score.

Activity Behaviors

Items from the Youth Risk Behavior Survey (CDC, 2004b) and two questions from a previous study (Ayala et al., 2005) were used to measure physical activity, sedentary behaviors, and involvement in extracurricular activities. Respondents were asked on how many of the last seven days they participated in vigorous physical activity for 20 minutes or more, number of days per week they attend physical education classes at school, and number of hours they spend watching television and using the computer/internet in a typical day. All of these questions were closed-ended. Two questions assessed involvement in extracurricular activities at school and in the community from a list of 13 options.

Process Evaluation

Satisfaction with the program and generalization of the skills and knowledge acquired as peer leaders were assessed. The quantitative component was administered immediately post-training and the qualitative component occurred at post-intervention. Survey items included: satisfaction with the program content, structure, and manuals; and effort put into becoming a peer leader. All items were closed-ended. Several open ended questions assessed information shared with friends and family, whether there was anything more they wanted to learn, and the best and most difficult aspects of becoming a peer leader. Peer leaders were interviewed following implementation of intervention activities to assess generalization of skills learned, information shared, and overall satisfaction with the program. Interviews were conducted by telephone or in-person, audio-recorded, and transcribed. Key themes were identified by two independent coders.

RESULTS

Peer Leader Characteristics

We intended to recruit and train four peer leaders. Thirteen girls were invited to attend the informational session, and of these, eight returned their parental consent forms (62% response rate; four 8th graders and four 7th graders). An additional seventh grader requested permission to participate. Three of the eighth graders had participated in soccer the previous year.

Table 2. Peer leader characteristics at Pre-Training

	Pre-Training
Peer leader demographic characteristics	
Mean age (SD)	12.9 (1.1)
% on free or reduced meal program	89% (n=8)
% born in the Mexico	67% (n=6)
% self-describe as average student	89% (n=8)
Self-rated health	
Excellent to very good	44% (n=4)
Good to fair	56% (n=5)
Median # of days of vigorous PA in week	4.00
Median # of days of PE in week	4.00
Median hours of TV per day	2.00
Median hours of computer/game use	1.00
Peer leader extra curricular activity characteristics	
Percent of girls on school team or club	67% (n=6)
Percent of girls involved in community activities	44% (n=4)

The peer leaders' mean age was 13 (SD=1.1). Six girls (67%) were born in Mexico and three were born in the United States of Mexican parents. Of those who were born in Mexico, the average length of residence in the U.S. ranged from 3 to 14 years (M=7.2; SD=2.0). Nearly all girls (89%, n=8) were enrolled in the free or reduced-price breakfast and lunch program. Most of the girls (89%; n=8) described themselves as average students and 44% (n=4) rated their health as very good to excellent. Table 2 provides a description of the peer leaders demographic and activity characteristics.

Participation in Organized School Sports During the Spring Season

During the year preceding the peer leader program, 13% of 7th and 8th grade females in the control school participated in spring sports, compared with 11% in the intervention school. During the 2004-2005 academic year, 14% and 12% of 7th and 8th grade females in the control and intervention schools respectively, participated in spring sports. Thus overall, no significant increases were observed in the proportion of middle school girls who participated in spring sports.

Table 3. Latina representation in the schools and participation in school sports

	2003-2004	2004-2005
Female student population		
Size of 7th and 8th grade student population		
Control school	230	200
Intervention school	244	247
Percentage of 7th and 8th graders of Latina descent		
Control school	16% (n=37)	20% (n=40)
Intervention school	23% (n=56)	30% (n=74)
*Female student athletes during **spring season***		
Percentage of 7th and 8th graders who were athletes		
Control school	13% (n=30)	14% (n=28)
Intervention school	11% (n=27)	12% (n=30)
Percentage of athletes who were Latina		
Control school	10% (n=3)	0% (n=0)
Intervention school	15% (n=4)	27% (n=8)

With respect to Latinas, significant increases were observed in the proportion of Latinas who participated in spring sports (see Table 3). In 2003-2004, 10% of the athletes were Latina compared with 15% in the intervention school. During the 2004-2005 school year, when the intervention took place, the control school experienced a decrease in the number of Latina girls who participated in school sports and the intervention middle school experienced an increase. The control school had no Latina participation in girls' school sports during the 2004-2005 school year despite the fact that Latina girls represented 20% of all 7th and 8th grade girls. The intervention middle school increased its percentage of all female athletes who were Latina to 27%, comparable to the proportion of Latina girls in the school. Participation increased in soccer but not volleyball.

Changes in Confidence, Knowledge, and Self-Esteem, among Peer Leaders

Using non-parametric tests given the small sample size, statistically significant improvements were observed in knowledge between baseline and post-training, and in confidence between baseline and post-intervention (see Table 4). Reported self-esteem decreased between baseline and post-training; however following involvement in intervention delivery, self-esteem increased though this change was not statistically significant.

Table 4. Self-esteem, confidence, and knowledge among peer leaders at three points

	Pretest	Post training	Post-Intervention	
	N=9	N=9	n=6	Sig.
Mean Self Esteem Score (SD)[1]	2.84 (0.37)	2.69 (0.34)	2.97 (0.46)	n.s.
Mean Confidence Score (SD)[2]	2.51 (0.58)	2.58 (0.54)	3.20 (0.40)	<.05
Mean Knowledge Score (SD)[3]	7.25 (1.98)	8.56 (2.55)	not assessed	<.05

[1]Self-esteem measured on a four-point scale, with higher scores indicating higher self-esteem;
[2]Confidence measured on a four-point scale with higher scores indicating greater confidence in being a peer leader;
[3]Knowledge measured on a 12-point scale with higher scores indicating more accurate knowledge.

Process Evaluation

The post-training survey assessed satisfaction with the program content, structure, and manuals. Satisfaction with the program content was moderate to high. Five of the peer leaders reported that the training sessions were very helpful in making them feel like peer leaders, yet only three found them very interesting. In terms of structure, six of the peer leaders reported that the training sessions were just the right length at 30 minutes. Similarly, seven peer leaders reported that the training manuals were easy to understand. The peer leaders reported putting in a moderate degree of effort in becoming a peer leader (M=7.5, SD=2.07, Range 5-9), and 7 reported sharing new knowledge gained with friends and family.

In the open-ended questions, the peer leaders stated that they enjoyed being part of a group, being with friends, and learning new information. In addition, several girls noted that they liked the training content on peer communication styles. These results parallel those found in the open-ended interviews conducted at post-intervention. Three themes emerged from the interviews: positive communication skills, importance of participation in sports, and the importance of building relationships. A notable implication of the intervention was the strengthening of relationships between the peer leaders, school personnel, and peers as suggested in these two quotes: "*I talk to them [teachers] and they talk to me. I didn't want to ask questions of them, but now I do.*" "*At first I didn't listen to other people's problems, they'd be upset and I didn't care, but now I listen to my friends and those who aren't my friends...they can trust me.*"

CONCLUSION

Researchers have noted disparities in physical activity and participation in organized school sports (CDC, 2003). These disparities in part explain racial/ethnic differences in the prevalence of overweight among children and adolescents (Hedley et al., 2004). Research extols the benefits of organized sports (Richman & Shaffer, 2000) and school-based interventions are designed to promote physical activity among adolescents (McKenzie et al., 2004); yet to our knowledge no studies have attempted to bridge the two. The purpose of this study was to design and test a peer leader intervention to increase participation in organized school sports among middle school Latina girls. The intervention doubled participation in organized school sports during the spring semester, compared with a control school that experienced a reduction to zero in the same year. Our study also found significant increases in peer leader confidence and knowledge, but no significant changes in self-esteem between pre-training and post-intervention activities. This is consistent with other research (Milburn, 1995) as is the informal sharing of new information with friends, sometimes referred to as the cascade effect (Cuijpers, 2002).

Unlike most peer leader programs where the intervention was created by a health educator, for example, a set curriculum (Story et al., 2002), a play (Starkey & Orme, 2001), or a series of public behaviors (Lombard et al,, 1991), the peer leaders were encouraged to work together to develop their own intervention to achieve their goals. This methodology is consistent with community based participatory research (Minkler & Wallerstein, 1996). It also followed the Society of Adolescent Health's recommendations for working with youth by encouraging participation on all levels of the research project, especially in the intervention development phase (Litt, 2003).The peer leaders were quick to identify potential targets for the intervention (parents, peers, and school personnel), as well as appropriate methods and messages to reach their target audiences. Their decision to give away t-shirts and bracelets reflected their preference for informal communication because it fit with their normal social patterns at school. Their decision to use the theme "Believe in Yourself – *Cree en Tí*" reflected the importance they placed on self-esteem among Latina girls. Peer leaders used the skills they learned in training to organize a meeting with the principal. The peer leaders grew increasingly more comfortable interfacing with the school system and proposed ongoing meetings. These experiences are hoped to have a long-term positive effect.

Limitations

These results need to be considered within the context of its limitations. This was a quasi-experimental study with only two schools and peer leaders within one school setting.

Generalizability is an issue at many levels. We matched schools on size and number of Latina athletes during the spring season prior to project implementation to control for potential confounders. Nevertheless, as a small demonstration study, it can only suggest areas where we might build a larger intervention. A second limitation of this type of intervention is the cap placed on the number of girls who can actually participate on a team. School teams are normally limited to 20 athletes and are usually smaller given limited school resources. An equally important consideration is the grade requirement to participate in school sports. In this study, the soccer coach reported that 12 Latina girls tried out for soccer, but only 8 made the team, two of whom were ineligible due to low grades. An examination of school policy is needed to better understand the potential value of increasing the size or number of teams in a school and/or using sports participation as an incentive to achieve versus a reward for good grades. A fourth limitation was the duration of the intervention. All activities (training, intervention, evaluation) occurred within one academic year, thus we were only able to evaluate the impact of the intervention on spring sports. Most peer leader programs run an entire academic year, and often become integrated into the school system for two or more years (Mellanby et al., 2000). Nevertheless, this intervention was successful at increasing participation in a short period of time with limited resources.

Future Directions

The question lingers as to why more adolescent physical activity interventions do not explicitly encourage involvement in organized school sports. As the literature shows, the opportunity to participate on sports teams can benefit girls' psychosocial development in ways broader than physical activity alone. Promoting involvement also attempts to address parent-reported barriers to physical activity (e.g., safety issues, lack of opportunities, expense; CDC 2003). In Story's analysis, eight factors within the school setting were identified as areas for nutrition and physical activity interventions, however, none of them pertained to organized after-school sports (1999). While Title IX has helped expand sports opportunities to girls, there is still ground to cover. More research is needed on the potential value of removing barriers to greater school sports participation, for example, how best to increase resources to schools to create more opportunities for adolescents to be physically active (CDC, 2004).

Further research should be conducted as to what motivates teenage girls, and particularly minority girls to participate in sports activities. Research is also needed on how sports programs at schools can be expanded to become more inclusive to all girls, regardless of cultural and socioeconomic background, and how schools can reduce barriers to participation. This study revealed that using peer leadership is one method to encourage Latina girls, who are often underrepresented in sports, to try out and consequently participate. School sports may be an underutilized area in population-based intervention research and an area which holds potential for preventing childhood obesity.

REFERENCES

Allen, J.B. (2003). Social motivation in youth sport. *Journal of Sport and Exercise Psychology, 25,* 551-567.

Ayala, G.X., Maty, S., Cravey, A., & Webb, L. (2005). Mapping social and environmental influences on health: A community perspective, (pp. 188-209). In Israel et al (Eds) '*Multiple methods for conducting community-based participatory research for health*'.

Backett-Milburn, K., & Wilson, S. (2000). Understanding peer education: Insights from a process evaluation. *Health Education Research, 15(1),* 85-96.

Baumert, P.W., Henderson, J.M., & Thompson, N.J. (1998). Health risk behaviors of adolescent participants in organized sports. *Journal of Adolescent Health, 22,* 460-65.

Brustad, R.J. (1996). Attraction to physical activity in urban schoolchildren, parental socialization and gender influences. *Research Quarterly for Exercise and Sport, 67,* 316-23.

Centers for Disease Control and Prevention. (2003). Physical activity levels among children aged 9--13 Years --- United States, 2002. *Morbidity and Mortality Weekly Report. 52 (33).* Retrieved from *http://www.cdc.gov/mmwr/preview/ mmwrhtml/mm5233a1.htm* on March 8, 2005.

Centers for Disease Control and Prevention (2004a). School health policies and programs study. Retrieved from *http://www.cdc.gov/HealthyYouth/shpps/factsheets/pe.htm* on March 17, 2005.

Centers for Disease Control and Prevention. (2004b). Youth Risk Behavior Surveillance– United States, 2003. *Morbidity and Mortality Weekly Report 53*(SS-2). Retrieved from *http://www.cdc.gov/mmwr/preview/mwrhtml/ss5302a1.htm* on March 8, 2005.

Cuijpers, P. (2002). Peer-led and adult-led school drug prevention, a meta-analytic comparison. *Journal of Drug Education. 32(2),* 107-119.

Elder, J.P., Ayala, G.X., Campbell, N.R., Slymen, D., Lopez-Madurga, E.T., & Engelberg, M. (2005). Interpersonal and print nutrition communication for a Latino population. *Health Psychology, 24(1),* 49-57.

Ference, R. & Muth, K.D. (2004). Helping middle school females form a sense of self through team sports and exercise. *Women in Sport and Physical Activity Journal, 13(1),* 28-35.

Forshee, R.A., Anderson, P.A., & Story, M.L. (2004). The role of beverage consumption, physical activity, sedentary behavior, and demographics on body mass index of adolescents. *International Journal of Food Sciences and Nutrition, 55(6),* 463-478.

Gortmaker S.L., Peterson K., Wiecha J., Sobol A.M., Dixit S., Fox M.K., & Lair, N. (1999). Reducing obesity via a school-based interdisciplinary intervention among youth: Planet Health. *Archives of Pediatric and Adolescent Medicine, 153(4),* 409-18.

Hall, M., Cross, D., Howat, P., Stevenson, M., & Shaw, T. (2004). Evaluation of a school-based peer leader bicycle helmet intervention. *Injury Control and Safety Promotion, 11(3),* 165-74.

Heaney CA & Israel BA. (2002). Social networks and social support. In K Glanz, FM Lewis, & B Rimer (Eds), *Health behavior and health education: Theory, research, and practice,* 2nd ed., San Francisco, Jossey-Bass Publishers. Pp. 185-209.

Hedley, A.A., Ogden, C.L., Johnson, C.L., Carroll, M.D., Curtin, L.R., & Flegal, K.M. (2004). Prevalence of overweight and obesity among US children, adolescents, and adults, 1999-2002. *JAMA.* 291, 2847-50.

Laiho, M., Honkala, E., Nyyssonen, V., & Milen, A (1993). Three methods of oral health education in secondary schools. *Scandinavian Journal of Dental Research, 101,* 422-27.

Lindsey, B.J. (1997). Peer education: A viewpoint and critique. *Journal of American College Health, 45(4),* 187-9.

Litt, I.F. (2003). Research *with,* not *on,* adolescents: Community-based participatory research. *Journal of Adolescent Health, 33,* 315-16.

Lombard, D., Neubauer, T.E., Canfield, D., & Winett, R.A. (1991). Behavioral community intervention to reduce the risk of skin cancer. *Journal of Applied Behavior Analysis, 24(4),* 677-86.

McKenzie, T.L., Sallis, J.F., Prochaska, J.J., Conway, T.L., Marshall, S.J., & Rosengard, P. (2004). Evaluation of a two-year middle-school physical education intervention, M-SPAN. *Medicine and Science in Sports and Exercise, 36(8),* 1382-8.

Mellanby, A.R., Rees, J.B., & Tripp, J.H. (2000). Peer-led and adult-led school health education: A critical review of available comparative research. *Health Education Research, 15(5),* 533-545.

Melnick, M.J., Sabo, D.F., & Vanfossen B. (1992). Educational effects of interscholastic athletic participation on African-American and Hispanic youth. *Adolescence, 27(106),* 295-308.

Milburn, K. (1995). A critical review of peer education with young people with special reference to sexual health. *Health Education Research, 10(4),* 407-20.

Minkler, M. & Wallerstein, N. (1996). Improving health through community organization and community building: A Health education perspective. In K Glanz, FM Lewis, & B Rimer (Eds), *Health behavior and health education: Theory, research, and practice,* 2nd ed., San Francisco, Jossey-Bass Publishers.

National Center for Educational Statistics (2005). Information on schools. Retrieved from http://nces.ed.gov/fastfacts/display.asp on March 17, 2005.

Pate, R.R., Trost, S.G., Levin, S., & Dowda, M. (2000). Sports participation and health related behaviors among US youth. *Archives of Pediatrics and Adolescent Medicine, 154(9),* 904-11.

Prochaska, J.J., Rodgers, M.W., & Sallis, J.F. (2002). Association of parent and peer support with adolescent physical activity. *Research Quarterly for Exercise and Sport, 73,* 206-210.

Richman, E.L. & Shaffer D.R. (2000). If you let me play sport, How might sport participation influence the self-esteem of adolescent females?" *Psychology of Women Quarterly, 24,* 189-199.

Rosenberg, M. (1965). *Society and the adolescent self-image.* Princeton, NJ, Princeton University Press.

Sabo, D., Miller, K.E., Farrell, M.P., Melnick, M.J., & Barnes, G.M. (1999). High school athletic participation, sexual behavior and adolescent pregnancy. A regional study. *Journal of Adolescent Health, 25,* 207-216.

Society for Adolescent Medicine. (2003). Position Paper. Guidelines for Adolescent Research. *Journal of Adolescent Health, 33,* 396-409.

Starkey, F., Moore, L., Campbell, R., Sidaway, M., & Bloor, M. (2005).Rationale, design and conduct of a comprehensive evaluation of a school-based peer-led anti-smoking intervention in the UK: the ASSIST cluster randomised trial. *BMC Public Health,* 22, 43.

Stevens, J., Murray, D.M., Catellier, D.J., Hannan, P.J., Elder, J.P., Young, D.R., Simons-Morton, D.G., & Webber, L.S. (2005). Design of the Trial of Activity in Adolescent Girls (TAAG). *Contemporary Clinical Trials, 26(2),* 223-233.

Story, M. (1999). School-based approaches for preventing and treating obesity. *International journal of obesity and related metabolic disorders, 23(2),* 43-51.

Story, M., Lytle L.A., & Birnbaum A.S. (2002). Peer-led, school-based nutrition education for young adolescents: Feasibility and process evaluation of the TEENS. *Journal of School Health, 72 (3),* 121-127.

Therrien, M. & Ramirez, R.R. (2000). *The Hispanic population in the U.S: March 2000.* Current Population Reports, P20-535, U.S. Census Bureau, Washington, D.C.

Veugelers, P.J. & Fitzgerald, A.L. (2005). Effectiveness of school programs in preventing childhood obesity: a multilevel comparison. American Journal of Public Health, 95(3):432-5.

Wiist, W.H., Jackson, R.H., and Jackson, K.W. (1996). Peer and community leader education to prevent youth violence. *American Journal of Preventive Medicine 12(5),* 56-64.

Yin, Z. & Moore, J.B. (2004). Re-examining the role of interscholastic sport participation in education. *Psychological Reports, 94(3),* 1447-54.

Zibalese-Crawford, M. (1997). A creative approach to HIV/AIDS programs for adolescents. *Social Work in Health Care, 25(1-2),* 73-88.

In: Health Education Research Trends
Editor: P. R. Hong, pp. 211-225

ISBN: 978-1-60021-871-2
© 2007 Nova Science Publishers, Inc.

Chapter VII

PROCESS-ORIENTED TRAINING IN BREASTFEEDING ATTITUDES AND CONTINUITY OF CARE IMPROVE MOTHERS PERCEPTION OF SUPPORT

Anette Ekström[1,] and Eva Nissen[1,2]*

[1]School of Life Sciences, University of Skövde, Skövde Sweden;
[2]Department of Woman and Child Health, Division of Reproductive and Perinatal Health Care, Karolinska Institutet, Stockholm, Sweden.

ABSTRACT

The over all objectives of this study was to map factors of importance for breastfeeding such as maternal perception of breastfeeding support, breastfeeding attitudes of health care professionals, and to investigate whether a training intervention within the team of the antenatal care (ANC) and child health centers (CHC) would improve maternal perception of support.

Material and method: A questionnaire was sent to mothers when their babies were 9-12 months old with questions regarding mothers perception of support and duration of breastfeeding (n=540). Thereafter an attitudinal instrument was developed to measure breastfeeding attitudes in health care professionals (n=168). Thereafter ten municipalities was paired and randomized to intervention or control. Thus, all midwives and postnatal nurses working at the ANC or CHC in a randomized municipality were asked to participate in the study (n=81). Health professionals in the intervention group had a process-oriented training in breastfeeding counseling including planned continuity in family education and development of a common breastfeeding policy within the caring team. Thereafter mothers were recruited from the maternity and were allocated to

---

* Correspondence concerning this article should be addressed to: Dr. Anette Ekström, RNM School of Life Sciences, University of Skövde, Box 408, SE 541 28 Skövde, Sweden. Tel. +46 500 44 84 54, fax + 46 500 44 84 99, E- mail: anette.ekstrom@his.se.

intervention- or control group according to the randomization of municipalities in an earlier study (n=565). Questionnaires were sent out at three days, 3 and 9 months post partum to investigate how the care and counseling skills acquired by the health care professionals would be reflected in maternal perception of breastfeeding support.

Results: Mothers were dissatisfied with the breastfeeding information they got from the ANC and CHC. This induced the idea to develop an attitude instrument and start a training intervention for the care team at ANC and CHC. The attitudinal dimensions identified by the factor analysis were: The regulating factor comprising statements scheduling breastfeeding; the facilitating factor comprising statements showing confidence in the ability of the mother-infant dyad to breastfeed on their own; the disempowering factor comprising statements that objectified the woman and ascribed her no ability to breastfeed without guidance of the health care professional and the breastfeeding hostility factor comprising statements that showed unwillingness and failing knowledge about breastfeeding. After training the health care professionals became less regulating and more facilitating. Family classes provided the intervention mothers with better breastfeeding information, more knowledge about their social rights, the needs of the baby and a stronger social network than the control mothers. The postnatal nurse gave a better over all support, was a better listener, showed more understanding and provided the mother with better information about breastfeeding and the needs of the baby.

Keywords: Breastfeeding, support, health professional, significant other, process-oriented training, WHO, BFHI.

TRAILER

The over all objectives of this chapter is to describe the background, development and results of a research program which was designed after obstacles to breastfeeding had been identified in a baseline study where breastfeeding and breastfeeding counseling were mapped in southwestern Sweden. In this research programme a breastfeeding attitude scale was developed and tested on health professionals before and after a process oriented training program in breastfeeding techniques and counseling had been carried through. The training program, its goals and the attitude scale will be described in depth as well as the effects of training on the health professionals and maternal experiences of received support as well as their feeling for the baby.

INTRODUCTION

The protection, promotion and support of breastfeeding is a public health priority. Low rates and early cessation of breastfeeding have important adverse health and social implications for women, children, the community and the environment. It can result in greater expenditure on national health care provision, and increase inequalities in health (European Commission & Assessment, 2004).

The Global Strategy on Infant and Young Child Feeding, adopted by all WHO member states at the 55th World Health Assembly in May 2002 provides a basis for public health initiatives to protect, promote and support breastfeeding. It is necessary that health workers have accurate and up-to-date information about infant feeding policies and practices, and that they have the specific knowledge and skills required to support caregivers and children in all aspects of infant and young child feeding in exceptionally difficult circumstances. Health professional bodies, which include medical faculties, schools of public health, public and private institutions for training health workers should have the responsibilities towards their students or membership to educate in protecting, promoting and supporting appropriate feeding practices (WHO, 2003). If care routines in healthcare organizations during childbirth change in a positive way it may have great advantages to the parents, the child, the profession and the future healthcare organization (Eriksson, 2005).

Blueprint for Action, written by breastfeeding experts representing all EU and associated countries and the relevant stakeholder groups, including mothers, is a model plan that outlines the actions that a national or regional plan should contain and implement. Specific activities for the protection, promotion and support of breastfeeding should be supported by an effective plan for information, education and communication, and by appropriate pre- and in-service training. Monitoring and evaluation, as well as research on agreed operational priorities, are essential for effective planning. Under six headings, the Blueprint recommends objectives for all these actions, identifies responsibilities, and indicates possible output and outcome measures.

1. *Policy and planning*; A comprehensive national policy should be based on the Global Strategy on Infant and Young Child Feeding and integrated into overall health policies. The Health care system should access to the quality of care during antenatal care, delivery, the first few days, postnatal maternal and child health care.

2. *Information, education, communication;* Expectant and new parents have the right to full, correct and optimal infant feeding information, including guidance on safe, timely and appropriate complementary feeding, so that they can make informed choice provided by adequately trained health workers.

3. *Training;* Pre- and in-service training for all health worker groups needs improvement.

4. *Protection, promotion and support;* Based on the full implementation of the International Code, access for all women to get breastfeeding support provided by appropriately qualified health workers.

5. *Monitoring;* The implementation of an action plan to protect, promote and support breastfeeding.

6. *Research:* Research needs to do interventions studies, and in general, of public health initiatives (European Commission & Assessment, 2004).

Associations between the social support given by professional caregivers and the duration of breastfeeding have been established in the literature. Mothers are dissatisfied with the breastfeeding counseling provided both by the antenatal-, and maternity midwives and by the postnatal nurses at the child health centers. Too little attention is paid to the women's psychosocial problems and their satisfaction with counseling is not checked by the caregivers. (Giugliani, Caiffa, Vogelhut, Witter, & Perman, 1994; Humphreys, Thompson, & Miner, 1998; Review., 2007; Women & Gynecologists., 2007).

Social Support During Childbirth

In stressful events in life or transition periods like childbirth, social support has been described as an interactive process that is protective. Social support is affected by the persons involved, their age, personality and earlier experiences, as well as by the context in which it takes place (Kahn, 1980). Oakley has described social support as an attitude where a non judgmental approach is important (Oakley 1994).

Further trials are required to assess the effectiveness of professional support in different settings, particularly those with low rates of breastfeeding initiation, and for women who wish to breastfeed for longer than three months. Trials should consider timing and support interventions and relative effectiveness of intervention components, and should report women's views. Research into appropriate training for supporters (whether lay or professional) of breastfeeding mothers is also needed (Britton, McCormick, Renfrew, Wade, & King, 2007).

Social Support Given by Professional Caregivers

In our baseline study the aim was to describe breastfeeding support and feeling of confidence in relation to the duration of breastfeeding in primi- and multiparous women. The result shows that both primiparas and multiparas experienced low satisfaction with the breastfeeding information they got from the health professionals in the care team around childbirth. However mothers were more content with the breastfeeding information they got from the midwives at the maternity wards, compared with the breastfeeding information they got from the antenatal midwives and the postnatal nurses ($p < 0.001$) (Ekström, Widström, & Nissen, 2003 b). It is possible that the woman is most receptive to information at the maternity ward during her early establishment of lactation and therefore remembers this information better than the information acquired from the antenatal centers and the child health centers. Yet another explanation is that antenatal midwives and the postnatal nurses may provide contradictory and less sensitive counseling. In either case the antenatal midwives and postnatal nurses do not provide effective counseling for breastfeeding mothers (Ekström, Widström, & Nissen, 2003 b). This has also been shown in previous studies (Bergman, Larsson, Lomberg, Möller, & Mårild, 1993; Tarkka & Paunonen, 1996). The difficulties may arise not only from lack of knowledge in caregivers but also from their harmful, personal experiences of breastfeeding support. Most of the caregivers had their own children during the sixties and seventies when the breastfeeding rates were very low in Sweden. This implies that there is a generation of nurses and midwives who had little support themselves or a sad experience of breastfeeding. We can thus not exclude the possibility that some of the breastfeeding counselors of today may have to overcome unpleasant memories of their own breastfeeding in order to become good counselors (Ekström, Widström, & Nissen, 2003 b).

WHO has issued directives as to how health professionals in the care teams around the breastfeeding mother should protect, promote and support breastfeeding. It has been emphasized that breastfeeding knowledge is not enough –a positive breastfeeding attitude is a condition to provide good breastfeeding support. A number of studies has evaluated the effects of breastfeeding training of caregivers according to the Breastfeeding Friendly Hospital Initiative (BFHI) proposed by the WHO (WHO, 1989, 2003).

Breastfeeding Attitudes and Development of an Attitudinal Scale

Bernaix, studied the relationship between postnatal nurses' attitudes to breastfeeding, their knowledge, their intentions to provide support to mothers and found that the nurses' intention to provide support did not influence their actual behavior in a positive way (Bernaix, 2000). Short training in breastfeeding for caregivers resulted in better knowledge and increasing exclusive breastfeeding rates among the mothers, but no change in attitudes to breastfeeding among the caregivers was found (Kools, Thijs, Kester, van den Brandt, & de Vries, 2005; Martens, 2000). Thus, it may be difficult to alter adverse breastfeeding attitudes. If nurses and midwives lack knowledge or have less friendly attitudes to breastfeeding, this may result in inaccurate or inconsistent counseling (Sikorski J, Renfrew MJ, Pindoria S, & A, Issue 3, 2002). In general attitudes to breastfeeding are shaped by individual experiences, especially during sensitive periods of transition to motherhood, and seem to be deeply rooted among mothers and possibly also among caregivers (Raphael-Leff, 2001). Unfavorable attitudes may bring about non-supportive counseling (Zanna, 1986). It may therefore be valuable to antenatal midwives and postnatal nurses involved in breastfeeding counseling to reflect upon their own breastfeeding experience in a process oriented, training program (Raphael-Leff, 2001).

Our purpose in a following study was to developed a breastfeeding attitude instrument based on WHO standards managing breastfeeding (WHO, 1989) . This instrument was used in order to describe and measure breastfeeding attitudes in a group of antenatal midwives, maternity- nursing staff and postnatal nurses. The study took place in the south west of Sweden, during 2000. Caregivers at the largest antenatal, child health centers and at the maternity were asked to participate in the study. Four factors were identified by the factor analysis in order of importance; Regulating, Facilitating, Disempowering and Breastfeeding hostility factors (Table 1 and 2). Harmful attitudes were identified and suggested a need for educational programmes to help caregivers to reconcile damaging values, in order to improve breastfeeding counseling (Ekström, Matthiesen, Widström, & Nissen, 2005a). Caregivers with high scores on this *facilitating factor* are likely to empower the mother to manage on her own and avoid disturbing the baby's feeding behavior. The counselors scoring high on the *regulating factor* are likely to instruct the mother how to organize her breastfeeding on a routine basis, instead of being sensitive to the baby's needs. Caregivers scoring high on the *disempowering factor* put much emphasis on the guiding responsibilities of the care-giver and have no or little trust in the mothers' ability to take in breastfeeding information during the pregnancy and they consider the newborn baby as a nuisance to the mother. Caregivers scoring high on the regulating and the disempowering factor may be unable to provide individualized care for the mother and her baby in a sensitive way. Caregivers scoring high on the *breastfeeding hostility factor* are ignorant of breastfeeding techniques and are not likely to promote breastfeeding, and are unable to feel empathy with the mother and her baby. Thus, caregivers scoring high on this factor are likely to be very harmful when counseling breastfeeding (Ekström, Matthiesen, Widström, & Nissen, 2005a).

Table 1. Factor loadings in the factor analysis. An item was included if the factor loading was > 0.33. Statement numbers are referred to in Table 2 (Ekström, Matthiesen, Widström, & Nissen, 2005a)

Statements number	Factor loadings			
	Factor 1 Cronbach alpha: 0.80	Factor 2 Cronbach alpha: 0.60	Factor 3 Cronbach alpha: 0.62	Factor 4 Cronbach alpha: 0.29
30	0.89			
45	-0.57			
40	0.56			
4	-0.55			
12	0.51			
25	0.48			
11	0.44			
38	0.39			
36	0.37			
24		0.69		
5		0.46		
41		0.46		
20		0.45		
22		-0.43		0.37
10		0.42		
37		-0.41		
27		0.38		
23		-0.34		0.34
3			0.60	
42			0.53	
1			0.52	
13			0.49	
7	0.43		0.47	
43			0.46	
6			0.40	
33				-0.55
2				-0.46
9				0.45
46				-0.38
21				-0.36
31				-0.36
14				0.35

The attitude scales need further refinement. More statements can be removed without and greater effort should be made to capture the breastfeeding hostility scale which had low loadings, The scales should be tested by a confirmatory factor analysis in a new sample (Raykov & Marcoulides, 2000).

Attitude instruments, even good ones, bring about a very shallow understanding of attitudes and changes of attitudes. Nothing is learned about the process taking place through the interactions prior to a change in attitudes. It would be worth while to delve deeper into the processes lying behind changes in attitudes and consequencies on mother and child care. Thus a process oriented training program was developed (Ekström, Matthiesen, Widström, & Nissen, 2005a; Ekström, Widström, & Nissen, 2005).

Table 2. The items of the four different factors identified and their factor loadings.
Statements in italics indicate the items have negative loadings
(Ekström, Matthiesen, Widström, & Nissen, 2005a)

Statement number	Regulating factor
30	It is appropriate to introduce taste portions when the baby is 4 months old.
45	*It is appropriate to introduce taste portions when the baby is 6 months old.*
40	I think it is appropriate to recommend mothers to prolong breastfeeding intervals during the night.
4	*A baby who shows no willingness to be nursed in the first 24 hours should be left in peace.*
12	It is not good if the baby starts to use the breast as a pacifier.
25	I know what I need to know about breastfeeding.
11	Breastfeeding at night is tiring for mothers.
7	The majority of mothers are not receptive to information about breastfeeding before the 24 th week of pregnancy.
38	The care-team provides mothers with the breastfeeding advice they need.
36	Babies who are breastfed for a long period of time are not willing to eat/try other kinds of food.
	Facilitating factor
24	A breastfeeding mother whose baby needs extra food is recommended to give it with a cup or a spoon.
5	It is important that the mother and baby stay together at all times.
41	I feel absolutely positive about breastfeeding on demand without regard to any time schedules.
20	Breastfeeding protects the baby from diseases.
22	*There is too much debate about breastfeeding.*
10	I teach the mothers to express milk by hand.
37	*I think mothers should be encouraged to stop breastfeeding when the baby is 1 year old.*
27	The maternity ward should offer the partner the opportunity of staying over night.
23	*I do not discuss breastfeeding so much, since mothers who have not breastfed might feel bad about it.*
	Disempowering factor
3	Most babies need assistance from care-givers to be nursed for the first time.
42	On the maternity ward mothers can be disturbed when their room mates babies cry.
1	Most mothers are not receptive to breastfeeding information during pregnancy.
13	Most mothers are not receptive to breastfeeding information during the 35-40th weeks of pregnancy.
7	Most mothers are not receptive to breastfeeding information before the 24th weeks of pregnancy.
43	Once the mother starts to give supplementary feeding she will stop breastfeeding.
6	It is tiring for mothers to have their babies stay with them during the night at the maternity ward.
	Breastfeeding hostility factor
33	*Milk stasis is often caused by a wrong sucking technique.*
2	*It is important that the baby should be nursed within the first 2 hours after birth.*
9	The baby's position at the breast has nothing to do with sore nipples.
46	*It is easy for me to feel empathy with the mother about her breastfeeding.*

Table 2. (Continued)

Statement number	Regulating factor
22	There is too much discussion about breastfeeding.
21	*The bonding between the mother and her child is promoted by breastfeeding.*
31	*Mothers who feel insecure need extra support from the care- teams.*
14	After childbirth most mothers do not feel strong again until they have stopped breastfeeding.
23	I do not discuss breastfeeding so much, since mothers who have not breastfed might feel bad about it.

A Process-Oriented Training Program in Breastfeeding Counseling

In Sweden, first-time expectant parents are offered family classes, which aim, among other things, is to increase their knowledge about parenthood and forming a parental network. Family classes begin at the antenatal center during the 25th week of pregnancy and are conducted by the midwife. Family classes are also offered after childbirth, but are then conducted by the postnatal nurse at the child health center. Thus, the standard routine care still provides family classes, which are usually discontinued at birth (The National Board of Health and Welfare, 1997). In 1997, the National Board of Health and Welfare in Sweden issued new guidelines to promote breastfeeding by means of new directives for conducting family classes. This action promoted extensive collaboration between the antenatal and child health center to strengthen support and continuity of family learning and help parents take on their new roles (The National Board of Health and Welfare, 1997). Special attention should be given disadvantaged women in terms of socio-demographic background and feelings about the approaching birth in order to adapt their specific needs (Fabian, Radestad, & Waldenstrom, 2004). In addition, it was believed that this model for family classes would improve social support, which is very important for the success of breastfeeding (Bergman, Larsson, Lomberg, Möller, & Mårild, 1993; Ekström, Widström, & Nissen, 2003 b; The National Board of Health and Welfare, 1997). Previous studies showed that mothers found breastfeeding counseling by health professionals unsatisfactory at both antenatal and child health center (Bernaix, 2000; Ekström, Widström, & Nissen, 2003 b). One reason for this dissatisfaction might be that health professionals were not sufficiently supportive toward mothers and their breastfeeding (Bernaix, 2000).

In the intervention group the midwives and the postnatal nurses worked with a common breastfeeding strategy where the family classes should be continued during pregnancy and the first year after the babies were born. It is not far fetched to believe that this effort led to concordance in breastfeeding counseling between the midwives at the antenatal clinics and the postnatal nurses at the child health centers as reported. Extended co-operation about family classes may form the basis for a coherent counseling for mothers seeking breastfeeding advice and is quite in line with the recommendations to strengthen the cooperation between the antenatal clinics and the child health clinics made by the National Board of Health and Welfare (The National Board of Health and Welfare, 1984).

Antenatal midwives and postnatal nurses were randomized (on municipality level) to have this training program (intervention group (IG) and the controlgroup received no training (CG)

The study took place in a county in the southwest of Sweden. The antenatal clinics and child health centers served both an urban/ suburban district and a rural district. (Ekström, Widström, & Nissen, 2005).

The process oriented training program (Jerlock, Falk, & Severinsson, 2003), consisted of seven days lectures on breastfeeding management and promotion (WHO, 1989), and discussions about lived experience of breastfeeding and counseling. Half of the time was spent on reflection in following areas.

The main theme which were brought up was own breastfeeding experiences (both private and professional), breastfeeding attitudes, cooperation and communication between antenatal centre and child health centre in order to get a common breastfeeding policy. Midwives and postnatal nurses from the same municipality got homework to reflect about different areas around breastfeeding support. The examination was to develop a common breastfeeding policy in the caring chain including antenatal and postnatal care which should be used in family classes. The family classes should start in the middle of the pregnancy and should continue during the first year of the baby. Each group had a "group leader". The group leader had a profession as a midwife at the delivery or maternity ward or a postnatal nurse from the neonatal ward. Physicians from the obstetric and neonatal clinics participated. The health professionals were all experienced and practiced breastfeeding support in different ways.

The group leaders at the training program were chosen to strengthen the process between the health care centers ant the hospital wards. The following topics were chosen by the groups as home work.

How do we:
o   Protect, promote and support breastfeeding.
o   Inform about parenthood and family life.
o   How do we broaden our minds to help parents with another cultural background?
o   How can you share parental leave on equal bases? Or should we not?
o   What is attachmnent and the how do parents best support attachment?
o   What happens if postnatal depression occurs?
o   Relations with health professionals and significant others.
o   How to discuss complicated deliveries?
o   How do we best support parent-infant interaction when the infant is cared for at the neonatal ward?
o   How do we talk about lifestyle proplems?
o   How do we approach single parents?

During the training program the participants were encouraged to develop a common breastfeeding policy between the antenatal clinic and the receiving child health centers. In addition, the participants were asked to develop a system where the parents were kept together in family classes before and after birth of the baby improving the continuity of care was guaranteed. The participants in both the intervention and the control groups were asked to fill in the attitude instrument before the training in the intervention group and one year after the training had ended. In addition, the attitude instrument was administered immediately after the end of training in the intervention group (Ekström, Widström, & Nissen, 2005).

The perception of concordance in breastfeeding counseling between the midwives at the antenatal clinic and the postnatal nurses at the child-health centers was rated by the participants on a visual analogue scale (VAS) before the intervention and one year after the intervention. The VAS ranged from 0.0 to 10.0 cm, where 0.0 indicated no concordance at all and 10.0 indicated satisfactory concordance.

RESULTS

The results showed that a process-oriented training promote caregivers breastfeeding attitudes.

Before the intervention there was no significant differences in any of the attitude scales between the intervention and the control group, but one year after the intervention the participants in the intervention group scored significantly lower on the regulating scale than did the control group (p <0.001). This difference remained also after controlling for profession (Ekström, Widström, & Nissen, 2005). The scores on the facilitating scale increased significantly in the intervention group (p = 0,003) and in the control group (p = 0.037). There were no significant changes in the scores over time either in the intervention group or in the control group on the disempowering scale and the breastfeeding hostility scale. In other studies, few or no sustainable changes in attitudes have been reported (Coreil, 1995). In this study a small but sustainable change was found in the regulating scale, suggesting that the caregivers become less dependent on scheduling breastfeeding and possibly become better listeners to the mothers' breastfeeding problems and may as a consequence provide them with more appropriate advice. Indeed, this change could be related to the character of the training, involving reflection upon both professional and personal experience of breastfeeding counseling. It has been suggested that the nurse or midwife who introduces the mother to "the art" of breastfeeding brings her own feeding history into the situation. In effect, the facilitating nurse or midwife is giving guidance and support to the mother, which in turn helps the mother to feel replenished and good enough to take care of and feed her own baby. If the caregiver has been able to reflect upon her own breastfeeding experience, she may be able to distance herself from negative, compromising memories and this insight may help her not to transfer bad experience to the breastfeeding mother seeking her advice (Ekström, Widström, & Nissen, 2005).

Differences between Professions in Breastfeeding Attitudes

The *postnatal nurses* significantly decreased their scores on the regulating scale (p = 0.001) and on the disempowering scale (p = 0.038) over the first year after intervention and increased their scores on the facilitating scale (p = 0.008) over the first year after intervention. The scores of the *midwives* in the intervention group remained stable in all scales except for the breastfeeding-hostility scale, where they significantly decreased their scores over the first year after training (p = 0.014) (Ekström, Widström, & Nissen, 2005). Thus, it seems that the training had more effect on the postnatal nurses than on the midwives. The reason for this may have been that the postnatal nurses were more receptive to training, since they are confronted with mothers and infants and their breastfeeding problems on a daily basis, while the antenatal midwives' main focus in breastfeeding issues was to promote breastfeeding before it has actually started and the confrontation with practical breastfeeding problems is not imminent. In a previous study (Ekström, Matthiesen, Widström, & Nissen, 2005a) we also found that midwives scored lower on the regulating scale and higher on the facilitating scale than the postnatal nurses did even before the training started. Thus, there was less scope for altering attitudes during the training. Some changes also took place in the control group: The scores on the facilitating scale increased and the midwives in the control group received lower scores on the disempowering scale one year after the time of training in the intervention group. These changes may have been caused by a spill-over effect from the intervention units, by other interventions in society outside the scope of this study, or be an effect of knowing they were included in a study on this subject (Ekström, Widström, & Nissen, 2005).

Caregivers Perceived Concordance in Breastfeeding Counseling

The perceived concordance in breastfeeding counseling was measured on a VAS in the intervention and control group before the breastfeeding training started and one year after the time of the training. There were no significant differences in the perceived concordance in breastfeeding counseling between the intervention group and the control group, before the training of the intervention group started (p = 0.250). One year after training, the intervention group tended to score concordance on breastfeeding counseling to be more satisfactory (p = 0.066). Both groups increased their scores on concordance significantly over time (p=0.002 for the intervention group and p=0.023 for the control group) (Ekström, Widström, & Nissen, 2005).

Continuity of Care by Well-Trained Breastfeeding Counselors Improve Mothers' Perception of Support

The present study was a follow-up investigation of mothers' feelings for their babies (Ekström & Nissen, 2006) and perception of support in relation to the kind of care they received (Ekström, Widström, & Nissen, 2006). The sampling frame was based on women cared for at either intervention or control clinics (Ekström, Widström, & Nissen, 2005). Mothers at the control clinics had received standard routine care, and had attended family classes through the time of birth. Data collection for control group A started before effects of the intervention could be studied. Data for control group B was collected simultaneously with data collection for the intervention group. This methodological approach with different data collection time points for the two control groups was used so as to detect effects of the intervention. Eligibility for the study was defined as Swedish-speaking mothers who gave birth to singleton, healthy, full-term babies delivered spontaneously, by vacuum extraction, or by cesarean section. Of the total of 584 mothers, 540 gave their informed consent to participate in the study (Ekström, Widström, & Nissen, 2006).

This longitudinal study was based on 3 questionnaires developed for the purpose of this study. All 3 questionnaires enquired about mothers' perceptions with respect to the family classes and their encounters with the antenatal midwife and the postnatal nurse. The mothers were asked to consider two aspects of social support, namely, emotional support (reflects the individual's emotional experience of receiving care) and informative support (refers to practical advice given by health care professionals (Oakley, 1994).

During pregnancy, intervention group mothers perceived that they received better breastfeeding information compared with control group B mothers.

At *3 months postpartum*, the intervention group mothers were still significantly more satisfied with the breastfeeding information than control group B mothers and they perceived overall support provided by postnatal nurses significantly better than did both control groups. The intervention group mothers perceived that postnatal nurses were more sensitive and understanding than did both control groups.

At *9 months postpartum*, intervention group mothers had increased their social network significantly more, and they were more satisfied with information about their social rights and with their knowledge about the baby's needs when compared with control group B mothers. The intervention group mothers perceived that postnatal nurses were significantly more sensitive and more understanding than did both control groups (Ekström, Widström, & Nissen, 2006).

This study investigated the effects of a breastfeeding counseling program for health care professionals and an intervention plan that aimed to guarantee continuity of care during the first 9 months postpartum. In the intervention group, family classes started early in the pregnancy and the postnatal nurses in this group attended antenatal classes more often. Thus, the intervention was successful in respect with nurses' compliance with the intervention. In contrast, the midwives did not attend the family classes after childbirth to the same extent as the postnatal nurses, and the midwives' compliance with the design of the intervention was therefore less successful (Ekström, Widström, & Nissen, 2006).

At 3 through 9 months postpartum, intervention group mothers rated postnatal nurses as being more sensitive and understanding than did the mothers in both control groups, and they also felt better prepared to take care of the babies' needs and better informed about breastfeeding. The results of the questionnaires at 3 and 9 months clearly point to improvement of postnatal nurses' supportive behavior and skills. The finding that encounters with postnatal nurses were so well assessed in the intervention group is in line with our previous study, in which postnatal nurses altered their attitudes toward a more facilitating and less regulating direction than did the midwives (Ekström, Widström, & Nissen, 2005). It is possible that behaviors such as sensitivity and understanding are aspects of good counseling that are developed by the process-oriented training program. This program allowed the counseling midwives and nurses to reflect and work on their past breastfeeding experience, both in private and in counseling (Ekström, Widström, & Nissen, 2006).

The Improvement of the Social Network for the Intervention Group Mothers in the family Classes when compared with Control Group

Postnatal nurses in the intervention group participated in family classes significantly more often during pregnancy than postnatal nurses in the control groups. In contrast, midwives in the intervention group did not participate significantly more often during postnatal family classes when compared with control groups. Family classes started significantly earlier in the intervention group when compared with control groups, but the mothers of both control groups attended family classes more often during the pregnancy compared with the intervention group. After the birth through the baby's first 9 months, more intervention group mothers participated in family classes, and the intervention group was more often kept in the same group. Intervention group mothers participated more often than mothers from the control groups. No significant difference was found among the 3 groups with respect to partner participation rate in the family classes (Ekström, Widström, & Nissen, 2006).

Improvement of the parents' social network is a primary objective in guidelines for conducting family classes (The National Board of Health and Welfare, 1984), and is often neglected in Sweden today due to financial cutbacks in the community health care program's. A supportive network may help the inexperienced mother in her transition to motherhood and relieve stresses and worries about the baby (Ekström, Widström, & Nissen, 2003 b). Supportive behaviors of the postnatal nurse, such as those observed in the intervention group, may lead to empowerment and better self-esteem in mothers. Indeed, this finding was reported in other studies about support during childbirth (Hodnett, 2002). New parents are extremely vulnerable to critical judgments about their caretaking abilities. Therefore, supportive health professionals and experienced parents could be particularly powerful role models during the emergence of self-image of new parents, and these influences could greatly enhance (Ekström, Widström, & Nissen, 2006).

The finding that intervention group mothers also perceived that family classes provided better breastfeeding information when compared with perceptions of control group B mothers supported a primary aim of the study. This outcome was indicated early, already during pregnancy through the first 3 months post partum (Ekström, Widström, & Nissen, 2006).

CONCLUSION

These studies showed that a process-oriented training in breastfeeding counseling alters attitudes of health care professionals in a positive way. The trained health care professionals organized continuity of family classes and developed a common breastfeeding policy and were more supportive in their encounters with the mothers. A model to provide continuity of family classes, conducted by trained antenatal midwives and postnatal nurses should thus be practiced within the caring team around first time parents.

REFERENCES

Bergman, V., Larsson, S., Lomberg, H., Möller, A., & Mårild, S. (1993). A survey of Swedish mothers' views on breastfeeding experiences of social and professional support. *Scand J Caring Sci., 7*, 47-52.

Bernaix, L. (2000). Nurses' Attitudes, Subjective Norms, and Behavioral Intentions Toward Support of Breastfeeding Mothers. *Journal of Human Lactation, 16*, 201-209.

Britton, C., McCormick, F., Renfrew, M., Wade, A., & King, S. (2007). Support for breastfeeding mothers. *Cochrane Database Syst Rev.*

Coreil, J., Bryant, CA, Westover, BJ, Bailey, D. (1995). Health professionals and breastfeeding counseling: client and provider views. *Journal of Human Lactation, 11*, 265-271.

Ekström, A., Matthiesen, A., Widström, A., & Nissen, E. (2005a). Breastfeeding attitudes among counselling health professionals. *Scand J of Public Health, 33*(5), 353-359.

Ekström, A., & Nissen, E. (2006). Maternal feelings for her baby are strengthened by excellent breastfeeding counseling and continuity of care. *Peadiatrics, 118*(2), 309-314.

Ekström, A., Widström, A.-M., & Nissen, E. (2003 b). Breastfeeding Support from Partners and Grandmothers: Perceptions of Swedish Women. *Birth, 30*(4), 261-266.

Ekström, A., Widström, A.-M., & Nissen, E. (2005). Process-oriented Training in Breastfeeding Alters Attitudes to Breastfeeding in Health Professionals. *Scand. J of Public Health, 33*(6), 424-431.

Ekström, A., Widström, A.-M., & Nissen, E. (2006). Does continuity of care by well trained breast-feeding counsellors improves the mothers' perception of support. *Birth, 33*(2), 123-130.

Eriksson, N. (2005). *New Dawn is Breaking in Medical service. Support and hinders for change in professional organisation.*, Göteborg universitet, Göteborg.

European Commission, & Assessment, D. P. H. a. R. (2004). *EU Project on Promotion of Breastfeeding in Europe. Protection,promotion and support of breastfeeding in Europe: a blueprint for action.* Luxembourg.

Fabian, H., Radestad, I., & Waldenstrom, U. (2004). Characteristics of Swedish women who do not attend childbirth and parenthood education classes during pregnancy. *Midwifery*(20), 226-235.

Giugliani, E., Caiffa, W., Vogelhut, J., Witter, F., & Perman, J. (1994). Effect of Breastfeeding Support from Different Sources on Mothers' Decision to Breastfeed. *Journal of Human Lactation, 10*(3), 157-161.

Hodnett, E. (2002). Caregiver support for women during childbirth (A Cohrane Review). *Oxford: Update Software: The Cohrane Library.*

Humphreys, A., Thompson, N., & Miner, K. (1998). Intention to breastfeed in low-income pregnant women: the role of social support and previous experience. *Birth, 25*, 169-174.

Jerlock, M., Falk, K., & Severinsson, E. (2003). Academic nursing education guidelines: tool for bridging the gap between theory, research and practice. *Nurs Health Sci, 5*, 219-228.

Kools, E., Thijs, C., Kester, A., van den Brandt, P., & de Vries, H. (2005). A breastfeeding promotion and support program a randomized trial in the Netherlands. *Prev Med, 40*(1), 60-70.

Martens, P. (2000). Does Breastfeeding Education Affect Nursing Staff Beliefs, Exclusive Breastfeeding Rates, and Baby-Friendly Hospital Initiative Compliance? The Experience of a Small, Rural Canadian Hospital. *Journal of Human Lactation, 16*, 309-318.

Oakley, A. (1994). Giving support in pregnancy: the role of research midwives in randomised controlled trail. In *Midwives, Research and Childbirth* (pp. 30-63). London: Chapman & Hall.

Raphael-Leff, J. (2001). Psychological Processes of Childbearing. Revised edition. In (pp. p.342). London: Chapman & Hall.

Raykov, T., & Marcoulides, G. (2000). *A first course in structural equation modelling. p. 94.* London: Lawrence Erlbaum Associates.

Review., A. C. (2007). Breastfeeding: Maternal and Infant aspects. *4*(1).

Sikorski J, Renfrew MJ, Pindoria S, & A, W. (Issue 3, 2002). *Support for breastfeeding mothers (Cohrane Review)*. Oxford: Update Software: The Cohrane Library.

Tarkka, M., & Paunonen, M. (1996). Social support provided by nurses to recent mothers on a maternity ward. *Journal of Advanced Nursing, 23*(6), 1202-1206.

The National Board of Health and Welfare. (1984). *Family classes* (No. 1984:12). Stockholm, Sweden.

The National Board of Health and Welfare. (1997). *Support in parenthood.* Stockholm, Sweden.

WHO. (1989). *Protect, Promoting and Supporting Breastfeeding.* Geneve: World Health Organization.

WHO. (2003). *Global Strategy for Infant and Young Child Feeding.* Geneva: World Health Organization.

Women, C. o. H. C. f. U., & Gynecologists., A. C. o. O. a. (2007). ACOG Committee Opinion No. 361: Breastfeeding: maternal and infant aspects. *4*(1).

Zanna, M., Rempel, JK. (1986). Attitudes, a new look at an old concept. In D. Bar-Tal, Kruglanski, A (Ed.), *The social psychology of knowledge.* NY, Cambridge: University Press.

In: Health Education Research Trends
Editor: P. R. Hong, pp. 227-239

ISBN: 978-1-60021-871-2
© 2007 Nova Science Publishers, Inc.

Chapter VIII

THE USE OF COMPUTER-GENERATED TAILORED MATERIALS IN HEALTH EDUCATION

Tammy Hoffmann

Division of Occupational Therapy, School of Health and Rehabilitation Sciences, The University of Queensland, Brisbane Queensland, Australia.

ABSTRACT

Written health education materials are frequently used as a method of educating patients, and offer unique benefits. For health education materials to be effective, their readability level and design characteristics must be appropriate and they need to provide information that the patients want. Conventional written health education materials are generally designed to include as much information as possible for as many potential readers as possible. Because of this, the resulting material can be long and complex, and is likely to contain information that is irrelevant to many readers. In recent years, the application of computer technology to health education has led to the expanding use of computer-generated written health education materials that are tailored to the individual.

The majority of studies that have examined the effectiveness of tailored print information have had a health promotion focus and have been attempting to change participants' health-related lifestyle behaviours. A small number of recent studies have evaluated the effectiveness of using computer-generated tailored written information with people with chronic conditions such as arthritis and stroke. Heterogeneity in the patient populations studied, purpose of the interventions, study designs, and the outcome measures used prevents overall conclusions about the effectiveness of tailored health education materials from being drawn. It appears that patients prefer to receive information that is tailored to their individual situation, are more satisfied with tailored information, and are more likely to read and remember tailored information than non-tailored information. In some studies, patients who received tailored information were more likely to alter certain health behaviours than patients who received non-tailored information, however, in other studies, the provision of tailored information had no effect on health behaviours or other patient outcomes.

Overall, evidence regarding the effectiveness of tailored health education materials is inconclusive and it appears that tailored materials are only more effective than non-tailored materials under certain circumstances. What these circumstances are and the reasons why tailored materials are sometimes effective remain unclear. The potential for tailored materials to enhance patient health and well-being is high, however further studies that rigorously evaluate the effectiveness of well-designed tailored materials with various patient populations are urgently needed.

INTRODUCTION

Providing education to patients should be an integral component of all health professional-patient encounters and is important for the successful management of acute and chronic conditions as well as effective health promotion and prevention efforts. Health professionals commonly use written health education materials when educating patients. This chapter will briefly discuss the advantages of written health education materials and some of the common problems with them. As there is potential for overcoming one of the major problems through the use of tailored materials, this chapter will explore the various methods by which written health education materials are able to be generated to provide individuals with tailored information, review studies that have examined the use of computer-generated tailored health education materials, and discuss broader implications for the use of tailored health education materials.

ADVANTAGES OF WRITTEN HEALTH EDUCATION MATERIALS

Although it is common practice for health professionals to educate patients verbally, it is recommended that written materials be used to supplement or reinforce information that is presented verbally (Hill, 1997) as this reinforcement can have a positive impact on the effectiveness of patient teaching (Theis & Johnson, 1995). Raynor (1998) concluded that the combination of verbal and written information has the potential to maximise a patient's knowledge and adherence to treatment.

According to Bernier (1993), printed education materials have a number of advantages such as: message consistency, reusability, portability, flexibility of delivery, permanence of information, and they are economical to produce and update. Patients frequently forget information that is provided orally (Kitching, 1990). Written materials have the advantage of being available to refresh one's memory as needed (Ley, 1988). Tang and Newcomb (1998) conducted a patient focus group exploring patient education and found that patients sought answers to their questions at the time they formulate their questions. This usually occurred after the patient had seen the health professional, not during the encounter. To some extent, written materials may be able to assist patients in answering the questions that occur when they are not interacting with a health professional. A further benefit of written materials may be that patients can choose the level and amount of information that best suits them as their level of coping changes (Weinman, 1990). A randomised trial found that readers with an eighth grade or lower reading level who were provided with simplified written information could recall more information than readers who were provided with the information via a video (Campbell, Goldman, Boccia, & Skinner, 2004). The authors hypothesised that the difference may have been a consequence of the written information requiring more active involvement from participants than the video did. Ley (1988) reviewed numerous studies that provided patients with written information and concluded that the majority of patients who receive written information have a favourable attitude towards it. Webber (1990) also concurred that patients desire and appreciate written materials, pointing out that the reading levels of the materials must be appropriate to the intended audience.

COMMON PROBLEMS WITH WRITTEN HEALTH EDUCATION MATERIALS

Written information can only be useful if the recipients can read and understand it. Written materials should be written simply and at the lowest reading level possible while still conveying the information accurately. There are a growing number of studies finding that the written health education materials received by patients often have a readability level that is too high for the majority of the intended audience (Beaver & Luker, 1997; Eames, McKenna, Worrall, & Read, 2003; Estrada, Hryniewicz, Higgs, Collins, & Byrd, 2000; Hoffmann & McKenna, 2006; Sarma, Alpers, Prideaux, & Kroemer, 1995). When the reading ability of the target group cannot be predetermined, it has been suggested that a 5th-6th reading grade level is an appropriate goal for most health care materials (Doak, Doak, & Root, 1996; Estey, Musseau, & Keehn, 1991).

In addition to ensuring an appropriate readability level, consideration should also be given to other design characteristics of the written material in order to enhance readers' attention to and understanding and recall of the information. This includes factors such as the type and style of language, organisation, layout and typography, illustrations and presentation, and features that facilitate learning and motivation (Doak et al., 1996; Hoffmann & Worrall, 2004).

However, even if written health education materials are designed according to the recommended readability and design principles, the majority of readers may still disregard the materials. This may occur because conventional written health education materials are generally designed to include as much information as possible for as many potential readers as possible. Because of this, the resulting material is long and dense and likely to contain information that is irrelevant to most readers (Strecher et al., 1994). One potential advantage of computer-based patient education resources is the ability to tailor the information to individual needs. Tailoring refers to adapting the content of the material or the way it is presented according to the needs of the individual (Bental, Cawsey, & Jones, 1999).

Tailoring and the Use of Computers in Patient Education

As computer technology has advanced, the use of computers in patient education has also increased (Skinner, Siegfried, Kegler, & Strecher, 1993). Although computers cannot replace contact with health professionals, it is generally agreed that they can play a complementary role in patient education (Bental et al., 1999). There are a variety of computer applications in patient education, including computer programs with which the patient interacts, computer programs that are used to produce tailored information for patients, and computer networks that enable patients to communicate with one another and with health professionals. Computer systems that assist patients in making health-related decisions have also been developed and trialled (Gustafson et al., 1998). The focus of this chapter is the use of computer-based systems to generate tailored print health education materials for patients.

As discussed later in this chapter in more detail, studies have shown that patients prefer tailored information (Jones et al., 1999; Tang & Newcomb, 1998) and that tailored messages are more likely to be read and remembered (Brug, Steenhuis, van Assema, & De Vries, 1996; Campbell et al., 1994). The effectiveness of tailored print information has only been examined in a small number of studies and while the results of most studies are promising, the evidence about the outcomes of tailoring remains inconclusive.

Also lacking is information about which mechanisms are responsible for the anticipated effectiveness of tailoring. Tailoring allows for the removal of irrelevant information and it may be the increased relevancy of tailored information to a reader and the reader's perception that the information applies to him or her that increases the likelihood tailored materials will be read (Bental et al., 1999; Strecher et al., 1994). Indeed, having patients perceive the information as applying to only them is one of the goals of tailored intervention (Revere & Dunbar, 2001). It has also been suggested that tailoring may be effective because personalisation, such as putting the reader's name on the material, increases his or her attentiveness to the information (Bull, Holt, Kreuter, Clark, & Scharff, 2001; Kreuter & Strecher, 1996). In addition to facilitating the production of tailored health education materials, an additional advantage of computer-generated materials is that they have the potential to overcome two barriers to the use of written education materials by professionals, namely storage and access problems and the need to keep the materials up to date (Treweek, Glenton, Oxman, & Penrose, 2002).

To provide tailored information, the system must first capture information about the patient. The capture of information can be done in a variety of ways from linking the system to the patient's computerised medical record, to having the patient fill out a computer-based questionnaire, an online checklist, or a paper-based questionnaire from which the details are then entered manually into the system. The type of information that is captured will vary depending on the goal of the system. For example, some systems may only require information about the patient's age, gender and diagnosis, whereas others may require information such as the patient's health beliefs or level of readiness to change health behaviours (Bental et al., 1999). In studies where the aim is to influence people to change a lifestyle behaviour, such as smoking or exercising, it is common for the initial questionnaire to contain questions that will elicit information about the person's readiness to change, self-efficacy to undertake certain behaviours, and beliefs about causes of previous failures on similar tasks. Once this information is entered into the system, it will produce tailored information that is relevant to participants' responses.

The granularity of tailoring will also vary between systems. Granularity refers to the degree to which the text content is tailored (Bental et al., 1999). An example of coarse-grained tailoring is a system where patients select the information that they wish to receive from pre-written 'units' of material (Bental et al., 1999). In a system where the tailoring is more finely grained, individual words and phrases will be adapted according to information about the individual (Bental et al., 1999). Systems that use fine-grained tailoring typically use artificial intelligence techniques. An example is an interactive system designed for people who experience migraines (Buchanan et al., 1995). The system contains extensive knowledge about medical terminology, triggers, symptoms, and treatment of migraines. The interactive system collects information about the person's migraine history, produces a summary of the person's status for his or her doctor and a tailored information sheet written in simplified language, and is able to intelligently respond to follow-up questions about topics covered in the information sheet (Buchanan et al., 1995). Disadvantages of fine-grained tailoring systems are that the computer-generated text produced often lacks naturalness and creating these systems requires a level of effort and expense that often precludes them from being used in many situations (Bental et al., 1999).

REVIEW OF STUDIES EVALUATING COMPUTER-GENERATED TAILORED HEALTH EDUCATION MATERIALS

To date, the majority of studies that have examined the effectiveness of tailored print information have had a health promotion focus and have been attempting to change participants' health-related lifestyle behaviours such as quitting smoking, losing weight, or improving dietary behaviour. Only a few studies have used tailored print information with people who have a chronic medical condition which is surprising as patient education is an integral component of the management of chronic disease. The management of chronic disease requires the patient to take an active role and assume responsibility for the day-to-day management of their health. Education can teach patients the knowledge and skills they need to self-manage their condition, and this self-management can contribute to reducing disease burden and enhancing the patient's quality of life (Cooper, Booth, Fear, & Gill, 2001).

In an early study of computer-generated tailored information, 801 outpatients were randomised to either an enhanced education group or a control group (Osman et al., 1994). The 397 patients in the enhanced education group had four written booklets about asthma management, individualised on the basis of their medication, mailed to them at monthly intervals. There were 404 patients in the control group and they received conventional oral education at outpatient visits. The individualised booklets were associated with a reduction in hospital admissions for patients who were judged most vulnerable (severe asthma) on entry to the study. There was no significant relationship with any of the other outcome measures, which included prescription and use of medications, days of restricted activity, and number of general practitioner consultations for asthma. A weakness of this study is that it did not compare the effect of individualised booklets with generic booklets, and therefore any significant findings cannot be attributed to the tailored information.

Strecher et al. (1994) conducted two studies in a family practice setting that evaluated the effect of computer-tailored letters on smoking cessation. In the first study, 72 adults who smoked cigarettes, regardless of interest in quitting, were randomised to receive either a tailored or generic health letter. The tailored letters were created according to participants' responses to questions about his or her health-related beliefs, smoking stages, and attributions for previous failures in smoking cessation. The authors attempted to minimise the differences in appearance between the tailored and generic letters by using the same typeface and stationery, personalising each letter, and ensuring the letters were of similar length. Four months later, 51 participants were followed-up by telephone and asked if they had smoked a cigarette in the last seven days. A significant effect was found for participants who were moderate to light smokers, with 30.7% of participants in the tailored letter group reporting that they had quit smoking, compared to 7.1% of the people in the generic letter group. The methodology of this study is weakened by the low follow-up rate of 70.8%, with no reasons given for participants who were unable to be followed-up.

In the second study, 296 people who had indicated that they were interested in quitting smoking in the next six months, were randomised to receive either a tailored health letter or no letter (Strecher et al., 1994). Six months later, 197 people (67% follow-up rate) were followed up by either telephone or a postal questionnaire. Of the participants in the tailored letter group who were moderate to light smokers, 19.1% reported that they had quit smoking, which was significantly different to the 7.3% of participants in the control group who were moderate to light smokers that reported quitting. Education was also associated with cessation, with participants with higher levels of education more likely to report having quit. These two studies revealed that regardless of whether participants were interested in quitting smoking, tailored health letters were more effective than a generic letter or no letter in assisting people who were moderate to light smokers to quit smoking. The authors hypothesised that to assist people who are heavy smokers to quit smoking, nicotine replacement therapies would need to be used in addition to information that is tailored according to cognitive and behavioural factors (Strecher et al., 1994).

In a study that examined the provision of information that was individualised using patients' medical records, 525 oncology patients were randomised to receive either general computer-based information (n=167), individualised computer-based information that was linked to their medical record (n=178), or traditional printed booklets (n=180) (Jones et al., 1999). Patients in the two computer-based groups spent time with the computer system and were then sent printouts of the information that they had viewed. Patients who received individualised information were more likely to have a high information satisfaction score and to show the printouts to their family than patients who received the general computer information or the traditional booklets. Patients who received traditional booklets were significantly more likely to feel overwhelmed with information than patients in either of the computer-based groups. However, compared to patients in the two groups that received computer printouts, more of the patients who received the traditional booklets used the material at home. The authors hypothesised that this may have been because the booklets were more attractive than the computer printouts. At the three month follow-up, 19% of patients in the individualised information group were anxious compared with 37% of patients in the general computer information group.

Using a three-group randomised trial design, Kreuter and Strecher (1996) evaluated whether tailored behaviour change messages enhanced the effectiveness of health risk appraisal. Participants were 1317 patients who agreed to complete a health risk appraisal (HRA) questionnaire while they were waiting at a family medical practice to see a doctor. The questionnaire collected information about participants' risk factors, such as blood pressure and weight; health-related behaviours, such as smoking; preventive screening practices, such as cholesterol testing; depressive symptomatology; interest in changing behaviours; and perceived barriers to and benefits of changing behaviour. Participants were randomised to receive no feedback, typical HRA feedback, or enhanced HRA feedback. The enhanced feedback contained information about patients' positive and risky health-related behaviours and computer-generated, individually tailored behaviour change information. Patients in the typical feedback group received only risk information, not the behaviour change information. A six month follow-up, by either telephone interview or postal questionnaire, was completed for 1131 participants (86%). The follow-up questionnaire contained the same items as the baseline questionnaire.

Patients who received enhanced feedback were 18% more likely to have changed at least one risk behaviour than patients in the typical feedback or no feedback groups. Behaviour change was significant for only certain behaviours, namely cholesterol screening and reducing dietary fat, and near significant for engaging in regular aerobic exercise. There were no significant differences in behaviour change between the control and typical feedback group, which enabled the authors to attribute the behavioural changes to the tailored messages. The methodology of this study was strong, although it was not explicitly stated if allocation to the groups was concealed or if the results were analysed on an intention-to-treat basis.

In one of the few studies that has evaluated the effectiveness of tailored messages in promoting physical activity, tailored and personalised materials were compared to materials that were personalised but not tailored (Bull, Kreuter, & Scharff, 1999). Personalisation referred to putting the patient's name on the top of the first page of the information, whereas tailoring referred to providing information on the basis of patients' responses to questions such as their exercise goals, motives, perceived barriers, and stage of readiness to change. Participants were recruited as they waited in their physicians' offices and completed a baseline questionnaire. There were 882 patients recruited and randomised into four groups, but only 272 met the eligibility criteria and were retained in the study. The majority of patients were excluded as exercise was contraindicated. The four groups were: tailored and personalised material, general and personalised material, general and not personalised material, and usual care group (no material). Three months later, 75% of the participants completed a follow-up postal questionnaire. At follow-up there were no differences between the groups in terms of keeping, reading or sharing the materials. There were no significant differences in total exercise or leisure time activities between the groups, however participants in the tailored group were more likely to have increased physical activities of daily living (such as 'yard work' and 'work in the home') than participants in the other three groups. Bull et al. (1999) proposed that the inconclusive results of the study might have been due to the similarity between the messages in the general and tailored materials. For example, 'lack of time' is a common barrier to increasing physical activity and it is likely that information about this barrier would be contained in both the general and tailored materials.

Campbell et al. (1994) evaluated the effectiveness of tailored dietary information by randomising 558 family practice patients to receive tailored nutrition messages, non-tailored nutrition messages, or no nutrition messages. The tailored information was individualised on the basis of baseline food frequency and readiness to change information that participants provided in a survey, and the tailored and non-tailored information was mailed to the participants. Participants were surveyed four months later by either a postal questionnaire or a telephone interview with an assessor who was blinded to group membership. The follow-up rate was 82%. Seventy-three percent of participants in the tailored information group recalled receiving information compared to 33% of the participants in the non-tailored group. Participants in the tailored information group were more likely to report having read the entire message than participants who received the non-tailored information. Participants in the tailored information group also had significantly reduced total fat and saturated fat intakes compared with those in the control group, however statistical analyses of the difference in fat reduction between participants in the tailored information group and those in the non-tailored information group were not reported.

In an effort to identify which features of tailored education materials enhance specific outcomes, Bull et al. (2001) recruited 198 overweight participants via a newspaper advertisement and randomised participants to receive either tailored weight loss information ($n=72$), a generic booklet ($n=73$), or generic information with the same format and appearance as the tailored information ($n=53$). A baseline questionnaire assessed intention to change behaviour, stage of change, and self-efficacy to undertake change behaviours. Immediately after reading the assigned material, participants rated the booklet using a series of Likert items and re-answered the baseline questionnaire items. One month later, 189 (95%) participants completed a follow-up telephone interview where recall of information, change in motivation, self-efficacy, and behaviours were recorded. The tailored information was positively associated with heightened attention to the material and showing the material to others. Perceiving the material as applying to one's life was in turn significantly associated with liking and understanding the material, learning new information, remembering concepts, and attitudinal change. Participants with higher self-efficacy to undertake change behaviours or those in the action stage of behaviour change were more likely to remember more of the material's content at follow-up. Perceiving the material to contain new information was also associated with higher recall. Despite the bias that accompanies participant self-selection and the short follow-up time, this study was able to provide support for the importance of using education materials that individuals perceive as applying to them.

As mentioned earlier in this chapter, very few studies have evaluated the use of tailored written materials in people with chronic disease. However, a recent randomised controlled trial compared a traditional small group arthritis self-management program ($n=161$) with a mail-delivered, tailored, printed self-management intervention ($n=180$) (Lorig, Ritter, Laurent, & Fries, 2004). Outcome measures were self-efficacy, doctor visits, disability, pain, depression, role function, and global severity of arthritis. Participants in the tailored print intervention group received a tailored letter and action plan every four months, along with other resources such as brochures and a relaxation tape. Participants in the small group intervention group attended the group for two hours per week for six weeks. Participants were reassessed every six months for three years. The follow-up rates were 90% at one year, 83% at two years, and 73% at three years. At one year, participants in the tailored print intervention group had statistically significantly greater decreases in disability and increases in self-efficacy than participants in the group program. At two years, there were no significant differences between the groups, and at three years, participants in the group program had a significantly greater improvement in role function and reduction in doctor visits than participants in the tailored print intervention group. Lorig et al. (2004) concluded that the tailored print intervention was as effective as the traditional group program, with slightly better results in the first year, and a more rapid decrease in gains made in the following two years. The difference at one year may reflect that participants in the tailored print intervention group were still receiving the intervention at that time, whereas the intervention for participants in the other group had concluded after six weeks.

As part of the above trial, a second randomised controlled trial that compared the tailored print intervention (n=522) with usual care was conducted (n=568) (Lorig et al., 2004). The outcome measures and follow-up times were the same as the previously described trial. The follow-up rates were 81% at one year, 74% at two years, and 68% at three years. At one year, participants in the tailored print intervention group had a statistically significant improvement in role function and self-efficacy and decrease in disability compared to participants in the usual care group. At two years, participants in the tailored print intervention group had a statistically significant improvement in self-efficacy and decreases in global severity and doctor visits compared to participants in the usual care group. There were no significant differences between the groups at three years.

Only one study has explored the use of computer-generated tailored materials with people who have had a stroke (Hoffmann, McKenna, Worrall, & Read, 2007). In this study, patients were randomised to receive either computer-generated tailored written information about stroke (n= 69) or generic written information (n=69) while in hospital. Tailoring features of the computer system enabled patients in the tailored information group to identify which topics (34 topics available) they would like to receive information about, the amount of information (detailed or shortened) that they would like about each topic, and the font size that they would like the information to be printed in. Three months following discharge from hospital, a blinded assessor conducted a face-to-face interview with patients and evaluated the outcomes of knowledge about stroke, self-efficacy, anxiety and depression, perceived health status, satisfaction with content and presentation of the written information received, and desire for additional information. The follow-up rate was 96%. Patients who had received the tailored information were significantly more satisfied with the content and presentation of the information received than patients who received the generic information. Significantly fewer patients in the tailored information group desired additional information about stroke at follow-up than patients in the generic information group, indicating that the tailored information was better at meeting patients' informational needs than the generic information Although anxiety change scores improved slightly more in favour of the group that received the generic information, the size of the change was not of clinical significance. No significant differences between the groups were observed for any of the other outcome measures.

ADDITIONAL CONSIDERATIONS REGARDING THE USE OF COMPUTER-GENERATED TAILORED MATERIALS

Even though computer-based health education resources have the potential to produce large quantities of tailored information relatively easily and cost-effectively (Bental et al., 1999), very few studies have explicitly addressed the issue of the cost-effectiveness of tailored information systems. Even though the initial set-up cost of a tailored information system will be greater than when non-tailored materials are used, the per-patient cost is usually minimal (Bental et al., 1999) and a computer-based patient information system has the potential to strengthen the existing health education and learning environment (Lewis, 1999). However, a recent study has cautioned against implementing a computer-based patient information system without first assessing what the users of the system actually need and want, as a system will be rejected by users if their needs are not taken into consideration during the design phase (Stoop, van't Riet, & Berg, 2004). The authors concluded that computer-based patient information systems should be considered as a valuable supplement to, not a substitute for, traditional methods of patient education (Stoop et al., 2004).

CONCLUSION

When receiving health information, it is important that patients receive only information that is relevant to them. Using written materials that are computer-generated and tailored according to the individual's informational needs is a relatively new method of achieving this. The studies that have evaluated computer-generated tailored materials have found that compared to non-tailored materials, tailored materials are more likely to be: attended to, read, shown to others, perceived as containing personally relevant information, satisfying to the patient, successful in meeting the patient's informational needs, and effective in changing certain behaviours. However, the evidence is not conclusive and it appears that tailored materials are only more effective than non-tailored materials under certain circumstances. What these circumstances are and the reasons why tailored materials are sometimes effective remain unclear. Only one of the studies described the design characteristics of the written material that was evaluated and subsequently evaluated the effectiveness of a well-designed tailored written health education material. It is unclear if important factors such as the content and design characteristics of the written materials were considered in the other studies. As these factors could impact on the effectiveness of tailored written materials it is important that any tailored health education material is designed according to the recommended content and design principles. Further research into the effectiveness of well-designed tailored education materials is needed, as is research regarding the cost-effectiveness of developing and using computer-generated tailored written health education materials.

REFERENCES

Beaver, K., & Luker, K. (1997). Readability of patient information booklets for women with breast cancer. *Patient Education and Counselling, 31,* 95-102.

Bental, D., Cawsey, A., & Jones, R. (1999). Patient information systems that tailor to the individual. *Patient Education and Counselling, 36,* 171-180.

Bernier, M. J. (1993). Developing and evaluating printed education materials: A prescriptive model for quality. *Orthopaedic Nursing, 12*(6), 39-46.

Brug, J., Steenhuis, I., van Assema, P., & De Vries, H. (1996). The impact of a computer-tailored nutrition intervention. *Preventive Medicine, 25,* 236-242.

Buchanan, B. G., Moore, J. D., Forsythe, D. E., Carenini, G., Ohlsson, S., & Banks, G. (1995). An intelligent interactive system for delivering individualised information to patients. *Artificial Intelligence in Medicine, 7,* 117-154.

Bull, F. C., Holt, C. L., Kreuter, M., Clark, E., & Scharff, D. (2001). Understanding the effects of printed health education materials: Which features lead to which outcomes? *Journal of Health Communication, 6,* 265-279.

Bull, F. C., Kreuter, M., & Scharff, D. (1999). Effects of tailored, personalised and general health messages on physical activity. *Patient Education and Counselling, 36,* 181-192.

Campbell, F., Goldman, B., Boccia, M., & Skinner, M. (2004). The effect of format modifications and reading comprehension on recall of informed consent information by low-income parents: A comparison of print, video, and computer-based presentations. *Patient Education and Counselling, 53,* 205-216.

Campbell, M. K., DeVellis, B. M., Strecher, V. J., Ammerman, A. S., DeVellis, R. F., & Sandler, R. S. (1994). Improving dietary behaviour: The effectiveness of tailored messages in primary care settings. *American Journal of Public Health, 84,* 783-787.

Cooper, H., Booth, K., Fear, S., & Gill, G. (2001). Chronic disease patient education: Lessons from meta-analyses. *Patient Education and Counselling, 44,* 107-117.

Doak, C. C., Doak, L., & Root, J. (1996). *Teaching patients with low literacy skills* (2nd ed.). Philadelphia: J.B. Lippincott Company.

Eames, S., McKenna, K., Worrall, L., & Read, S. (2003). The suitability of written education materials for stroke survivors and their carers. *Topics in Stroke Rehabilitation, 10*(3), 70-83.

Estey, A., Musseau, A., & Keehn, L. (1991). Comprehension levels of patients reading health information. *Patient Education and Counselling, 18,* 165-169.

Estrada, C. A., Hryniewicz, M. M., Higgs, V. B., Collins, C., & Byrd, J. C. (2000). Anticoagulant patient information material is written at high readability levels. *Stroke, 31,* 2966-2970.

Gustafson, D., Hawkins, R., Boberg, E., Pingree, S., Serline, R., Graziano, F., et al. (1998). Impact of a patient-centered, computer-based health information / support system. *American Journal of Preventive Medicine, 16,* 1-9.

Hill, J. (1997). A practical guide to patient education and information giving. *Baillieres Clinical Rheumatology, 11,* 109-127.

Hoffmann, T., & McKenna, K. (2006). Analysis of stroke patients' and carers' reading ability and the content and design of written materials: Recommendations for improving written stroke information. *Patient Education and Counselling, 60*(3), 286-293.

Hoffmann, T., McKenna, K., Worrall, L., & Read, S. (2007). Randomised trial of a computer-generated tailored written education package for patients following stroke. *Age and Ageing, 36*, 280-286..

Hoffmann, T., & Worrall, L. (2004). Designing effective written health education materials: Considerations for health professionals. *Disability and Rehabilitation, 26*, 1166-1173.

Jones, R., Pearson, J., McGregor, S., Cawsey, A. J., Barrett, A., Craig, N., et al. (1999). Randomised trial of personalised computer based information for cancer patients. *BMJ, 319*, 1241-1247.

Kitching, J. B. (1990). Patient information leaflets: The state of the art. *Journal of the Royal Society of Medicine, 83*, 298-300.

Kreuter, M. W., & Strecher, V. J. (1996). Do tailored behaviour change messages enhance the effectiveness of health risk appraisal? Results from a randomised trial. *Health Education Research, 11*, 97-105.

Lewis, D. (1999). Computer-based approaches to patient education: A review of the literature. *Journal of the American Medical Informatics Association, 6*, 272-282.

Ley, P. (1988). The use of written information for patients. In P. Ley (Ed.), *Communicating with patients* (pp. 110-124). London: Chapman and Hall.

Lorig, K., Ritter, P., Laurent, D., & Fries, J. (2004). Long-term randomised controlled trials of tailored-print and small-group arthritis self-management interventions. *Medical Care, 42*, 346-354.

Osman, L., Abdalla, M. I., Beattie, J., Ross, S. J., Russell, I. T., Friend, J. A., et al. (1994). Reducing hospital admissions through computer supported education for asthma patients. *BMJ, 308*, 568-571.

Raynor, D. K. (1998). The influence of written information on patient knowledge and adherence to treatment. In L. Myers & K. Midence (Eds.), *Adherence to treatment in medical conditions* (pp. 83-111). London: Harwood Academic.

Revere, D., & Dunbar, P. (2001). Review of computer-generated outpatient health behaviour interventions. *Journal of the American Medical Informatics Association, 8*, 62-79.

Sarma, M., Alpers, J. H., Prideaux, D. J., & Kroemer, D. J. (1995). The comprehensibility of Australian educational literature for patients with asthma. *Medical Journal of Australia, 162*, 360-363.

Skinner, C. S., Siegfried, J. C., Kegler, M. C., & Strecher, V. J. (1993). The potential of computers in patient education. *Patient Education and Counselling, 22*, 27-34.

Stoop, A. P., van't Riet, A., & Berg, M. (2004). Using information technology for patient education: Realising surplus value? *Patient Education and Counselling, 54*, 187-195.

Strecher, V., Kreuter, M., Den Boer, D., Kobrin, S., Hospers, H., & Skinner, C. (1994). The effects of computer-tailored smoking cessation messages in family practice settings. *Journal of Family Practice, 39*, 262-270.

Tang, P., & Newcomb, C. (1998). Informing patients: A guide for providing patient health information. *Journal of the American Medical Informatics Association, 5*, 563-570.

Theis, S. L., & Johnson, J. H. (1995). Strategies for teaching patients: A meta-analysis. *Clinical Nurse Specialist, 9,* 100-105.

Treweek, S. P., Glenton, C., Oxman, A. D., & Penrose, A. (2002). Computer-generated patient education materials: Do they affect professional practice? A systematic review. *Journal of the American Medical Informatics Association, 9,* 346-358.

Webber, G. C. (1990). Patient education: A review of the issues. *Medical Care, 28,* 1089-1103.

Weinman, J. (1990). Providing written information for patients: Psychological considerations. *Journal of the Royal Society of Medicine, 83,* 303-305.

In: Health Education Research Trends
Editor: P. R. Hong, pp. 241-252

ISBN: 978-1-60021-871-2
© 2007 Nova Science Publishers, Inc.

Chapter IX

The Impact of a Culturally Grounded Male Development Program on Reducing Health Risk Behaviors Among Minority Male Adolescents

Ruth S. Buzi[1], Peggy B. Smith[1], Maxine L. Weinman[2]
and Mahasin F. Saleh[3]

[1]Baylor College of Medicine, Houston, TX 77030, USA;
[2]Graduate College of Social Work, University of Houston, Texas 77204-4492, USA;
[3]School of Social Work, University of Nevada, Reno, NV 89557-0068, USA.

Abstract

The purpose of this descriptive study was to analyze longitudinally health risk behaviors of young males who were enrolled in a pregnancy prevention program. The Rites of Passage (ROP) project included 177 adolescent males between the ages of 12-22 and used a culturally grounded approach. Outcomes for the program included sexual and contraceptive behaviors, cigarette smoking, substance use, and antisocial behavior. The study also included open-ended questions that captured participants' expectations from the program and perceived benefits. Data were collected at intake, three months, and six months. Changes over time occurred in several risk behaviors. The results of the open-ended questions also indicated that participants felt that the program benefited them in the areas of self development, heritage awareness and risk reduction. Implications for future culturally grounded interventions are suggested.

Keywords: Hispanic Youth, Risk Behaviors, Culturally Grounded Interventions.

INTRODUCTION

Large ethnic disparities exist in regard to risk taking behaviors among adolescents. Hispanic males in particular were identified as a high-risk group. According to the 2005 Youth Risk Behavior Surveillance Survey (YRBSS) (Centers for Disease Control and Prevention, 2006), Hispanic males reported higher rates of lifetime cigarette use (62.1%) than either white or black males (54.9% and 56.3%, respectively). This report also suggests that lifetime alcohol use was also greater among Hispanic male students than among male students of other ethnic groups, at 79.9% for Hispanics compared to 75.0% for whites and 66.5% for blacks. Furthermore, Hispanic males reported more high risk sexual behavior than did white teens. For example, 57.6% of Hispanic males reported having had sexual intercourse, compared to 42.2% of white teens. Hispanic males were also more likely than white males to have had four or more sexual partners in their lifetime (21.7% and 11.6%, respectively), and to have used drugs or alcohol before their last sexual encounter, at 32.2% compared to 29.9% of whites and 15.4% of blacks. Finally, only 65.3% of Hispanic males reported to have used a condom during the last sexual encounter compared to 70.1% of whites and 75.5% of blacks.

As young males in general, and minority males in particular, are involved in multiple risk behaviors including early sexual activity and pregnancy, they need ready access to services that promote positive and responsible behaviors (Armstrong et al., 1999, Brindis et al.., 1998). The need to target young males encouraged the development of programs for this group such as initiatives funded by the Department of Health and Human Services, Office of Population Affairs/ Office of Family Planning (OPA/OFP) (OPA/OFP, 2000).

Recent programs targeting high risk teens advocate the use of youth development programs. For specific minority groups, culturally grounded approaches are recommended. Youth development models are based on the philosophy that resiliency and competency building are essential in order to influence adolescents' healthy development (Roth & Brooks-Gunn, 2003). Zeldin (2000) discusses the paradigm shift that occurred in youth programs from a focus on prevention of risk behavior to the promotion of healthy and positive behavior. This new focus stresses the importance of a holistic approach that addresses not only the individual but also the community and social network. This has influenced the growth in programs that work to foster youth leadership, activism, community service, and partnerships with adults. For example, Keating, Tomishima, Foster and Alessandri (2002) evaluated the impact of a six-month mentoring project on risk behaviors among young males and females 10 to 17 years of age. Significant differences between the treatment and matched control groups were found in problematic behaviors, suggesting that exposure to caring adults helped youth feel better about themselves and engage in less destructive behaviors. Specifically, the project seemed to keep those young people beginning to evidence behavioral and emotional problems from developing worse behaviors. Such findings may be attributed to the pro-social attitudes modeled by the mentor or to the development of more effective life skills for problem management.

Culturally Grounded Interventions

Despite the growing number of Hispanics in the US and the health disparities associated with this group, Pantin, Prado, Schwartz, and Sullivan (2005) have noted a lack in research on prevention programs specifically for Hispanics. Culturally grounded prevention programs have been advocated as effective in preventing risk behaviors among youth. The authors suggest two major reasons culturally-specific intervention programs are important. Such programs are not only more likely to retain non-whites, but these programs can also target specific risk or protective factors associated with a particular ethnic group. All programs, they suggest, should address cultural, ethnic, linguistic, and socioeconomic realities of the individuals and families they are serving. The authors point out that interventions may be more successful if they target specific cultural variables that may act as risk factors for unsafe behavior. These variables include acculturation to American culture, the discrepancies in acculturation between adolescents and families, and the lack of communication between parents and adolescents about drugs and sex.

Other researchers also suggest that as rates of risk factors vary by ethnicity, response to treatments may be different as well (Adam, McGuire, Walsh, Basta, & LeCroy, 2005; Gil, Wagner, & Tubman, 2004). Therefore, interventions that convey culturally appropriate and sensitive information increase the relevance of the material and affect participants' ability to avoid risky behavior and to make healthy choices. It is suggested that in essence, culturally grounded interventions can improve the effectiveness and relevance of the curriculum content (Mize, Robinson, Bockting, & Scheltema, 2002). Overall, cultural interventions have also been found beneficial to youth. For example, Spencer, Dobbs, and Swanson (1988) found that interventions promoting a minority group's own cultural identity, rather than the dominant group's identity, resulted in greater resiliency as well as improved academic and mental health outcomes for the minority group.

In a major review of the literature, Prado et al. (2006) found that there were a limited number of eco-developmental interventions specifically for Hispanic adolescents and little research on their efficacy. While the authors found several studies on intrapersonal interventions for minorities, they did not find published articles specifically about these programs for Hispanic adolescents. Based on their examination of current research and the state of intervention programs, the authors recommend that even studies designed specifically for Hispanics need to be flexible to allow for the wide range of diverse subgroups. They also note that some specific aspects of Hispanic culture can cause increased risk for sexual risk taking, including Machisimo, a heightened sense of masculinity, that has been linked to multiple sexual partners and sexual risk taking. Benavides, Bonazzo, and Torres (2006) also noted that if those leading interventions were not aware of and educated about aspects specific to Hispanic culture, they could limit the outcomes of the intervention. When designing programs for Hispanics, it is especially important to take into account aspects of their culture including allocentrism, familialism, personal space, time orientation, gender roles, and fatalism.

Villarruel, Jemmott, and Jemmott (2006) conducted a study on the efficacy of a prevention intervention for Latino adolescents. The program included 553 Latino adolescents aged 13 to 18. The program presented abstinence and condom use as culturally-accepted ways to prevent sexually transmitted infections (STIs). Adolescents in the HIV-prevention group were less likely to have had sexual intercourse in the three months following the program than those in the general health promotion prevention group. Adolescents in the HIV-prevention group were also more likely to have used condoms consistently during the follow-up period than those in the other group. The authors argue that this study illustrates the effectiveness of intervention programs that are based on behavioral theories and are culturally adapted.

Hecht, et al. (2003) describe culturally grounded intervention programs as interventions that start with the culture and develop the intervention from there. Such interventions require not only appropriate images and language, but must also take into account cultural values. In this study, the *keepin' it R.E.A.L. (Refuse, Explain, Avoid, and Leave)* curriculum was developed for three cultures, including Mexican-American. During development, narratives were collected from Mexican-American adolescents and were incorporated into performance-based aspects of the curriculum. The Mexican-American curriculum also emphasized family orientation, action orientation, respect, personal treatment (preference for being treated as an individual rather than according to categories) and niceness. The Mexican-American program was more effective in reducing substance use than the control program, suggesting infusing programs with cultural elements is beneficial.

Based on the review of the literature, it appears that young Hispanic males engage in high risk behaviors. The literature also emphasizes the need for prevention programs that take into consideration the cultural milieu of this group. Therefore, the purpose of this study was to compare longitudinally health risk behaviors of young males who were enrolled in a culturally grounded pregnancy prevention project.

METHODS

Project Description

This 5-year Rites of Passage (ROP) pregnancy prevention project was funded by the Texas Department of State Health Services (TDSHS) through a grant provided by the Office of Population Affairs/Office of Family Planning (OPA/OFP). The main objective of this pregnancy prevention project was to develop personal and social competencies and reinforce messages of pregnancy prevention. A culturally grounded approach guided program components.

The goal of the ROP was to provide an environment where young males would experience a culturally rooted process through mentorship, education, and spiritual components that encourage young men to assume responsibilities of manhood. The project offered a traditional rite of passage for young males and provided a model and experience for accepting the responsibilities of manhood and fatherhood. The young males participated in 10-week two-hour sessions of the Joven Noble curriculum that is divided into four stages of development. The four stages of development are Conocimiento (Acknowledgment), Entendimiento (Understanding), Integracion (Integration), and Movimiento (Movement). The curriculum is designed to include the physical, emotional, mental, and spiritual aspects of each stage as a basis for direction. Each stage utilizes various interactive activities and teaching experiences related to the individual, family, and community of the young man's life. Young males also participated monthly in Circulo de Hombres, a support group for men. This component integrated adult male role models with the young men to offer advice, support and guidance toward manhood.

Participants

The target population for the ROP was youth between the ages of 12 and 22 who resided in two large geographical areas in the southwest part of the US. The two areas are major centers of the Mexican American population, encompassing centers of commerce and residency for this group. These areas also have a high concentration of individuals below the poverty level, unemployed males, teenage high school dropouts, households receiving public assistance, and female-headed households.

Instruments

The assessment instrument recorded demographic information, language preference, fatherhood status, marital status, and school status. Six measures were used to record participants' involvement in risk behaviors: contraceptive use, a history of STIs, cigarette smoking, alcohol use, substance use, and problems with the law. These measures assessed participation in health risk behaviors in the last three months. To track behavioral changes among project participants, the assessment was administered upon enrollment in the project and at subsequent follow-up in three month increments. The assessment was tailored to a seventh grade reading level. In addition to collecting quantitative data pertaining to risk behaviors, participants were asked to complete a qualitative assessment. At program entry they were asked to describe in their own words their expectations from the program and at three and six months to describe how the program helped them. A thematic analysis was used to group and analyze these responses.

Procedure

Project staff administered the assessment instrument to participants upon enrollment to the project and was also responsible for collecting follow-up data. Each participant signed an informed consent prior to entering into the project. The project protocol was approved by the affiliated Institutional Review Board. Following the assessment, all the young males who enrolled in the project were assigned a case manager who was responsible for coordinating the services needed, providing referrals, and monitoring progress.

RESULTS

Demographic Profile

Table 1 provides information on the demographic profile of participants. One hundred seventy-seven males participated in the program. The mean age of the males was 16.9 (SD=2.42; Range 12-22). The majority (89.5%) of the participants were Hispanic, 6 (3.5%) were African American, 5 (2.9%) were Caucasian, 4 (2.3%) were Asian, and 3 (1.7%) were Native American.

Table 1. Socio-demographic Description of Target Population

Variable	Distribution	Rites of Passage
Age		Mean= 16.9 (SD=2.42; Range 12-22)
Ethnicity	Hispanic	154 (89.5%)
	Caucasian	5 (2.9%)
	Asian	4 (2.3%)
	African American	6 (3.5%)
	Native American	3 (1.7%)
Living Arrangements	Both parents	75 (46.0%)
	Single parent	64 (39.3%)
	Grandparents	10 (6.1%)
	Extended family	5 (3.1%)
	Girlfriend's parents	1 (.6%)
	Mother and stepfather	3 (1.8%)
	Girlfriend	2 (1.2%)
	Friends	1 (0.6%)
	Self	N/A
	Spouse and children	2 (1.2%)
Fatherhood Status	Has child/children	29 (17.8%)
	My girlfriend is pregnant	16 (9.8%)
	I have no children	118 (72.4%)
Language Spoken at Home	English	109 (64.5%)
	Spanish	20 (11.8%)
	English and Spanish	38 (22.5%)
	Other	2 (1.2%)
Primary Language	English	148 (89.2%)
	Spanish	5 (3.0%)
	English and Spanish	13 (7.8%)
School Status	In school	148 (85.6%)
	Not in school	23 (13.5%)

* Some variables have missing data

Substance Use Behaviors

Table 2 provides a longitudinal description of risk behaviors of the participants. At intake, the youth participating in the program reported several risk behaviors. For example, 37.6% reported cigarette use and 39.4% reported alcohol use. At three months follow-up, cigarette use declined from 37.6% at intake to 29.7%. Drug use decreased only slightly from 25.9% at intake to 23.1% at three months. However, changes between intake to six months were more remarkable. For example, cigarette use dropped from 37.6% at intake to 24.6% at six months and drug use dropped from 25.9% to 21.1%. Alcohol use dropped from 39.4% at intake to 29.8%. Overall, rates of risk behaviors at six months were lower than at intake.

Table 2. Comparison of Risk Behaviors

Variable	Response	Intake	3 Months	6 months
		N= 177	N=91	N=57
Contraceptive use past 3 months	Always	42 (24.9%)	17 (18.9%)	18 (31.6%)
	Sometimes	38 (22.5%)	25 (27.8%)	9 (15.8%)
	Never	22 (13.0%)	4 (4.4%)	1 (1.8%)
	Abstinent	67 (39.6%)	44 (48.9%)	29 (50.9%)
Type of contraception past 3 months	Birth control pills	2 (1.4%)	3 (3.6%)	1 (1.9%)
	Condoms	63 (62.9%)	28 (33.7%)	21 (40.4%)
	Depo	3 (2.0%)	3 (3.6%)	1 (1.9%)
	Foam	N/A	1 (1.2%)	N/A
	None	14 (9.5%)	6 (7.2%)	N/A
	Not sexually active	65 (44.2%)	42 (50.6%)	29 (55.8%)
STIs past 3 months	Yes	4 (2.4%)	4 (4.5%)	0
	No	161 (97.6%)	84 (95.5%)	57 (100%)
Cigarette use past 3 months	Yes	64 (37.6%)	27 (29.7%)	14 (24.6%)
	No	106 (62.4%)	64 (70.3%)	43 (75.4%)
Drug use past 3 months	Yes	44 (25.9%)	21 (23.1%)	12 (21.1%)
	No	126 (74.1%)	70 (76.9%)	45 (78.9%)
Alcohol use past 3 months	Yes	67 (39.4%)	27 (29.7%)	17 (29.8%)
	No	103 (60.6%)	64 (70.3%)	40 (70.2%)
Problems with the law past 3 months	Yes	35 (21.3%)	7 (7.8%)	6 (10.5%)
	No	129 (78.7%)	83 (92.2%)	51 (89.5%)

* Some variables have missing data

Sexual Risk Behaviors

Some sexual risk behaviors were noted at intake. Sixty (35.5%) participants reported sometimes or never using contraceptives and only 24.9% of the participants indicated they always used condoms. At intake abstinence was reported by 39.6% of the participants. Only 2.4% of the participants reported having had an STI in the last three months.

Some of the sexual risk behaviors showed improvement at three months. Abstinence increased from 39.6% at intake to 48.9% at three months. Consistent contraceptive use showed mixed results and STIs increased at three months. However, all sexual risk behaviors showed improvement between intake to six months. Consistent contraceptive use increased from 24.9% at intake to 31.6% at six months. Inconsistent contraceptive use declined from 35.5% at intake to 17.6% at six months. Abstinence also increased from 39.6% at intake to 50.9% at six months.

Anti-Social Behaviors

At intake, 21.3% reported problems with the law. Rates of problems with the law decreased at three months to 7.8%. At six months there was a slight increase compared to three months (10.5%, vs. 7.8%, respectively). Rates of problems with the law were still lower at six months as compared to intake (21.3%, vs. 10.5%, respectively).

Program Expectations

At program entry, there were 143 responses to the question "describe your program goals." Young men indicated expectations related to self-development, risk reduction and engaging in recreational activities. Expectations regarding self development included areas such as getting guidance on the right direction, learning how to form relationships with family and peers, and developing leadership skills and self-confidence. Participants also expressed a desire to get help with reducing risk behaviors such as unsafe sexual practices, drug use and anger. Expectations regarding recreational activities included the desire to have fun in the wilderness, have something to do over the summer, learn how to camp, and participate in art classes. Participants also noted a desire to connect to their heritage.

Program Benefits

There were 79 responses at three months and 51 at six months related to program benefits. Participants' statements reflected their accomplishments related to self-development, risk reduction, and excitement about program recreational activities. They indicated that they became more responsible in family, job and parenting duties, learned how to become better persons, and learned to be proud of their heritage. They also indicated that they learned how to make better choices related to safe sex practices and avoidance of cigarette, alcohol and drug use. It was clear that these young males enjoyed the opportunities to work with other young males and had fun with the different recreational activities including camping and art.

DISCUSSION

The purpose of this study was to examine longitudinally health risk behaviors of young males who were enrolled in a culturally grounded pregnancy prevention project. The findings of the study revealed notable risk behaviors among participants at intake. For example, 37.6% reported cigarette use, 39.4% reported alcohol use and 25.9% reported drug use. Some sexual risk behaviors were also noted with 60 (35.5%) of participants reporting inconsistent contraceptive use at program entry. The majority of participants in this program were Hispanic youth. Additionally, based on the language preference of these teens it can be assumed that they can be defined as acculturated. Numerous studies have documented high-risk behaviors among Hispanic youth, especially among those who are acculturated (Cervantes & Pena, 1998; Johnston, O'Malley, & Bachman, 2002).

The trend of risk reduction occurred in all behaviors. Consistent contraceptive use increased and the prevalence of abstinence also increased. Substance abuse behaviors such as cigarette, drug, and alcohol use also improved. It is important to note that the reduction in risk behaviors were more noticeable in the six months follow-up than in the three months follow-up. This may suggest that participants have to be exposed to the intervention for a longer period of time in order to adopt healthier behaviors.

The results of the study indicate that acculturated youth can modify risk behaviors when engaged in a culturally grounded intervention. It is possible that culturally grounded interventions such as the ROP are powerful in increasing cultural identity and can also be effective in reducing risk behaviors. Researchers have suggested that acculturation-related problems among Latino adolescents result from their difficulties in dealing with multiple cultural demands. Therefore, focusing on ethnic identity while addressing aspects related to mainstream culture might help adolescents to integrate these influences. Additionally, some researchers have argued that since the Hispanic population is very diverse, there may be a need for culturally grounded programs to be more sensitive to the unique characteristics of each group (Gil et al., 2004).

The responses to the open-ended questions also support the contribution of a culturally grounded intervention to the well-being of the participants. While the quantitative assessment was focused on outcomes related to risk behaviors, the responses to the open-ended questions revealed outcomes related to self development and connectedness to culture and heritage. Participants identified as program benefits aspects such as becoming more responsible in family and job, acquiring skills to prepare for the future, and learning about making better choices. Participants also appreciated the opportunity to learn about their heritage. The impact of the program on risk reduction was also identified by several participants in the open-ended questions.

Although this program was designed as culturally grounded, it included many elements of youth development programs. A youth development approach has been identified as powerful in decreasing risk behaviors. For example, Kirby's (2002) review of 733 studies that presented approaches to reducing high-risk sexual behaviors among youth demonstrated that intensive youth development programs with multiple components had reasonable success. The ROP also included some of the successful components identified by Kirby.

Several methodological and design limitations should be noted. The data were generated by self-administered surveys, a method that can be subject to social desirability bias. In addition, the project experienced significant attrition over time. Despite these limitations, the results of this descriptive study indicate that engaging at-risk adolescents in prevention programs with structured interventions that focus on culture and heritage can assist in reducing high risk behaviors and increasing abstinence among acculturated youth.

PRACTICE IMPLICATIONS

The findings of this descriptive study suggest that a culturally grounded intervention was successful in reducing risk behaviors and developing various competencies among acculturated youth. This emphasizes the importance of culturally competent practice. However, practitioners across disciplines are concerned about translating cultural competency as a conceptual definition into actual practice. For example, Singh, Williams and Spears (2000) describe a culturally competent practitioner as one who has skills and knowledge to appreciate culturally diverse groups, and to acknowledge, accept, and value cultural differences. The essence of cultural understanding begins with knowledge of one's own cultural origins. Choi (2002) notes among nurses who work with adolescent depression, culturally competent care should encompass a fluid view of cultural awareness in which nurses first assess their own biases and then develop skills in an interactive and dynamic process in which there is continuous modification. On the other hand, social workers have a different perspective. According to Yan and Wong (2005), a social worker's perspective of cultural awareness cannot just include self-awareness since it assumes social workers are subjects capable of being neutral and impartial, culture-free agents while clients are objects who stay within the limits of their culture. Within this framework, such a model is viewed as a panacea for problems related to cross-cultural social work practice rather than a set of professional and ethical responsibility. The authors suggest that cultural competency be viewed as a dialogue between client and social worker in which they both negotiate and communicate to create new meanings and relationships. This dialogue should include sensitivity, knowledge, attitudes, and skills that reflect our multicultural society.

Some researchers indicate that culturally grounded programs lack specific operationalization (Russell & Lee, 2004). Therefore, culturally grounded programs should make an effort to identify specific program components that fall under this approach. It appears that these programs should focus on increasing cultural identity as researchers have suggested that acculturation-related problems among Latino adolescents result from their difficulties in dealing with multiple cultural demands. However, focusing only on ethnic identify, without addressing aspects related to mainstream culture and risk behaviors, might not be sufficient to help adolescents to integrate these influences.

In order for intervention to be effective, clinicians must obtain an accurate understanding of the specific values, beliefs, strengths, and unique needs of ethnic/racial groups. Despite different professional perspectives, it is important that all practitioners realize that we are still in the process of defining culturally competent care. As the adolescent population living in this country undergoes numerous changes in their acculturation and assimilation, understanding their specific needs is crucial for program success.

REFERENCES

Adam, M.B., McGuire, J.K., Walsh, M., Basta, J., & LeCroy, C. (2005). Acculturation as a predictor of the onset of sexual intercourse among Hispanic and White teens. *Archives of Pediatric Adolescent Medicine, 159*, 261-265.

Armstrong, B., Cohall, A. T., Vaughan, R. D., Scott, M., Tiezzi, L., & McCarthy, J. F. (1999). Involving men in reproductive health: The young men's clinic. *American Journal of Public Health, 89*, 902-905.

Benavides, R., Bonazzo, C., Torres R. (2006). Parent–Child Communication: A Model for Hispanics on HIV Prevention. *Journal of Community Health Nursing, 23*(2), 81–94.

Brindis, C., Boggess, J., Katsuranis, F., Mantell, M., McCarter, V., & Wolfe, A. (1998). A profile of the adolescent male family planning client. *Family Planning Perspectives, 30*(2), 63-6, 88.

Centers for Disease Control and Prevention. (2006). 2005 Youth Risk Behavior Surveillance Survey. Retrieved on March 14, 2007 from *http://www.cdc.gov/HealthyYouth/yrbs/*

Cervantes, R. C., & Pena, C. (1998). Evaluating Hispanic/Latino Projects: Ensuring cultural competence. *Alcoholism Treatment Quarterly 16*(1/2), 109-131. *www.samsha.gov/oas/2k2/HispanicTX/HispanicTX.htm*

Choi, H. (2002) Understanding adolescent depression in ethnonocultural context. *Advances in Nursing Science, 25*(2), 71-85.

Gil, A. G., Wagner, E. F., Tubman, J. G. (2004). Culturally sensitive substance abuse interventions for Hispanic and African American adolescents: Empirical examples for the Alcohol Treatment Targeting Adolescents in Need (ATTAIN) Project. *Addiction, 99* (suppl.2), 140-150.

Hecht, M.L., Marsiglia, F.F., Elek, E., Wagstaff, D.A, Kulis, S., Dustman, P., & Miller-Day, M. (2003). Culturally Grounded Substance Use Prevention: An Evaluation of the keepin' it R.E.A.L. Curriculum. *Prevention Science, 4*(4), 233-248.

Johnston, L.D., O'Malley, P.M., & Bachman, J.G. (2002). *Monitoring the future National Survey Results on Drug Use, 1975-2001, Volume 1: Secondary School Students. Table 4-9.* Bethesda, MD: National Institute on Drug Abuse.

Keating, L. M., Tomishima, M. A., Foster, S., & Alessandri, M. (2002). The effects of a mentoring Project on at-risk youth. *Adolescence, 37*(148), 717-734.

Kirby, D. (2002). Effective approaches to reducing adolescent unprotected sex, pregnancy and childbearing. *The Journal of Sex Research, 39*(1), 51-57.

Mize, S. J.S., Robinson, B. E., Bockting, W. O., & Scheltema, K. E. (2002). Meta analysis of the effectiveness of HIV prevention interventions for women. *Journal of AIDS Care, 14*, 163-180.

Office of Population Affairs/Office of Family Planning. (2000). *Male Involvement Projects-Prevention Services.* Washington, DC: U.S. Department of Health and Human Services

Pantin, H., Prado, G., Schwartz, S., Sullivan, S. (2005). Methodical Challenges in Designing Efficacious Drug Abuse and HIV Prevention Interventions for Hispanic Adolescent Subgroups. *Journal of Urban Health, 82*(2,3) iii92-iii102.

Prado, G., Schwartz, S., Pattatucci-Arag´on, A., Clatts, M., Pantin, H., Fernandez M.I., Lopez, B., Briones, E., Amaro, H., & Szapocznik, J. (2006). The prevention of HIV transmission in Hispanic adolescents. *Drug and Alcohol Dependence, 84S*, S43-S53.

Russell, S. & Lee, F. (2004). Practitioners' perspective on effective practices for Hispanic Teenage pregnancy prevention. *Perspectives on Sexual & Reproductive Health, 36*(4), 142-149.

Roth, J.L. and Brooks-Gunn, J. (2003). What exactly is youth development Project? Answers from research and practice. *Applied Developmental Science, 7*(2): 94-111.

Singh, N. Williams, E, & Spears, N. 2002). To value and address diversity: From policy to practice. *Journal of Child and Family Studies, 11*(1), 35-45.

Spencer, M.; Dobbs, B.; Swanson, D. (1988). AfroAmerican adolescents: Adaptational processes and socioeconomic diversity in behavioral outcomes. *Journal of Adolescence, 11*: 117-137.

Villarruel, A.M., Jemmott, J.B., Jemmott, L.S. (2006). A Randomized Controlled Trial Testing an HIV Prevention Intervention for Latino Youth. *Archives of Pediatric and Adolescent Medicine, 160*, 772-777.

Yan, M.C. & Wong, Y.L.R. (2005). Rethinking self-awareness in cultural competence; toward a dialogic self in cross-cultural social work, *Families in Society, 86*(2), 181-188.

Zeldin, S. (2000). Integrating research and practice to understand and strengthen communities for adolescent development: An introduction to the special issue and current issues. *Applied Developmental Science, 4*(1): 2-10.

INDEX

B

H

I

J

K

L

M

N